AF423746

Thomas A. Ban: Lithium in Psychiatry in Historical Perspective

With contributions from

Jules Angst, Barry Blackwell, Samuel Gershon, Paul Grof, Magda Malewska-Kasprzak, Agneszka Permoda-Osip, Janos Radó, Janusz Rybakowski and Johan Schioldann

Introductory comment by Edward Shorter

With comments from

Robert H. Belmaker, William E. Bunney Jr., Aitor Castillo, Gordon Johnson, Bruno Müller-Oerlinghausen, Leonardo Tondo and Antonio Torres-Ruiz

Edited in English, Formatting, and Artwork by

Olaf Fjetland, Carlos A. Morra and Lucrecia Álvarez

INHN Publisher

Córdoba, Argentina

2021

Thomas A. Ban

DEDICATION

To Gyorgy (George) Sandor, my service chief and teacher in 1955 at the National Institute of Nervous and Mental Diseases in Budapest. It was from Sandor that I first heard about the therapeutic potential of lithium in manic-depressive patients. Far ahead of his time, he had already used lithium in the treatment of some of his patients with monitoring blood levels to keep the substance in the safe therapeutic range.

CONTENTS

Preface

Lithium in Historical Perspective is a collection of selected postings from INHN's website. To provide readily accessible information on the history of the clinical development of the substance in psychiatry, the postings are presented under eight headings: 1. Discovery, 2. Introduction, 3. Verification, 4. Controversy, 5. Re-evaluation, 6. Safety, 7. Action and 8. Indications.

The potential use of lithium in "mania" was discovered by William T. Hammond (1871) and in "periodic depression" by Carl Lange in the mid and late-19th century, respectively. There are two postings included in the collection relevant to this topic: 1. Johan Schioldann's comment on William T. Hammond and 2. Carl Lange's speech, "On Periodical Depressions and Their Pathogenesis," in Johan Schioldann's translation from Danish into English. Schioldann's comment on Hammond was posted in Books on September 20, 2018, and Lange's speech in Perspective on August 16, 2018.

Instrumental to the introduction of lithium into treatment was Edward Trautner's determination of the effective dose range in which lithium can be used safely. He carried out the crucial study with Charles Noack, his junior associate, and their paper was published in 1951, two years after John Cade's (1949) report of successful treatment of manic patients with lithium. There are four postings in the collection relevant to this topic: John Cade's and Edward Trautner's biographies, written by Samuel Gershon, posted in Profiles on August 1, 2013; Sam Gershon's autobiographic account, "Events and Memories," posted in Biographies on June 25, 2015; and Gershon' s "Lithium History" posted in Controversies on May 1, 2018.

The therapeutic effect of Lithium in "mania" was verified by Mogens Schou and his associates (1954) in the mid-1950s. Their findings set the stage for the clinical development of the substance. There are three postings in the collection relevant to this topic: Mogens Schou's autobiography, "My journey with Lithium," presented by Johan Schioldann in Biographies on August 10, 2018, and Paul Grof's and Janusz Rybakowski's comment on it posted on January 10, 2019, and October 24, 2019, respectively.

Acceptance of lithium treatment was delayed by a controversy in the mid-1960s, triggered in 1968 by Blackwell and Shepherd's paper in the Lancet in which they referred to Baastrup and Schou's (1967) findings that lithium has prophylactic effect in manic depressive patients as "another therapeutic myth." The controversy concluded with Baastrup and Schou's reply published in 1968 in which they provided further substantiation to lithium's prophylactic effect (Baastrup and Schou 1968 a,b). There are four postings in the collection relevant to this topic: Barry Blackwell's essay, "The lithium controversy, a historical autopsy," posted in Controversies on June 14, 2014; Paul Grof's and Jules Angst's comments on it, both posted on January 22, 2015; and Blackwell's reply to both posted on February 5, 2015.

In the 1980s lithium was re-evaluated and its place in the treatment of bipolar disorder (manic-depressive psychosis) consolidated. There are three postings in the collection relevant to this topic: Paul Grof's comment, "More hindsight thought," on Barry Blackwell's comments on Mogens Schou's "My journey with lithium," posted in Biographies on November 7, 2019; Barry Blackwell's review of Johan Schioldann's (2009) "History of the Introduction of Lithium into Medicine and Psychiatry: Birth of Modern Psychopharmacology 1949" posted in Books on September 14, 2017; and Johan Schioldann's comment ("Ripostes and Annotations") on Blackwell's review posted on February 15, 2018.

By the time the re-evaluation concluded, lithium had become lifetime treatment for patients with "bipolar disorder" and with the prolonged use of the substance its anti-vasopressin action, causing polyuria and nephrogenic diabetes insipidus in vulnerable patients, had become a safety concern. Spearheaded by the research of Janos Radó, by the end of the second decade of the 21st century renal toxicity of lithium could be successfully treated and prevented; the safety concerns about the chronic use of lithium, at least in terms of its renal toxicity, had been resolved. There are five postings by Radó included in this collection relevant to this topic. One, "Mechanism of lithium—induced polyuria in historical perspective," posted in Perspective on July 4, 2019; and four, "Calcitonin in nephrogenic diabetes insipidus," "Renal toxicity of lithium in historical perspective with special reference to nephrogenic diabetes insipidus," "Desmopressin may counteract polyuria in lithium-induced nephrogenic diabetes insipidus. Review of the literature" and "Use of modern antidiuretic agents in lithium-induced nephrogenic diabetes insipidus," posted in Controversies on January 25, 2018, September 13, 2018, May 2, 2019, and July 18, 2019, respectively.

Throughout the years the mode of action of lithium has been extensively studied. Yet, in this selection, information on its possible mode of action is restricted to its effect on the "purinergic system" presented in two postings: 1. Magda Malewska-Kasprzak, Agnieszka Permoda-Osip and Janusz Rybakowski's (2018) treatise on the "Disturbances of the purinergic system in affective disorders and schizophrenia" and 2. Janusz K. Rybakowski's "Additional information: A commentary on Walter Felber's paper on Lithium prevention of depression 100 years ago -- an ingenious misconception, published in 1987." Both were posted in Controversies on December 13, 2018, and February 21, 2019, respectively.

The therapeutic indication of lithium extended after its introduction from the treatment of "manic excitement" to the acute, maintenance and prophylactic treatment of "manic-depressive psychosis," referred to by that time as "bipolar disorder" in consensus-based classifications. The heterogeneity in responsiveness to lithium in bipolar patients was recognized early but it has remained an open question whether populations derived by psychiatric nosology and psychopathology would provide more homogenous populations in terms of responsiveness to lithium than the consensus-based diagnosis of "bipolar disorder." There are two postings by Thomas Ban which provide relevant information to this topic: 1. "Development of the diagnostic concept of Manic-Depressive Psychosis in Emil Kraepelin's classifications" posted in Archives (Ban Collection) on November 5,

2015, and "From Emil Kraepelin's Manic-Depressive Psychosis to Karl Leonhard's Phasic and Cycloid Psychoses" posted in Courses (Central Office) on April 16, 2016.

References:

Baastrup PC, Schou M. Lithium as a prophylactic agent: Its effect against recurrent depressions and manic-depressive psychosis. Arch Gen. Psychiatr. 1967; 16:162-72.

Baastrup PC, Schou M. Prophylactic lithium. Lancet 1968a; I:1419-22.

Baastrup PC, Schou M. Prophylactic lithium. Lancet 1968b; II:340-50.

Blackwell B, Shepherd M. Prophylactic lithium: Another therapeutic myth? An examination of the evidence to date. Lancet 1968; I: 968-71.

Cade JF. Lithium salts in the treatment of psychotic excitement. Med J Aust 1949; 2: 349-52.

Hammond WA. Treatise on Diseases of the Nervous System. London: Lewis, 1882.

Malewska-Kasprzak M, Permoda-Osip A, Rybakowski J. Disturbances of the purinergic system in affective disorders and schizophrenia. Psychiatr Pol 2018; 52.

Noack D, Trautner EM. The lithium treatment of maniacal psychosis. Med J Austr 1951; 2: 218-22.

Schioldann J. History of the Introduction of Lithium into Medicine and Psychiatry. Birth of Modern Psychopharmacology 1949. Adelaide: Adelaide Academic Press; 2009.

Schou M, Juel-Nielsen N, Strömgren E, Voldby H. The treatment of manic psychoses by the administration of lithium salts. J. Neurol. Neurosurg. Psychiatr. 1954; 17:250-60.

CHAPTER 1.

DISCOVERY

JOHAN SCHIOLDANN'S COMMENT ON WILLIAM T. HAMMOND

In the early 1980s Arvid Carlsson drew the attention of Amid Amdisen (1985, 1987 a,b) and Steven Tyrer to that of Yeragani and Gershon (1986, 1987) that William Hammond of Bellevue Hospital, New York, was possibly the first to have reported, in 1871 on the exclusive use of lithium in the treatment of acute mania in his: Treatise On Diseases of the Nervous System (Schioldann 2009). Hammond considered acute mania to be "the more common species of mental aberration" manifested as 1) acute mania with exaltation and 2) acute mania with depression.

Based on Hammond's view that cerebral congestion was the underlying cause, he wrote:

> "…latterly I have used the bromide of lithium in cases of acute mania and have more reason to be satisfied with it than any other medicine calculated to diminish the amount of blood in the cerebral vessels, and to calm any nervous excitement that may be present. The rapidity with which its effects are produced renders it especially applicable in such cases."

He emphasized that

> "the doses should be large, as high as sixty grains or even more – and should be repeated every two or three hours till sleep be produced, or at least till half a dozen doses be taken. After the patient has once come under its influence, the remedy should be continued in smaller doses, taken three or four times in the day, [whereas] in cases of cerebral congestion attended with illusions and hallucinations, but without mania the other bromides will answer the purpose – preferably the bromide of sodium. They may also be given in the more violent forms if the bromide of lithium cannot be obtained."

Thus, Hammond targeted mania without secondary features,

illusions and hallucinations, but when caused by cerebral congestion. He did not comment on any possible etiological causes, nor did he specify whether both type 1 and type 2 were treated, nor did he mention any inspirational sources. Most intriguingly, however, he did not mention use of lithium in his later works (1882, 1883 and 1890). In 1882 he wrote:

> "First among [internal remedies] must be placed the bromide of potassium. […] Latterly I have used the bromide of sodium […] instead of bromide of potassium. […] The bromide of calcium is also well adapted to the treatment of cerebral congestion and has the advantage over the other bromides of acting more promptly. […] Latterly I have made much use of arsenious acid in cerebral congestion, especially in cases which have been the result of mental exertion or anxiety."

Thus, he was not forthcoming with any comments on his having abandoned lithium therapy.

It must be speculated whether Hammond had ceased using lithium (the bromide!) due to lithium and/or bromide toxicity, in view of the "tremendously high doses" he had administered (Amdisen 1987a,b; Schioldann 2009; Yeragani and Gershon 1986, 1987). However, as we learn from his 1882 work, undeterred he continued to use salts of bromide. Although, as was established by Gowers, that weight for weight there is "much more bromine in the lithium salt than in any other salt of bromine, the percentage of bromine in the molecule being 92 per cent," it cannot be ascertained whether Hammond opined that lithium per se had specific anti-manic properties (Gowers 1881; Tuke 1892). He eliminated lithium from his treatment regime but not bromide, and he did not substitute carbonate or citrate for bromide.

As can be established from Carl Lange's 1886 depression treatise (Schioldann 2009), it was around 1874 that he had commenced prescribing lithium (carbonate), the year he opened his private neurology clinic in Copenhagen. He, as well as his brother, Fritz, discouraged the use of bromides.

References:

Amdisen A. Lithium as a pharmacological agent. Historical aspects.

Discovery

Topical aspects of monitoring of psychiatric lithium therapy. [Danish text]. Risskov, 1985:26.

Amdisen A. The history of lithium. Biological Psychiatry 1987:22:522-3.

Amdisen A. The first lithium era. In: Johnson FN. (ed.). Depression & mania. Modern lithium therapy. Oxford: IRL Press. 1987:24-8.

Gowers WR. Epilepsy and other convulsive diseases etc. London: Churchill, 1881:253.

Hammond WA. Treatise on diseases of the nervous system. New York: Appleton, 1871:358-66 ('Mania'), 380-1 ('Treatment').

Hammond WA. Treatise on diseases of the nervous system. London: Lewis, 1882:65-71.

Hammond WA. A treatise of insanity. New York: Appleton, 1883:744-745. ('Treatment').

Hammond WA. A treatise on diseases of the nervous system. New York: Appleton, 1890:66-7.

Schioldann J. History of the Introduction of Lithium into Medicine and Psychiatry. Birth of Modern Psychopharmacology 1949. Adelaide Academic Press, 2009:29-31, 100, 140, 147, 230-1, 275, 289. – Carl Lange, ibid. Appendix I:293-308.

Tuke DH. A dictionary of psychological medicine. London: Churchill, 1892: 1130-1 ('Bromide of Lithium').

Yeragani VK, Gershon S. Hammond and lithium: historical update. Biological Psychiatry 1986; 21:1101-2.

Yeragani VK, Gershon S. Response [to Amdisen]. Biological Psychiatry 1987; 22:523.

September 20, 2018

Thomas A. Ban

CARL LANGE: ON PERIODICAL DEPRESSIONS AND THEIR PATHOGENESIS SPEECH DELIVERED TO THE MEDICAL SOCIETY OF COPENHAGEN, JANUARY 19, 1886 TRANSLATED FROM THE ORIGINAL DANISH INTO ENGLISH BY JOHAN SCHIOLDANN*

Gentlemen,

Introducing the statements that I have the honor of making tonight with an apology for their shortcomings and weaknesses, I must ask you not to consider this as a token of customary modesty, but as a genuine expression of my all-too-full awareness that the investigations and observations, the results of which I am about to present to you, are lacking in no small degree the scientific exactitude and precision that nowadays are mandatory even within the clinical field. Perhaps I dare even hope that at the end of this presentation you might agree that the shortcomings do not entirely stem from my own deficiencies, nor from the conditions under which the observations have been collected, i.e., in private practice, but that, in essence, they stem from the nature of the subject, so that it has been beyond me to remedy them. Thus, the importance of these shortcomings has not diminished, and I should probably have delayed the matter still further than I have done before daring to bring up the subject in a scientific forum, had it not been for two reasons.

One reason is the great importance of the matter, as it is about an extremely frequent, often most serious form of illness which strangely enough has almost completely escaped any notice in the literature. The disease that in my announcement of this speech I have described as periodical depression is of such common occurrence that in my private practice, with which I have been occupied for a number of years, there is no other form of illness which by far occurs as frequently. Even the most common neuroses, such as epilepsy, hysteria, all the various forms of neuralgia taken together, are nowhere nearly so frequent. It is therefore that over the approximately 12 years during which I have particularly focused my attention on this disease, the material of my observations has grown to at least 7-800 cases. I suppose that I must be wary of drawing from my personal experiences definite conclusions regarding the relative frequency of the disease claiming that it really occurs more often than for instance epilepsy - although I am convinced that it does - for there are many ways in which a selection can easily happen concerning the cases that present to, or are referred to, a specialist. At any rate, my experience shows beyond doubt that the condition, at least in this country, is extremely common (Note 1). Moreover, that it is generally very serious will emerge in the following description which will illustrate to us a condition extremely painful both for the patient himself and for those surrounding him and which, despite remissions for major periods of life, often destroys or drastically reduces the happiness or capacity for work of its victim, causing him to waste his life, although rarely exposing him directly to danger.

The other factor that has contributed to my overcoming my reluctance to present to you such an insufficient account is my long and often rather urgent-felt need to make a report to those of my colleagues who have referred their patients of this kind to me, although I have not yet had the opportunity to contact them concerning my view on the nature of the cases and on the indications for their treatment. I am convinced and can fully understand that the advice with which their patients have been returning from me must usually have appeared enigmatic to them, at times even worse than that. I have often longed not only to make clear to these colleagues, who are not few, that I did have a definite opinion and plan concerning my prescriptions, but even, if possible, to win them over to my views.

That sufferings of such common occurrence and importance as those conditions of depression being dealt with here can be so little known that they have left but few sporadic traces in the literature, consequently leaving most doctors in the dark and unclear about them, might appear strange at first sight, but on closer scrutiny this is easily explained. Psychiatrists under whose field the illness really belongs, according to its nature, only seldom get to see it because the patients rarely seek the asylum. To the other doctors who, as a matter of fact, do not readily accumulate large numbers of definite cases for comparison, the illness does not commonly manifest in a particular form and for obvious reasons these patients are not among those with whom doctors in general practice prefer to occupy themselves.

Generally, they are considered odd, difficult and uncooperative rather than insane, which in fact they are, even in a distinct and very characteristic form.

It also happens often enough, of course, that the doctor when faced with these patients has to "make a diagnosis" or, in other words, give the illness a label, place it somewhere in the nosological system. It is then usually placed under one or another of the common illness concepts, many of which are sufficiently vague to allow for the inclusion of quite a number of heterogeneous features. Very often these patients have been referred to me as hypochondriacs, although hypochondriasis, sensu strictiori, the morbid worry over and theorizing about imagined illnesses, from a symptomatic viewpoint, has but a very superficial similarity with the periodical depression and concerning course and other nosological features, none at all. Others are labeled as melancholiacs and undoubtedly this is a defensible approach as the somewhat vague descriptions of melancholy other than the typical forms also include descriptions which to an acceptable degree are applicable to our patients. I dare say that it is important to consider whether this may be caused by a not entirely fortunate delineation of the concept of melancholy and if this concept would not gain in clarity and obtain a more homogenous content if it clearly excluded the cases that we are about to deal with here. I shall allude later to the relationship between melancholy and periodical depression. It is of some pathological interest to us, as will later become clear to you, that previously some number of these cases were undoubtedly subsumed under the concept of oxaluria (Golding Bird) with which the younger generation is hardly familiar but which was very popular 30-40 years ago, from a symptomatic viewpoint a poorly defined nosological entity which was identified only by means of the presence of oxalic acid in the patient's urine and which, therefore, had to be abandoned when it was shown that the presence of oxalic acid in the urine did not necessarily predict the presence of oxalic acid in the blood. Finally, I shall again briefly touch upon the fact that a number of cases of periodical depression nowadays are undoubtedly included in the modern "box room" for ill-defined and hitherto unclassified nervous sufferings, the so-called neurasthenia.

That a group of pathological phenomena of individual cases only late and with difficulty take the form of a pathological concept sui generis, is usually due to the fact that they occur either too rarely to allow the individual observer easily to obtain a large enough number of cases so that the characteristic common features leap to the eye, or because it is difficult to extract a typical pathological picture from the individual observations taken together because there is too much diversity amongst them. Regarding periodical depression, neither applies. I have already touched upon its frequency, at any rate, in a specialist practice and what constitutes the typical pathological picture is exceedingly easy to delineate. But it is not this common picture with which we are often faced, an abstract pathological picture, a kind of Galton photography that contains parts of all the components but without rendering any one of them clearly. Individual cases of periodical depression can, of course, vary according to the patients' mental inherent characteristics, their intellectual development, the degree of the illness, etc. Most of them are as like as two peas and one can often astonish patients by describing to them in detail all their sufferings once one has arrived at the main diagnosis.

As is suggested by the name that I have chosen for it, the illness manifests itself in distinct periods of very varying duration and intensity. However, the picture of the illness is in essence the same not only within the same period of depression but also in different periods.

The designation of the patient's condition as melancholy, depression, will at once bring forth in your mind a picture to which a verbal account cannot do justice but a picture which is certainly in need of a closer analysis in order not to be misinterpreted regarding its psychological conditions and significance. The pathognomonic characteristics of the illness, the patient's most constant complaints, the feeling of heaviness, weariness, weakness, of a burden, which is mentally and physically exhausting and of apathy towards the ambience of his surroundings, these are symptoms which, from a psychological viewpoint, could have been caused in many different ways. This is also the reason that it will not do to attach the very same pathological weight and significance to all the various clinical pictures one encounters.

Our patients, who under the influence of the "mental pressure" that weighs them down, have a tendency to abandon all their work and duties to live absorbed only by their thoughts or rather - for of thoughts there are hardly any - by the experience of their own misery, in real terms have not suffered an absolute break in their work capacity. They rather feel it as a great strain, thus as a great unpleasantness, to have to do something, to throw themselves body and soul into things and, therefore, they understandably try to shirk it, particularly when they must show initiative or make decisions. If they succeed in pulling themselves together to get started with work or are forced to do so, then it seems, as a rule, that it is carried out without deficiencies concerning quantity or quality. Indeed, it seems as if the initiative to stop again once they have got going with rather monotonous and routine work can prove just as difficult as the decision to start. For instance, I can recall patients who have indicated to me that once they had overcome their reluctance to go for a walk, then found it was "as if they had to walk to the end of the world."

Intelligent patients who strive to find appropriate expression for their subjective sensations often describe their condition as "a mental stiffness or paralysis" and thereby they probably give an apt expression of their feeling of exhaustion at, and thus displeasure with, any operation of thought, every decision, this loathing for all activity that is so characteristic of their condition. While one does not wish to read more into this expression than it actually yields, namely a picture, then I feel like saying that one cannot help getting the impression from these patients that the protoplasm in their brain cells has really congealed so that their molecular transformations, which are basic to mental activity, require an unaccustomed, at times impossible, impulse to occur. This feeling that "all has stiffened" in them results, of course, in the lack of spirits and joie de vivre that are their constant complaint. In the opinion of those surrounding them they cannot be bothered with anything, but according to themselves they are capable of nothing, are unfit for everything, their "lives are wasted." It is for the same reason that they usually shun human society. It is not the melancholiac's fear of or suspicion towards his fellow man, fear of persecution or the like that make him prefer solitude. The reason is simply that social intercourse demands more than he can cope with. When in the company of others, he has to talk, follow their train of thought, follow the rules of etiquette, etc., which cost him such a great effort and strain, it can seem only natural to us that he would rather evade it.

Therefore, when the depressed prefers to spend his days in solitude and idleness, then it is due neither to ruined working capacity nor to his being controlled by false ideas that inhibit his activities, nor fear of or abhorrence of his fellow man, but simply because he, like the tired or sorrow-stricken, feels most at ease where neither activity nor effort is demanded of him.

Yet, it is only relative well-being that he can procure by thus evading the painful effort that any demand on his activity causes him, for his suffering also spans other mental functions which are not within his power to suspend, as to some extent he can with regard to his "volitional" and reasoning power. This state of the nervous system, the "stiffening," if you like, which manifests itself as slowness, strain, fatigue at any operation of thought or decision-making, in the area of emotions manifests itself in analogous ways with a more or less marked indifference towards everything, an often total lack of interest and concern even about those persons who are closest and dearest to him and towards everything that happens around him. In intelligent patients, particularly in cultivated circles, this profound indifference towards the surroundings is often disguised by their ability to comply fairly well with usual conventional forms of mutual interest and sympathy, their lack of depth becoming evident only in more intimate relationships or in the unreserved confessions of the patients. In many cases it is this feeling of "mental emptiness," where neither other people nor events nor natural surroundings, are able to arouse any warmth in them, which is the most bitter complaint of these patients.

The very essence of the patient's mental difficulties and his sufferings is often characterized by himself as a feeling of sorrow or disaster. The picture he presents to the observer is certainly that of the mourning, the more so because he is inclined to burst into tears at the slightest provocation. At any rate, even the relatively few patients who do not have fits of crying feel a strong urge to cry, and they themselves have a feeling that tears would do them good, that it would unburden their souls - being something which is certainly not usual for them. In reality there is no other difference between the condition described here and what is usually described as sorrow other than that the latter has a psychological basis which, as we shall learn later, the depression lacks, or at least does not have to a degree adequate fully to account for it. Moreover, the patients are always, in contrast to the melancholiacs, fully aware that this feeling of misery is completely unrelated to, or at any rate insufficiently caused by, the trivial and passing worries that perhaps might have been the final straw in its development.

With regard to its physiological characteristics, sorrow is so closely related to anxiety that we are not surprised often to find in these patients' morbid mental state a more or less pronounced admixture of anxiety. This is not the rule, however, as anxiety is completely lacking in a great number of cases, while in other cases it can be so strongly pronounced that the depression, at any rate periodically, for instance during the night, is almost overshadowed by it. No more than sorrow and misery, does anxiety stem from any delusion not to mention hallucinations. The patient is terrified neither by imaginary persecutions nor threatening voices. He is as fully aware of the groundlessness of his anxiety as that of his sorrow; nor that it has any particular object. He is not afraid of this or that, but he has only an indescribable feeling of apprehension. As it is not rare to hear patients from the more unsophisticated social classes characterize this feeling as "agony," they are certainly not describing a fear of dying but rather giving an expression of the intensity of their feeling.

There are, of course, nuances in the illness picture, depending on whether inertia or apathy predominates and on whether the feeling of misery or of anxiety is especially pronounced. Generally speaking, the state of male patients is to a high degree marked by lack of initiative, strain and difficulty in deciding to work, whereas in the case of women it is often the obtuseness of their emotions that comes to the fore. This fact is probably more due to the difference between the normal and the morbid state than to any difference between the two sexes and is not marked to such a degree that the illness picture should generally manifest any particularly different character in men or in women.

The physical symptoms are generally less significant and less constant than the mental symptoms and they do not keep pace with them in such a way that one can generally say that they are most pronounced in those patients who suffer the most mentally. The depressed mental state is particularly evident, of course, in both physical appearance and facial expression so that the patients look "despondent" or unhappy. This is not, however, a constant feature and one cannot in any way flatter oneself by always being able to diagnose the condition going solely by the patient's appearance. This is partly due to the fact, which shall later be dealt with, that within the morbid period there often occur significant changes in well-being such that one can often encounter even a severely affected patient in a momentary state in which he does not appear to be unhappy. But this is also partly because many people, in particular those who are the most mentally developed, make great efforts to control themselves to such a degree that their appearance does not betray their mental state. Whereas it is often easy to read the illness from the facial expression of a patient of the peasantry - which yields a significant proportion of depressed people - it is the exception that in a patient from the "cultivated classes" one diagnoses the illness as he enters through one's door.

Now that I am describing the patient's behavior as presented to the doctor, it permits me to touch on another matter that is perhaps in itself quite inessential, but at the same time, quite characteristic of these patients and which can contribute to the difficulty of diagnosis. It is exceptional, at any rate in my practice, that a patient of the kind described here who when asked to indicate what his suffering is, when he presents for the first time, immediately admits to and complains of his low spirits, mental state or the like. Almost constantly one is confronted with complaints of some type of physical feeling: headache, dizziness, backache, abdominal discomfort, etc., etc., complaints which, as a rule, appear to have very little objective basis as it is very rare for further mention of them to occur once one has established the real nature of the illness with the patient. In this matter there undoubtedly exists a conscious reluctance in the patients to admit to or rather to accuse themselves of suffering from a mental illness. On the other hand, however, they usually clearly feel relieved when they feel they have been seen through and are asked directly if it is not rather a mental condition from which they are suffering of which they have always been fully cognizant and which they never try to deny.

It is fairly common that patients lose some weight during their morbid periods, but whether it is a matter of loss of actual substance or often rather the diminished turgor, this collapse, which in many patients manifests itself concomitantly with the onset of the illness, that is the real cause of this apparent diminution of flesh, is not always easy to determine. It is impossible, of course, to carry out really convincing weight studies in ambulatory patients in whom there occur only insidious weight variations. The collapse that is being referred to is often clearly pronounced. Thus, the patients become more pale than usual and they are frequently very sensitive to cold, and in particular they complain of cold hands and feet, though in many patients this condition is often interrupted by sudden paroxysms of heat, sometimes throughout the body, at times only in the head. There are also many patients in whom diaphoresis is a prominent symptom, partly as a general tendency to perspire, partly as sudden apparently inexplicable paroxysms of perspiration - especially with frequent nightly occurrence. The pulse shows nothing remarkably abnormal. Some self-observant patients claim that in their bad periods it throbs somewhat slower than when they are well.

Sleep is often disturbed, broken by anxious dreams and at times insomnia becomes a very tormenting symptom. One must not become misled by the answer that one generally gets to one's questions about sleep: "Well, it seems to me that I could sleep forever." This is but an expression of the mental and physical feeling of fatigue and weakness of these patients who, as closer examination shows, is not at all indicative of sound and unbroken sleep. Yet, on the other hand, it is not rare that patients, even in cases where the depression has become very pronounced, sleep well and calmly so that they long for the night as a refreshing intermission to their sufferings. Awakening is then all the more painful as the early morning hours, in the predominant number of cases, are the most tormenting part of the day. The feeling of misery and anxiety, often accompanied by the well-known oppressive epigastric feeling, at these hours reach their highest degree gradually abating during the day, in particular towards the evening - to the extent that the condition can be almost completely normalized later in the evening. This morning exacerbation and evening remission are extremely characteristic and very pronounced in well over half of the cases, although they appear to be lacking in a number of patients and a small number even state that the opposite occurs in them, but this never appears to reach such a pronounced degree as the contrast between the gloomy mornings and free easy-to-tolerate evenings.

Appetite is in many cases only moderate. Digestion appears to be somewhat sluggish in the majority of patients. There is often some constipation. Menstruation is undisturbed, also during the morbid periods and does not, as a rule, appear to have any influence as such on the patients' condition. Yet, a few women claim that they feel worse when they menstruate, whereas others claim quite the opposite, that they feel best during this time. These statements are, however, too vague and too sporadic to be given much significance. A small number of patients have vehemently claimed to have observed a pronounced periodicity in their illness, related to their menstruations, to a degree that they feel almost quite well during the days in between their periods of menstruation, yet increasingly unwell the closer they get to a period of menstruation or vice versa, but I have not had the opportunity to investigate the validity of these suggestions.

I shall later return to the matter of the urine to which I attach crucial importance in the understanding of the pathogenesis of the illness.

Gentlemen, there are perhaps among you those who would say that the illness picture which I have outlined to you here does not present anything peculiar as, at least concerning its main features, it gives us the picture of a melancholiac as he appears during the mildest degree of his illness and what I have called periodical depression is nothing but what some authors, at least in recent times, have described as the first stage of melancholia, the stage of depression. As I have already suggested, this is true in that in recent times the picture of melancholy has certainly been obscured and interfered with because psychiatrists who, as it has often been emphasized, "as a rule do not get to see this first stage," have undoubtedly placed depression under melancholia and regarded the former as the first phase of the latter due to a certain superficial similarity. But depression, as I have described it, has nothing to do with melancholia; the depressed never become melancholiacs and it is therefore quite inadmissible to categorize them as being in the first phase of melancholia simply because their illness, from a superficial viewpoint, shows a certain similarity with mild cases of melancholia. I have followed many of my patients over a considerable number of years and know of accounts of life-long pathological histories involving an even greater number of patients. Yet not a single one of the hundreds of patients I have had the opportunity to monitor is any closer to melancholia now than when his illness first afflicted him, perhaps 30 or 40 years before, and not a single one has developed either delusions or hallucinations (Note 2). Thus, if it is unjustifiable to place it under melancholia, using its course as a criterion, then it is, if possible, even more inadmissible to do so for psychological reasons - and certainly the psychiatric system is here psychologically based and, therefore, psychology must be the guiding principle in the delineation of these illness concepts. The distinctive feature of the melancholiac is that his feeling of misery, his anxiety stems from delusions, such as imaginary persecutions or tormenting and frightening hallucinations, and therefore he deems his sorrow and misery well-founded. In the depressed person, on the other hand, no matter how long his illness goes back and no matter how strongly it might have overwhelmed him, there is not the slightest suggestion of delusions or hallucinations.

Their illness is purely and simply an anomaly of mood and these persons are always fully aware that it has no external basis. This is, I suppose, a radical and decisive psychological difference. To this should be added the whole course of the illness which, as a rule, makes the course of the lives of the afflicted so very different in the two types of patients. In melancholiacs the periodicity is, if not unknown, always an exception to the rule and would possibly become even less common than is the case were the depressed that are assumed to be melancholic meticulously separated out from them. As opposed to this, in the depressed the periodicity is constant and is such a prominent feature that it certainly provides the basis to choose the name of the illness accordingly. This periodical course I shall now go on to describe.

As uniform as the illness picture generally must be considered to be within the limits of the periods of depression, just as varying it is concerning the periodicity itself, not only in such a way that it differs from patient to patient but also such that it is usually quite irregular within the individual patient. This irregularity occurs not only due to the fact that at times the morbid periods - as I shall later show - are hastened or precipitated by unfavorable external conditions and probably delayable or also preventable by more beneficial conditions, but to a significant degree appears to be inherent in the nature of the illness, as it is only exceptional that its course is influenced by external circumstances - or, at any rate, that such an influence can be established.

Accordingly, if one inquiries about the duration of the periods of depression and of the free intervals, then there exists no rule, no common picture. To be able to talk of what is common then, at any rate, one must allow considerable scope. One can probably say that the morbid period most often lasts three to six months, the good interval perhaps a little longer. However, it is not at all unusual that the period of depression lasts much longer: a year, even perhaps two years, and the free periods can spread over yet longer periods, three or four years, possibly more. On the other hand, one can also see cases in which the periods are very short lived. The depression may last for about one month, even for only a couple of weeks with similarly short intervals. On the whole, one can probably say that long periods of depression belong with long free periods and vice versa, but the individual cases show many exceptions to this rule.

Although it is impossible to establish any rule for most of the patients, either regarding the type of changeability or the duration of the individual periods, on the other hand, there exists a fair number in whom the illness in the above regards can occur with a certain regularity, at any rate for longer periods of their lives. As a rule, one can say that the shorter the periods of illness are, the greater is their tendency to occur in a regularly intermittent manner. Not a few patients for instance, over a number of years, have periods of depression lasting one to two months every six months, spring and fall or summer and winter. Others have only a single bad period each year. If this happens to occur during winter, of course they then assume that it is the cold that adversely affects them, whereas, in the opposite case, they think that it is the heat that is causing their troubles. However, I do not believe that temperature has any noticeable influence. Depression occurs during summer and winter alike. On the other hand, during summer, under more favorable conditions the patients generally feel more able to resist the morbid state and, therefore, perhaps manage it better at this time of the year than in winter. In the rare cases of the type with short periods, at least according to the claim of some patients, these can be so regular that they can predict on which day the depression will occur and on which day it will end. Here we are only dealing with periods of depression that last approximately one week with free intervals of a couple of weeks, although this is extremely rare, and as the disease persists this appears to be replaced by the usual irregularity.

The morbid period itself, at any rate when it is of longer duration, never passes evenly and uniformly, even disregarding the aforementioned common evening remissions. Much more common is a constant fluctuation in the patient's state such that weeks or months of profound illness alternate with similar periods of relative well-being and within these greater or longer swings one can, on the other hand, again observe numerous regularly small swings with a duration of days or just hours.

When one observes this continual rise and fall within the morbid periods, which certainly can vary to an extreme degree in different patients but which is hardly ever completely lacking, then one will necessarily have to ask the question if not all the changes during the course of the illness are due to similar swings and if these patients, once their illness has started, will ever again return completely to a normal level; in other words, whether these periods that I have described as the free intervals are really full intermissions or possibly just an expression of strong remissions with relative well-being which in contrast to the periods of suffering are described by the patient himself and those surrounding him as good health. Concerning the answer to this question one is, true enough, to a significant degree dependent on an estimation by the patient himself and the circle within which he moves daily and, in most cases, therefore, one has to leave the matter undecided. However, often enough one learns that never since the start of the illness or even never, as far as the patient can remember, has he felt completely free of a certain mental oppression, never has he had a confident or cheerful nature, yet without in his everyday life in any way having felt that he was abnormal or in a proper sense suffering. On the other hand, however, there are also many patients, and at times amongst them those who suffer the most in their bad times, who are described as, or who themselves testify that they are, "by nature" good-spirited and that before the manifestation of their illness they felt, and in the free intervals still feel, as easy and happy as anyone, although, and this should be emphasized, as far as my experience goes, between the periods of depression there never develop states of morbid "elevation" that could place the whole illness under the sphere of the cyclical forms of insanity. Even in cases where there are initially complete intermissions, particularly in persistent and protracted cases and on the whole in elderly people, these intermissions gradually appear to become less clear cut and I have experienced several elderly patients in whom the hope of obtaining an even tolerable remission of their sufferings appears to be very slim.

Under such constant swings between suffering and well-being, in absolute or relative terms, these miserable people drag on often for a large part of their lives and their deplorable condition becomes all the more burdensome, as it is only rarely considered to be morbid by those surrounding them, but rather much more frequently as evidence of oddity, uncooperativeness, moroseness, indifference or the like. They themselves often share this opinion to a degree and from this it follows that probably, on the whole, only a fraction of the patients think of seeking medical assistance for their sufferings. The one who has sharpened his eye to the manifestations of depression will have no difficulty in recognizing its milder forms in a great number of people who are accustomed to bearing their periods of "bad moods," "indisposition," as something which belongs with the vicissitudes of any human life. Indeed, perhaps one dares say that there are probably only few people who completely escape any taint of the illness described here.

The duration of the illness is very variable in individual patients and significantly dependent on the time of the manifestation of the first period of depression. For once a person has fallen victim to this illness, he is rarely rid of it until sometime into his advanced years. I believe, however, that I can say that the earlier in life the periods of depressions occur, the earlier they show a tendency to diminish. But I must admit that even with a good many years of experience it is difficult to be completely certain regarding this matter which, in all events, is in no way constant. The first pronounced period of depression in more than half of the cases probably manifests itself during the period from the ages of 25 to the age of 35, yet very frequently between the age of 20 and 25 as well, and even between puberty and the age of 20. I have never myself encountered children with typical and marked depression. But the accounts of quite a number of patients of their childhood make it obvious to me that children as well, albeit probably only rarely, can be afflicted by this illness. After the age of 35 the number of sufferers rapidly diminishes year by year so that it can be said that it is a rarity for people to develop the illness if they have not shown signs of it before the age of 50. Yet it can happen. I have even encountered patients who were adamant that they had never had the slightest trace of depression until they were 60-years-old and in these cases the illness has appeared to me to be particularly tormenting, the remissions short and incomplete, the treatment without result.

If the illness is left to itself then the regular course appears to be this: that for a number of years, commonly to about the 50th year, it worsens as the periods of depression gradually become longer, the depression deeper, the intermissions less clear cut. At a more advanced age, approximately after the 60th year, there appears to be, at any rate in many cases, a tendency towards spontaneous improvement. In earlier periods of life such a "spontaneous" improvement or recovery is extremely rare; yet, every now and then I learn from parents that in their children's illness they recognize conditions which they themselves experienced but had recovered from at a young age.

Here I shall mention that pregnancy does not appear to be compatible with depression (a view he corrected in his preface to the second edition of this treatise: translator's note). As far as my experience goes, it is an established rule that depression, if it is present, is interrupted with the commencement of pregnancy and it does not recur until after the period of gestation - and probably also that of lactation.

Regarding the causes of the illness as we first consider the predisposing factors, next to age, the significance of which I have already touched upon, it is only inheritability that is of importance, but this is certainly of decisive importance indeed. Gender is without significance except that women are perhaps afflicted at a slightly younger age than men. It appears that one need attribute little influence to profession, job and level of education. The significance in the development of nervous and mental illnesses that one so often ascribes to the hectic, restless life in big cities does not apply to periodical depression. It thrives as well among the rural population, even in the most remote regions as in the capital, and with the same frequency afflicts those individuals whose intellectual life is the least developed, the most monotonous and apathetic and those who live the most intensive business or intellectual life. Although all walks of life, both gender and practically all age groups, are equally exposed to the ravages of this illness, then in another way it is extremely limited in terms of the persons it afflicts. Regarding those who do not have an inhereditary predisposition it is powerless. There exists no other nervous illness, and very few illnesses at all, and then only such, as we shall learn later, which have a certain pathological affinity to periodical depression where inheritability has such a decisive significance as for the illness with which we are concerned here. It is only a rather small minority among my patients in whom it has not been possible to establish inheritability with certainty and only a few cases in whom it has been possible to exclude inheritability with certainty, and even in those cases where the parents of the depressed have been known not to have been victim of depression themselves, there has often been an inheritable predisposition present in another form as I shall demonstrate to you shortly.

Depression is inherited, it seems, equally from the father or the mother. At times it has been possible to recognize the heritable predisposition only because several siblings have fallen victim to the illness. This is something that is particularly often the case, although it has not been possible to establish with certainty that any of the parents have been afflicted. It is not easy to say if the children ever completely avoid the illness when one of their parents and particularly if both of them are suffering, as it is rare that it falls to one's lot to be able to keep an exact account of the pathological history of a whole generation for a sufficient length of time. It is certain, however, that it is not rare to come across families who down through several generations, in a tragic manner, have been burdened by this illness.

Yet, although it is firmly established that the great majority of patients from birth are predisposed towards this illness that manifests itself sooner or later in their lives, this does not mean that randomly occurring causes or the manner in which their lives take shape, their internal and external mode of living, can be considered to be without significance for the development of the illness or for the time when the depression first manifests itself and the subsequent morbid periods erupt. In a short while when I address the pathogenesis of the illness, it will occur to you that an appropriate diet in the widest sense of the word is of extreme importance in the fight against the inborn predisposition and it will become easily understandable that this can be kept under control for a long time, perhaps even throughout life, where the conditions of life are such that they constantly work against the morbid predisposition and where occasional triggering events are avoided. As mentioned before, the latter are certainly not necessary either for the development or for the manifestation of the individual periods of depression. In a significant number of cases, all searches for occasional factors have been entirely futile and the patients themselves remain adamant that their morbid periods occur "quite spontaneously." Yet there are quite a few exceptions to this rule. It is not rare at all that patients blame some kind of effort or another for the eruption of a period of depression, in particular when it has been connected with mental unrest or tension - as for instance vigil over very ill relatives - or a mental "shock" or finally, and frequently, a sorrow which to us would appear quite natural, as the effect of so-called sad experiences, as mentioned before, has an impact which appears to be consistent with the patient's state of mind during their morbid periods. Such periods of depression, which have been provoked by occasional events, often develop acutely so that the morbid state of mind very quickly, at times virtually immediately, reaches a pronounced degree, as opposed to the usual pattern of a slow and gradual development.

Concerning the pathogenesis of periodical depression, I must admit that I would probably have acquiesced with the same negative attitude which one usually assumes regarding mental illnesses, were it not for the reason that during my preoccupation with this illness reasons for a more positive viewpoint have gradually been forced upon me.

From the first, when experience taught me in periodical depression to recognize a peculiar form of mental disease and I thus started to separate out patients with this picture as a particular group, I became struck by how often I received from these patients the unsolicited message that they were suffering or had suffered from "gravel," an expression which among lay people usually means nothing else but the well-known 'sedimentum lateritium' (from later brick, brick-red, added by this writer) in the urine. When, as a result of these indications I systematically started investigating the patient's urine in this regard, I soon found that this was really the case and that there was generally a strong tendency in them to pass urine containing an abundant, often colossal sediment of urates and uric acid proper. Other than having investigated virtually all my depressed patients' urine regarding its content of uric acid, I have, for reason of comparison, made a similar investigation of an even far greater number of other patients' urine, and the difference has been extremely striking to the effect that when not one of the well-known factors - fever, profuse perspiration, considerable cooling down of the urine, rich meals and other factors - which in everybody could cause urine sediments, are present, then it is very exceptional for the average man's urine to be sedimentous, whereas the urine of the patients concerned here usually is. Of course, it can be free of sediment, partly for the reason that there is undoubtedly some periodicity regarding the content of uric acid in the urine, not to mention its metabolism in the body, and partly for the reason that a coincidental consumption of alkali, plenty of liquids or the like can momentarily make it disappear. Its presence, however, has been so common, and in those cases where I have only been able to do a few investigations in which it has been lacking, information from the patient or those surrounding him about the condition of the urine has usually been so confirmative that I dare assert with the greatest certainty that depressed patients generally, both in their sick periods and outside them, have a tendency to pass a strongly sedimentous urine even when at random common causes for the production of uric acid deposits are not present (Note 3).

No matter how certain and decisive this fact is, I need not mention that in itself it teaches us absolutely nothing as such about the pathogenesis of periodical depression. Although the constant tendency of the urine to deposit uric acid sediment can be considered proof that there is an ample production of it in the organisms or its metabolism insufficient - and there is hardly any reason to doubt this - then it is in no way certain that uric acid diathesis is the cause of periodical depression and although there is no doubt that there is, in one way or another, a relationship between the two phenomena then, a priori, this can be assumed to have been of a very different nature. The following possibilities, in particular, appear to me: 1) the uric acid in the individuals here concerned can have an analogous significance to phosphoric acid in so many other "nervous" patients; a significance, which is probably very disputable and which can never be considered such that the presence of phosphoric acid in the organism should be considered the cause of the nervous symptoms, but rather that the nervous disturbances in one way or another causes the phosphaturia; 2) the presence of a surplus of uric acid, particularly by precipitation, gives rise to uric acid infarcts and, consequently, an irritation in the kidneys that, one can imagine, can have a "reflex effect" on brain functions just as it is thought possible that these can be influenced by irritative conditions in the digestive tract and in other places; 3) the abnormally high blood uric acid content – "the uric acid diathesis" - directly affects the central nervous system structures and causes a modification of their function.

Of these three theories concerning the significance of the uric acid surplus in depressed patients, the former two, however, at closer scrutiny, soon turn out to be unsustainable. As proof of this I will particularly stress the fact, which I have already touched upon above, that the increased secretion of uric acid is not limited to the depressed periods, but occurs continuously, although always with interruptions - during normal periods as well, even if they last for several years. This has no analogy at all with "nervous phosphaturia" nor would it fit in with any "reflex theory." That the abnormal condition of the urine could in no way be considered as a secondary phenomenon to the nervous dysfunction is also demonstrated by another circumstance which, on the whole, regarding the pathogenesis, is very striking. When I spoke about the significant inheritability, I remarked that, at times, the condition is manifested other than for the reason that depressed persons were descendants of depressed parents. With this I wanted to point out that generally, where parents have not been depressed, it can be shown that they were carriers of a "uric acid diathesis" as they had suffered from either urine sediments or arthritis urica. Thus, the inheritable factor per se turns out to be the diathesis - the surplus of uric acid in the organism - and should be considered to be the primary, the basic illness, of which the depression is a function, similar to what uric acid arthritis or the production of sediments could be. This is a manifestation that at first glance could appear to be somewhat peculiar in an area where one is used to seeing stones and tophi as the products of the illness, but which, on the other hand, shows several very striking similarities with the other clinical forms of the diathesis. If one juxtaposes the pictures of the arthritic patient, the lithiasis sufferer and the one suffering from periodical depression, then on closer scrutiny the immediately obvious differences might carry but little weight in comparison with the similarities, such as the particularly significant inheritability and the spontaneous periodical occurrence. The dissimilarities are easily and simply explicable by the various localizations of the dyscratic manifestations, whereas periodicity and inheritability - and in addition inheritability between the various illness forms - in the sense and in the form in which we experience them in the conditions dealt with here - are hardly known in any other area of pathology (Note 4).

Therefore, if we dare rely on the assumption that states of depression, when they occur in the form and with the course that I have described here, bear testimony to the presence of a uric acid diathesis, and that they must be understood as effects of this diathesis, to which the predisposition, as a rule, is inborn, then this provides the basis for a rational treatment of the depression, a treatment that extends somewhat further than the exclusively symptomatic treatment or expectative or restrictive regime with which the mental illnesses usually have to make do. It is certainly true, however, that the rules for the rational treatment so far can only be given in the crudest outline. It is not yet possible to get closer to the matter than to the establishment of this general direction: to counteract the underlying diathesis. This is what we are limited to as long as we do not know anything about the way in which the diathesis affects or harms the nervous system. In this regard there exist different possibilities, but I shall not enter into a discussion of them as I do not believe that it is possible for me to judge between them with certainty.

Discovery

The treatment that I have already been using for a considerable number of years in cases of periodical depression has primarily consisted in the battle against the uric acid diathesis. It would be needless to give a special account of the remedies that I have applied in this regard, for I would not be able to communicate anything to you that is not well known to all of you. Indeed, you know as well as I do that the task is not only with medicaments to facilitate and accelerate the excretion of the uric acid but to an even larger extent it must be the task to prevent its abundant production by dietary measures and, finally, where there exists such a tendency to overproduction, by means of those remedies that we generally have at our disposal to accelerate the oxidation processes of the body, in order to increase its metabolism.

It is quite clear however, that along with these rational treatments there will generally be a need for remediation of symptoms. In this regard I believe, particularly concerning the somewhat unfortunate way in which these patients are often treated from a psychological viewpoint, I must emphasize that they must not be permitted to follow their own inclination to withdraw from the company of other people and from their usual occupation, only to live with their feeling of misery all by themselves. On the contrary, one must do all that is possible to provide them the mental stimulus of which the inertia of their nervous system is in need, so that to a reasonable degree it can assume its usual level of functioning. As far as it is possible the patients must be forced into being constantly active, doing something, and it does them good to be exposed to changing and strong stimuli. In endeavoring to accomplish this, one almost always faces considerable resistance from the patients for the reason that a concentrated effort is demanded from them and of which only a few have sufficient energy and perseverance to mount during the often-long period before improvement starts to show. Therefore, in this matter, it is rare that the doctor gets anywhere if he does not receive intelligent and unflagging support from those nearest and dearest to the patients.

There is one thing that I never neglect to strongly impress upon the patients as well as those around them, this being that the matter in question is neither a temporary measure nor a short-lasting treatment, but that the patients for the rest of their lives or, in all events, for a number of years, must adjust their whole lifestyle to counteract the morbid predisposition that they carry. When the uric acid diathesis is inherited it is based on peculiarities in the structure of the organism about which we have but very incomplete knowledge, but which we do know that we are unable to remove and that we must simply be satisfied when we are successful in neutralizing their effects. Of course, in far too many cases it is impossible to engender in the patient and those who are associated with him, the admittedly not insignificant amount of energy and perseverance that is necessary for the carrying out of such permanent measures, although these in no way upset the duties and activities of everyday life, for this often demands the abandonment of some habits and the acquisition of others - and, unfortunately, the habits which must be acquired are of a more active nature than those to be abandoned - a matter which makes them have little attraction for the patients to whom any demand of activity is so tormenting.

Gentlemen, if you would now ask me what results I have had with this therapy whose fundamental features I have described here, then you would put me into a very difficult situation, for it is in the nature of the matter that the therapeutic results, in all events, are in no way so striking or conclusive that they could not be disputed. As I have already stated, the issue cannot be to eliminate or to cure the inborn predisposition, which is fundamental to the illness, but only to counteract its effects. If treatment is ceased, be it dietetic or medicinal, then these effects recur, even if for some time one has been successful in removing them. Regarding the therapy, however, how can one decide whether one has achieved any influence on the course of the illness whose changing pattern in itself is so irregular and unpredictable? After a usually unpredictable duration of morbid periods they improve spontaneously, independently of any therapy. Also, the free intervals are of indefinite duration such that it is not easy to determine whether the treatment contributes in extending them. As for the course, variation occurs regarding the intensity of the illness. From a very pronounced intensity in one period one cannot with certainty conclude that there will also be just as great an intensity of the illness in the next. Therefore, apparent effects of treatment in this regard also become disputable. Along with this, as it is obvious that it is usually impossible in the course of time - often years - accurately to control the patient in terms of his compliance with the imposed measures, then one can easily understand that it is not possible to draw up anything that has the merest resemblance to statistics concerning the effects of the treatment and that one must make do with a completely subjective estimate. Therefore, I shall confine myself to a few brief remarks. In the course of years, I have arrived at the conviction, which has its best support that it is shared by a great number of patients, that it is possible, at any rate in younger persons, and in not too severe cases, to shorten and significantly alleviate the sick periods and to prolong the free intervals by means of a therapy that has had its indications pointed out earlier, whereas it is not possible to completely cure the illness.

Before I finish, I must very briefly mention the question of whether the pathogenetic interpretation that is being advanced here has ever before been advanced if not as a fully formed theory - for such has not been possible of course - as periodical depression has not hitherto been put forward as a nosological entity, then at any rate only as a tentative hypothesis. At the same time, I must readily admit that I have not attached great importance to tracing every statement concerning this matter which might have been dropped in passing from some author's pen. Therefore, it is very possible that I have overlooked something, although hardly anything of significance, as for a number of years, as a matter of course, I have paid attention to other observers' statements which might support my point of view. Unfortunately, my endeavors have yielded very little indeed. It is true that one often finds the statement that the arthritic diathesis may cause mental illnesses, but then it is emphasized that it is the sudden suppression of an attack of gout that is succeeded by an outbreak of insanity. Whether this can be cited in support of what has been claimed in my point of view is obviously doubtful. It gains more support from a statement by Maudsley who, in his renowned book on mental illnesses concerning their etiology, after having emphasized in general the great importance of the presence of excretory substances in the urine, reports that a couple of times he has observed "melancholia" in people with an arthritic diathesis and that he has seen the melancholy get cured by an efficient treatment of the gout. In some remarks about "neurasthenia" Huchard in l'Union médicale (1882) states that this illness - amongst the variegated elements of which, as already noted, one will certainly also find many cases of periodical depression - as a rule develops on an arthritic soil. This statement, however, is so casual and unsupported that it is easily explained that it has remained unnoticed. Also, Arndt in his thorough - almost too thorough - treatise on neurasthenia claims a kinship between this condition and not only arthritis, but also rheumatism, which he is even inclined to consider as one of the manifestations of neurasthenia (!).

As far as I know this is all that previous authors have stated or rather suggested concerning the pathogenetic factor which has been put forward here. Consequently, I have virtually nothing to rely on from previous observers; the more reason I have to hope that my understanding of this matter is going to be tested by future investigators, for in all events I dare expect that the remarks that I have had the honor of presenting here tonight, no matter how imperfect they may be in more than one regard, may contribute to drawing the attention of my colleagues to a very serious, very frequent and very neglected form of illness.

Notes:
1. Here I shall only talk about the more severe cases in which medical attention is being sought. As will be touched on later, there are surely very many people who suffer from milder forms of the illness which do not come to the attention of a doctor.
2. Three have committed suicide, but they were all patients whom I only knew very superficially. Perhaps, therefore, their diagnosis was wrong. It is possible that they were melancholics. Moreover, it would not be particularly remarkable if the often very profound sufferings of the depressed patients would sometimes drive them to suicide without paranoid ideas being involved. Nothing is more common than the (depressed patients) themselves harboring the feeling that their illness will end with suicide, but this risk is small or non-existent.
3. Not only would it be impossible to carry out exact quantitative assays of the uric acid amounts in outpatient, but also, even if they could be done, they would not be of any value. For the amount of uric acid in a single urine sample, or the daily excreted amount, or the amount excreted in a shorter period of time is, in the first place, under normal conditions so varying that one would have no norm with which to compare one's results. A normal person's daily excretion of uric acid is not known, partly because the amount is influenced by the varying conditions of daily life and partly because there undoubtedly exist individual differences concerning the quantitative factors of this substance to be excreted.

4. Direct proof that a uric dyscrasia exists, the presence of uric acid in the blood of the depressed patients, would, of course, be very desirable, but this is just as difficult to provide in these cases as in other forms of this dyscrasia. Boucheron found that saliva gave a positive murexide reaction in a number of patients in which he felt that he could assume the presence of uric acid diathesis (cf. l'Union Médicale 1881;121). The same appears to have been the case in several of my patients, whose saliva I have tested according to Boucheron's method. But lacking sufficient comparative investigations, I do not thus far attach any importance to these results.

* Johan Schioldann's translation of Carl Lange's speech "On Periodical Depressions and Their Pathogenesis" was included in:

1. Johan Schioldann: Commemoration of the Centenary of the Death of Carl Lange. The Lange Theory of 'Periodical Depressions.' A Landmark in the History of Lithium Therapy. Adelaide: Adelaide Academic Press; 2001, pp. 23-49.
2. Johan Schioldann: History of the Introduction of Lithium into Medicine and Psychiatry. Birth of Modern Psychopathology 1949. Adelaide: Adelaide Academic Press; 2009, pp. 293-308.
3. Periodical Depressions and their Pathogenesis. History of Psychiatry 2011; 22:116-30.

August 16, 2018

CHAPTER 2.

INTRODUCTION

JOHN CADE BY SAMUEL GERSHON

John Cade was born in 1912 in Murtora, Australia, and received his M.D. in 1933 from the University of Melbourne. He worked as House Officer at St. Vincent's Hospital and trained in psychiatry before joining the Australian Armed Medical Corps, where he rose to major, in 1941. After spending two years as prisoner of war, Cade retuned home and joined Bundoora Repatriation Hospital in Melbourne.

Influenced by Rolv Gjessing's reports that altered metabolism with the production of mescaline-like like substances was possibly responsible for a form of catatonia, and Albert Hofmann's discovery that lysergic acid diethylamide, an ergot alkaloid, has psychomimetic effect in minute amounts, Cade began his research in the mid-1940s at Bundoora. He assumed that manic-depressive illness is analogous to thyrotoxicosis and myxedema and hypothesized that mania is a state of intoxication by a normal product of the body in excess, and melancholia is a state of deficiency of the same substance. To test this hypothesis, he compared the effects of intra-peritoneally injected manic urine with urine from normal subjects in guinea pigs and found the former more toxic in killing the animals than the latter. Cade identified urea as the culprit that killed the animals; but when he administered lithium urate to establish uric acid's toxicity enhancing effect on manic urine, he found that instead of enhancing toxicity, it protected the animals from urea's toxic effects. He attributed the protective effect of the substance to lithium and when trying to determine whether lithium salts alone have any discernable effect, he found that after injecting them in large doses of aqueous solution into guinea pigs, the animals became lethargic and unresponsive. Since Cade's investigations had commenced in an attempt to demonstrate the presence of a toxic substance excreted in the urine of manic patients, he compared the effect of lithium in 10 manic, 6 schizophrenic and 5 depressed patients, after taking the substance himself for about two-weeks to ascertain its safety, in the dose at which it was used before in gout, epilepsy, etc. He found that lithium was effective in controlling psychotic excitement, especially in manic patients. The publication of his findings, in 1949, in the Medical Journal of Australia, signals the rediscovery of lithium treatment in psychiatry.

Cade recognized that lithium exhibited remarkable specificity for mania, that it was not sedating to patients and that the treatment could be continued with a possible prophylactic benefit. Yet, concerned about its toxicity, after the death of one of his patients included in his first experiment, he virtually stopped using lithium in his hospital and stopped experiments with the substance.

In 1953, Cade was appointed Medical Superintendent of Royal Park Hospital, in Melbourne. In the years that followed, he had done no further research with lithium but carried out investigations with protective foods in psychiatry and with high doses of thiamin in the prevention and treatment of memory disturbances in alcoholism. About fifteen years after the publication of his historical paper on lithium, he reported high magnesium levels in schizophrenia and during the 1960s, he studied the effects of manganese in mongolism.

Cade retired from his position at Royal Park, in 1977, and died at age 68, in 1980.

References:

Cade JF. Lithium salts in the treatment of psychotic excitement. Med J Aust 1949; 2: 349-52.

Cade JF. A significant elevation of plasma magnesium levels in schizophrenia. Med J Aust 1964; 1: 195-6.

Cade JF. The story of lithium. In: Ayd FJ, Blackwell B, editors. Discoveries in Biological Psychiatry. Philadelphia: Lippincott; 1970, pp. 218-29.

August 1, 2013

EDWARD TRAUTNER BY SAMUEL GERSHON

Edward Trautner was born, in 1886, in Germany and received his medical degree in his native country. He left Germany, in the 1930s, and after a short stay in Spain and England, he arrived in the 1940s, as a refugee to Australia, where he was invited by Professor Douglas Wright, head of the joint Department of Physiology and Pharmacology at the University of Melbourne, to join his faculty.

In 1949, John Cade published his report in the Medical Journal of Australia on "Lithium salts in maniacal excitement" that lead to the re-introduction of lithium therapy in psychiatry. Yet, the clinical use of the new treatment entailed difficulties because of lithium's toxicity that was to the extent that Cade himself prohibited the use of the substance in his own hospital. Recognizing the importance of rendering lithium feasible for clinical use, Trautner with his junior associates that included Charles Noack, Douglas Coats and Samuel Gershon, conducted a series of four studies, during the 1950s, that set the foundation for lithium therapy.

In the first of these reports, published in 1951, it was established that lithium, if administered in a dose, in which plasma lithium levels are kept within 0.6 mEq/l to 1.2 mEq/l, is a safe and effective treatment in manic depressive patients. Plasma level determinations in the study were carried out with the flame photometer, an instrument constructed by Victor Wynn at the University, just a year before. From the other three reports, one published in 1955, showed increase of lithium retention in mania and of lithium excretion, when mania is resolved; another, published in 1956, revealed possible use of lithium in maintaining manic depressive patients in remission; and the third, published in 1957, dealt with the treatment of lithium toxicity. Without Trautner's contributions, implementation of lithium treatment would have been considerably delayed. Trautner died in Queensland, in 1979, at age 93.

References:

Coats DA, Trautner EM, Gershon S. The treatment of lithium poisoning. Austr Ann Med 1957; 6: 11-5.

Gershon S, Trautner EM. The treatment of shock-dependency by pharmacological agents. Med J Austr 1956; 43: 783-7.

Noack D, Trautner EM. The lithium treatment of maniacal psychosis. Med J Austr 1951; 2: 218-22.

Trautner EM, Morris R, Noack CH, Gershon S. The excretion and retention of ingested lithium and its effect on ionic balance of man. Med J Austr 1955; 2: 20-91.

August 1, 2013

SAMUEL GERSHON: FIRST-HAND ACCOUNTS
1. EVENTS AND MEMORIES

I have been pressured by my colleagues in INHN to write about some of the events and memories of my professional life in psychopharmacology. Barry Blackwell has written a memoir titled "Bits and Pieces of a Psychiatrist's Life," a complete account of his personal and professional accomplishments. I could not do that, but Tom Ban suggested I contribute an account of each of the drugs I helped develop - "bits and pieces" - if not a full memoir. I have accepted the challenge and will stick mainly to professional aspects told through work events and scientific episodes.

I graduated from medical school at the University of Sydney in 1950 and then did a rotating internship. During 1951, I took a rotation through the psychiatric inpatient facility at the Royal Prince Alfred Hospital attached to the University. The psychiatrist in charge of the institute was a very liberal fellow, not convinced he knew all the answers and willing to admit we had very few. Australia at that time was a fairly isolated place, but we heard a lot about Dr. Cade including his talks in 1948 and article in 1949 on lithium treatment of mania and the enormous success he reported (Cade 1949). So, it was possible to use lithium therapeutically during this elective. In the few cases I treated, lithium seemed effective, using it cautiously over 7-10 days, since deaths from lithium had been reported by others in Australia.

The next year, 1952, I transferred to the University of Melbourne and joined the Department of Mental Health. I was assigned to the Royal Park Mental Hospital in Melbourne, where Cade was the Superintendent. At the same time, I enrolled at the University where mandated courses in psychiatry were given and exams over the next four years were administered. Unlike the boards in Psychiatry in the US, we had to pass every subject in the curriculum each year or do it again.

Royal Park Hospital was the acute receiving hospital for Melbourne. So, this seemed the greatest place in the world to actually study lithium - the first significant discovery in psychiatry.

At this point, I only wanted to evaluate and understand its therapeutic profile, clinical effects and process of improvement. So, I asked senior colleagues who I should speak to about getting supervision. They told me this was not a good idea as Dr. Cade had banned lithium in the hospital because of the deaths and serious toxicities that had occurred, including one of his own patients in the original 1949 report. This was not a great start, and after a lot of psychological turmoil, I decided I would have to find another route.

Also at this point, I only thought of personal observation of lithium's effects and course of treatment; I had done no research and did not know of anyone doing research. My choice of action was born of desperation; I contacted a Professor at the University of Melbourne known as approachable to students and faculty. This was Professor Wright, Chair of Physiology. I went without an appointment, a young dopey kid, but he was nice and kind. He elicited what I wanted to do and evaluated me carefully. After further questioning and discussion, the meeting ended when he said, "Well, you should go up and see "Trautie." So, I went upstairs and found Dr. Trautner in his lab with a couple of doctoral students… I had found my research mentor and a future friend.

Trautner was an elderly, wrinkled gentleman with a heavy German accent. I am ashamed to say I have no photo of him. We had a general discussion about his published 1951 study of 100 hospitalized psychiatric patients treated with lithium. An important feature was that it was the first lithium study in the world in which patients had their lithium assays monitored and no patients had died. Also, this was the first study to use flame photometry to monitor the plasma levels of sodium and potassium, the result of Dr. Victor Wynn's first use of the assay. Dr. Wynn was also a faculty member in the Department of Physiology at the University of Melbourne, so the University faculty played the main role in a broad range of studies on the physiology of lithium.

They established the procedures for safe use of lithium in humans, keeping it alive in psychiatry. As I mentioned, Cade banned the use of lithium in his hospital and Roberts and Ashburner at two other state hospitals in Victoria reported deaths of a patient at each hospital and that was the death knell for lithium therapy in Australia. However, two other psychiatrists (both new immigrants) in two other states in Australia also contacted Trautner and he advised them to carry out their own mania studies. Both Glesinger and Margulies, published papers confirming their findings in the large study by Noack and Trautner; both used plasma assays and had no untoward effects.

Thus, my encounter with Trautner generated enthusiasm for how one might treat and understand at least one psychiatric disorder. As a novice, I had no research funds or assistants but was encouraged and supported with help and advice by colleagues at the University of Melbourne who gave their knowledge and time unconditionally.

The first major lithium project (Trautner, Morris, Noack and Gershon 1955), was on the differential retention and excretion between manic and non-manic phase patients. We found that classic manic bipolar 1 patients would retain more of the lithium ion ingested over a one-week period than normal or control subjects, whose retention and excretion was more in daily balance. When the manic phase remitted, they excreted the retained lithium, exceeding their daily dose until they reached homeostasis. This new and exciting finding was state and trait dependent.

This study also gave us clues about other ionic effects, including sodium and potassium losses. This was time consuming, taking a couple of years, but provided the groundwork for later studies. Our findings also dictated we develop a treatment plan for lithium toxicity. Again, we went to our colleague at the University of Melbourne, Dr. Douglas Coats, an expert in electrolyte and renal physiology who agreed to work with us on this urgent and important topic. Our paper (Coats, Trautner and Gershon 1957) offered an explanation of the aberration in water and electrolyte balance found in bipolar disorder and proposed a treatment plan that followed logically from the previous study. We had occasion to use our results to help other psychiatrists deal with toxic patients to obtain positive outcomes.

The next lithium report came after I arrived in the U.S. at the University of Michigan on a scholarship awarded after an Australia-wide competition; it had a large grant to establish Schizophrenia and Psychopharmacology Research projects. This paper summarized laboratory and clinical experiences to date (Gershon and Yuwiler 1960). Art Yuwiler was head of the biochemistry research division. The views presented are still those I hold today. After an additional 55 years of study and observation, lithium is one of the few examples of psychopharmacological specificity in psychiatric treatment.

During this period, we established the efficacy of lithium in mania; demonstrated the effect of lithium on water and electrolyte physiology; reported the differential retention and excretion of lithium in the manic phase; elucidated the therapeutic range for treatment of mania; and also studied the clinical picture of lithium toxicity, as well as demonstrated an effective treatment plan for it.

The next issue we thought urgent was potential toxic effects to the embryo. Now that safe clinical usage was possible, we realized special risk could exist in pregnant women, but the best we could do was an animal study on the results of prolonged sub-toxic lithium in rats (Trautner, Pennycuik, Morris et al. 1958). All animals went through pregnancy with good weight and general health. On examination of the uterus near term, the one finding was that lithium-treated rats retained fewer intact fetuses than controls, indicating that some toxic effects would have to be studied in higher species. This was the case in humans, where a low incidence of some cardiac defects occurred. The authors were all University of Melbourne colleagues.

Our next study may seem esoteric by current standards. However, it demonstrated important findings. Maintenance ECT was used in many cases of patients who suffered from recurrent depression, recurrent bipolar disorder and resistant schizophrenia unresponsive to other treatments. This study examined the use of lithium in bipolar cases and found that it could provide a maintenance medication to replace the use of recurrent treatments with ECT (Gershon and Trautner 1956).

In Australia, we also did some experiments in Trautner's lab using Warburg brain biochemical techniques. With the simple belief that mania had an increase in brain cell activity, we embarked on our first experiment. We also knew that we could increase brain slice energy activity with di-nitro-phenol (DNP). Would the addition of lithium have an effect on this system? After a non-toxic concentration of lithium was added to the DNP activated system, we consistently found a decrease in metabolic activity. This was an exciting finding but due to the usual "circumstances beyond our control" we never continued with these experiments.

All of the studies cited were conducted without grants or research funds, contributed to by the faculty and the meager resources of their labs. They were all unblinded because we could not afford elaborate designs.

References:

Blackwell B. Bits and Pieces of a Psychiatrist's Life. United States; XLibris Corporation: 2012.

Cade J. Lithium salts in the treatment of psychotic excitement. Med J Austr 1949; 2: 349-52.

Coats DA, Trautner EM, Gershon S. The treatment of lithium poisoning. Austr Ann Med 1957; 6: 11-15.

Gershon S, Trautner EM. The treatment of shock dependency by pharmacological agents. Med J Austr 1956; 43: 783-7.

Gershon S, Yuwiler A. Lithium ion. A specific psychopharmacological approach to the treatment of mania. J Neuropsychiat 1960; 1: 229-41.

Glesinger B. Evaluation of lithium in treatment of psychotic excitement. Med J Austr. 1954; 41: 277-81.

Margulies M. Suggestions for the treatment of schizophrenic and manicdepressive patients. Med J Austr 1955; 1: 137-43.

Noack CH, Trautner EM. The lithium treatment of maniacal psychosis. Med J Austr 1951; 2: 219-22.

Trautner EM, Morris R, Noack CH, Gershon S. The excretion and retention of ingested lithium and its effect on ionic balance in man. Med J Austr 1955; 2: 280-91.

Trautner EM, Pennycuik PR, Morris RJH, Gershon S, Shankly KH. The effects of prolonged subtoxic lithium ingestion in rats. Aust J Exp Biol Med Sci 1958; 36: 305-21.

June 25, 2015

2. LITHIUM HISTORY

Introduction

Lithium preparations have been mentioned in medical writings since ancient times. They have, on occasion, been proposed as treatments for a variety of conditions. Sometimes these were accompanied by explanations of their possible modes of action. There have even been previous publications suggesting the usage in various forms of manic-depressive illness. However, for our purposes at this time, we plan to focus primarily on the period from 1947 to 2018.

Our focus on this 80-year period is selected because during this time lithium generated world-wide interest in its possible clinical utility and generated equally a real commitment to mode-of-action studies in the neurosciences. Of minor importance, this period coincides with my own professional life in psychiatry.

This 80-year period was marked by the publication of two seminal papers by Dr. John Cade, the first in 1947, the second in 1949. These two papers, **The Anticonvulsant Properties of Creatinine** (1947) and **Lithium Salts in the treatment of Psychotic Excitement** (1949), require careful evaluation and interpretation of what they stated and how clearly.

In order to present the scope of Cade's broader thinking, I would like to mention two other original papers he published: **The Etiology of Schizophrenia** (1956) and **Manganese and Mongolism** (1958). These reports were, I think, related to his earlier thoughts about diet and mental function. The former could derive its data from the admission sheets to Royal Park Receiving Hospital, which was the acute receiving hospital for the city of Melbourne. This data could provide patient names, last address for admission and admission diagnosis. This 1956 paper looked at the intake of stone fruits (peaches, etc.) and diagnosis. It showed that this patient population from the inner city did not seem to have access to this sort of fruit diet. It proposed that this lack in the diet could be causal of schizophrenia.

Significance of 1947 and 1949 papers

In presenting this discussion I wish to clarify the limitations of this section. As I mentioned, we are concentrating on a limited time frame of 80 years. In addition to that, we still have to set fixed parameters in which we can elaborate the questions that have been raised by other authors and the many INHN contributors.

Tom Ban, our editor in chief, asked me to try my hand at this resume. I therefore wish to state at the outset that our main marker is Johan Schioldann's masterly work: **History of the Introduction of Lithium into Medicine and Psychiatry; Birth of Modern Psychopharmacology 1949** (2009). The author is a Norwegian psychiatrist educated at the University of Copenhagen, living in

Australia since 1984 and now Emeritus Professor of Psychiatry at the University of Adelaide. This document became our foundation to present the rest of the story. Next, we asked Barry Blackwell to review Johan's book and publish his review on the INHN website. A brief correspondence then occurred between these two, Tom Ban and me.

The parameter of this review

Schioldann's book is a major compendium of most publications in the history of lithium. The author attempted to cover the entire world literature in English and several other languages in his volume. His book includes the citation of 1,245 references, going back to the 19th century. Thus, it became clear that this unique and massive work was our main cornerstone of discussion.

The secondary cornerstone for our exercise is Barry Blackwell's extensive review of Johan's book. Blackwell undertakes a careful, thorough and detailed review with a discussion of some of the questions raised by Schioldann about Cade's work and other comments and questions raised by contributors to the INHN network. For example, some of these touch on questions such as: Why Cade did not mention any prior publications on this general subject before his own?; How did Cade very quickly move from his guinea pig experiments to the use of lithium in man?; and especially, how was he able to develop an appropriate human dose from his work with these animals? One topic that has also been a matter of fundamental conjecture is the use of the word "serendipity" to describe Cade's discovery and the antipathy that this word is applied at all.

Schioldann responded to Blackwell's review of his book and did criticize Blackwell's acceptance of the term "serendipity" to adequately describe Cade's use of Lithium in man. My personal view is that it does matter who obtains the credit (full or partial) for a particular scientific discovery. The actual inventor has the responsibility to demonstrate the steps taken to build the structure necessary to explain the logic and thinking processes to achieve the endpoint.

I think it is necessary to deconstruct the details and specifics of some of these studies and attempt to reorder them so we can obtain a clear and more satisfying explanation of the events that have been recorded, reinterpreted and restated in different colors.

Now, we turn to the **Editors**.

Exhibit 1. 1947 Guinea Pigs

I quote from Schioldann's response to Blackwell: "Cade started by injecting urine from manic patients and, in way of control, urine from normal, schizophrenic and melancholic individuals, into the abdominal cavity of guinea pigs. All animals died… he [then] proceeded to inject the animals with the 'end-products' of protein metabolism, the nitrogenous constituents of urine: creatinine, urea and uric acid, and found that urea was the 'guilty substance.'… In his belief that the urine from manic patients was more or less more toxic than that from non-manic patients… he finally postulated a third toxic substance… At no later time did Cade make any mention of such a third substance… I concluded that Cade's observations cannot be considered to be documentation of scientific fact."

In addition, Schioldann hears directly from Schou that Schou could not replicate Cade's findings in these guinea pig experiments.

What behavioral observations did Cade record on these animals? He stated that after these IP injections of lithium carbonate to these previously active animals, they were seen lying quietly on their side in the cage for some time. It is also not clear why he used lithium carbonate for these IP injections as it is relatively insoluble. Thus, this quiet, apparently immobile behavior was the only behavior recorded by Cade. (This has been mostly interpreted as lithium intoxication.) He then rapidly moved on to his human experiments.

Exhibit 2. Human Studies

Cade began his patient experiments using a lithium dose of 1200 mg. of the citrate thrice daily or 600 mg. of the carbonate. With no references, on his part, to prior publications in the world literature and with no real ability to develop a dose for human patients with mania from these guinea pig experiments, it is extremely hard to understand how Cade could proceed to an appropriate human dose at all. Here, we have to consider that he had to determine, not one safe dose for one day in a manic patient, but the long-term dosage plan. As an aside, the Lange brothers and Hammond both published the actual prescriptions of lithium salt doses they had been using chronically in patients. Hammond even considered the need to increase the doses if the mania was not controlled.

To return to Cade's report. In his 1949 paper he stated he had included 10 manic patients, three with chronic mania and seven with recurrent episodes. He reported that within a couple of weeks all manic patients were recovered. At a later date, he reported that two patients diagnosed as schizophrenic also responded. This last observation is a little difficult to interpret, as generally schizophrenic patients do not do well on lithium treatment. After this 1949 paper was published, it was reported that the first patient (WB) subsequently died. The clinical notes indicate that "patient continued well with occasional biliousness." This is evidence of lithium toxicity. However, on March 8th, 1950, WB was readmitted with lithium toxicity and the drug was discontinued. These effects were not included in his 1950 lithium efficacy paper. At this time, Cade further commented: "Under all circumstances it seems that he would be better off as a care-free restless case of mania rather than the dyspeptic, frail little man he looks on adequate lithium… on May 12, 1950, Lithium was reinstituted because his manic state worsened. This state seems as much a menace to life as any possible side effects of lithium… on May 22, W.B…. died." Cade recorded the death as "toxemia due to Lithium salts therapeutically administered. This was the coroner's verdict in October 1950." (Cade never publicly admitted the cause of death and years later in four publications he portrayed the final outcome as successful.)

However, in 1950 Cade banned the use of lithium in his own hospital. In these toxic experiences, it seems that Cade may not have been aware of this possibility even though this had been published by Garrod in 1859. Furthermore, the FDA had received reports of lithium toxicity from a product marketed in the US as a substitute for sodium in cardiac patients. The FDA finally banned the sale of lithium-containing products in 1950.

In addition to this knowledge, there was an ongoing study underway in Melbourne, Australia, which reported on 100 manic patients treated with lithium. This study, conducted by Noack and Trautner, was published in 1951 and, at that time, it was the largest data base on lithium usage in mania. The other unique feature of this study was that it was it was done under regular lithium plasma assays and no deaths or serious deaths or serious toxicities were reported.

In summary, several reports by Schou (1992, 1996, 1996, 1998, 2001) and others, find Cade's work "indeed strange." The hypothesis that started his work was crude. His experimental design was not clear and, indeed, his interpretation of his animal data may well have been wrong, especially so as the behavioral changes in the animals to immobility may simply have been due to lithium toxicity. Also, and importantly, Schou's own attempts to replicate the guinea pig experiments failed.

When it came to the big jump into human studies, Cade says himself: "the original therapeutic dose, decided on fortuitously, proved to be the optimum, that is 1200 mg citrate twice daily or 600 mg carbonate."

This single statement rings loud as phenomenal since Cade did no dose range studies in animals or man.

To sum up, I conclude the simple recorded facts that:

1. The Lange brothers were the First to establish the use of lithium for the treatment of a depressive episode if occurring as a single manifestation or recurrently;

2. They also recorded a copy of a medical prescription for a standard dose and course of lithium. This is the dose that Cade himself uses in his human study. The Lange brothers continued and then reported that in many of these cases the depression was recurrent and then routinely recommended continued treatment to prevent a recurrence of the depression. Thus, the Langes are First to

introduce the concept of prophylactic therapy (at least) for recurrent depression; and

3. The report by Hammond describing, in his textbook, the use of lithium to treat manic excitement thus, Hammond, in 1871 in New York, becomes the First person to describe the therapeutic effects of lithium in mania.

Thus, after reviewing all the material available to me, I concluded that the animal experiments of Cade were not explained as a basis for any planned outcome related therapeutics. His clinical trial, therefore, raises as many questions as it answers, as do his reports that two schizophrenic patients were also given lithium treatment, yet both were reported to benefit. It is somewhat unusual for schizophrenics to gain any significant benefit from lithium.

Neither Schioldann nor I can reach a conclusion that Cade's work had the prior information necessary to plan the animal experiments and that he had no clear idea of what he intended to find out from these animal experiments. Yet he proceeded to a clinical trial with a lucky guess and to the correct initial safe therapeutic dose with no information as to the safety of continuing to treat at this dose long term.

It appears that there was no established claim developed for long-term treatment with lithium. The starting dose, as he himself states, was a fortunate guess. He was not aware of the reports on toxicity in the older literature or the more recent warnings from 1945/50 reported in the US ending with the complete ban of lithium salts by the FDA in 1950. During his clinical trial there was another major study going on in Melbourne by Noack and Trautner. However, I know for a fact that Cade never approached Trautner to discuss these concerns of toxicity. Trautner had a well-trained team of lithium researchers working with him at the University of Melbourne. Cade, as superintendent of Royal Park, could have readily obtained additional information on the serious concerns by contacting any member of this group, including the chairman Professor Wright.

Introduction

In summary, the reader has been presented with two documents by Schioldann and two by Blackwell, plus my document presented here.

Schioldann and I cannot offer our endorsement of the scientific pattern of Cade's two papers on lithium or that either one gave a clear and definitive presentation of rational, logical facts acquired in a methodical series of studies to establish it as an authentic original contribution.

However, as this entire set of papers has danced around the word "serendipity," we need to consider this aspect of the debate in more detail. Blackwell's response to Schioldann references is a very elegant and learned article on the 300-year history of the word by Tom Ban. His exegesis and discussion of serendipity diffuses, rather than clarifies, the attempts at factual evaluation presented in our discussion. One could also side-step specificity by offering a new word altogether: pseudo-serendipitous. Portmanteau words like serendipity are often used to provide a form of over-inclusion to bypass the specific problem of the debate. One could also add other words or descriptions, such as "scientifically serendipitous" or "serendipitous and deductive."

I must end with significant doubts as to how this history has become legend.

References:

Cade, JF. The Anticonvulsant Properties of Creatinine. Med. J. Aust. 1947; 2, 621-3.

Cade, JF. Lithium Salts in the treatment of Psychotic Excitement. Med. J. Aust. 1949; 2, 349-52.

Cade, JF. The Etiology of Schizophrenia. Med. J. Aust. 1956; 2, 135-9.

Cade, JF. Manganese and Mongolism. Med. J. Aust. 1958; 2, 848-9.

Schioldann, J. History of the Introduction of Lithium into Medicine and Psychiatry; Birth of Modern Psychopharmacology 1949. Adelaide Academic Press, c2009 xxv, 363 p.

May 3, 2018

CHAPTER 3.

VERIFICATION

Thomas A. Ban

MOGENS SCHOU:
MY JOURNEY WITH LITHIUM
PRESENTED BY JOHAN SCHIOLDANN*

I was born in Copenhagen on 24 November 1918 as second child of Margrethe Schou, née Brodersen (1887-1960), and Hans Jacob Schou, M.D. (1886-1952). Having graduated from High School in 1936 I vacillated between studying engineering and medicine. After six months at Askov Community College - where I met my later wife Agnete Jessen - I opted for medicine, and I graduated from the medical faculty of the University of Copenhagen in 1944.

My father was the medical director of two hospitals, one for epileptic and psychotic patients (kolonien filadelfia) and one for patients with neuroses and mild depressions (dianalund nervesanatorium). He took a special interest in manic-depressive illness. At the time patients were given supportive psychotherapy and the medications that were then available: barbiturates for mania and opium for depression. Unfortunately, both were quite ineffective. I have vivid memories of depressed patients wandering in the hospital park with bent heads and anguished faces, waiting and waiting for the depression to lift and fearing manic and depressive recurrences. It is difficult to imagine the torment of these drawn-out depressions.

In order to study possible biochemical and physiological changes in the manic-depressive patients my father established a research laboratory. He was very impressed by the longitudinal and extremely careful studies carried out by the Norwegian psychiatrist Rolv Gjessing who followed the nitrogen balance in patients suffering from periodic catatonia. Manic-depressive illness has also a periodic course and might reveal related biochemical changes. My father further shared the notion of a biological basis of moods and mood disorders with his countryman, the physiologist and neurologist Carl Lange. The fact that his 12 years older cousin, August Krogh, a Nobel laureate, was professor of zoophysiology, may also have been a factor.

In 1938-39 my father spoke to me with exhilaration about the advent of electroconvulsive therapy. Here was finally something that worked: within weeks both manias and depressions were brought to an end. When recurrences developed, electroconvulsive therapy was administered again, but the treatment was not given during symptom-free intervals.

Following my father's example, I trained in psychiatry and took three to four years of clinical psychiatry at Danish, Norwegian and Swedish hospitals. Because at that time the only effective treatment for mood disorders was electroconvulsive, I decided to turn to research. So, after having finished my clinical training, I studied experimental biology with Herman Kalckar in Copenhagen and Heinrich Waelsch in New York. In Kalckar's laboratory of cytophysiology I studied xanthopterin, a compound from butterfly wings with interesting chemical features. Waelsch worked at the New York State Institute of Psychiatry at Columbia University. He was a pioneer in neurochemistry, was brilliant and dynamic, and he taught me the experimental approach.

Among my professional mentors I count with gratitude Erik Strömgren, professor of psychiatry at Aarhus University and medical director of the psychiatric hospital at Risskov. He was a remarkable man, respected in international as well as in Danish psychiatry for his erudition and clarity of thought. Rather than taking a more prestigious chair in Copenhagen he chose to build up the Risskov hospital as a comprehensive psychiatric institution with clinical and research units (Schioldann and Strömgren 1996). He created a position for me as research associate and I founded and headed a laboratory of biological psychiatry and psychopharmacology. For some years I was associate professor of psychopharmacology at Aarhus University and in 1971 I was appointed to a newly created chair of biological psychiatry.

In 1952 (1951) Strömgren drew my attention to the Australian publications by Cade and by Noack and Trautner about the antimanic action of lithium. Here was a welcome opportunity to study a supposedly effective drug, but I felt that the studies reported until then were insufficiently stringent. I therefore devised a protocol for a trial that was partly open, partly randomized and placebo controlled (Schou, Juel-Nielsen, Strömgren and Voldby 1954). Together with two other clinicians, Niels Juel-Nielsen and Holger Voldby, Strömgren selected, treated and observed manic patients. I did not see the patients, but I threw a dice to allocate them randomly to lithium or placebo, carried out the serum lithium determinations with an old and often recalcitrant flame photometer, analyzed the data and wrote the final paper. This trial fully confirmed the antimanic effect of lithium and it was the beginning of my almost lifelong journey with the drug. Since the laboratory in Risskov could not compete with neurochemical institutes elsewhere with their surplus of expensive equipment, basic research on lithium's mode of action did not seem a promising avenue, but Risskov offered me some special advantages. In Danish hospitals patients were diagnosed according to Kraepelinian traditions and owing to the stability of the Danish population patients could be followed for many years. Our proximity to the clinical wards had benefits. Observations made in animals, for example concerning the treatment and prevention of side effects, were sometimes directly applicable to patients; clinical observations could immediately be tested in animals, mostly white rats, by administering larger doses under more extreme conditions.

At times my work proceeded smoothly, but I also experienced setbacks. There have been both tailwinds and headwinds on the way. By 1964 G. P. Hartigan, England (1963), P. C. Baastrup, Glostrup, Denmark (Baastrup 1964), and I (Schou 1956) had, independently of each other, made observations on small groups of patients, which seemed to indicate that prolonged treatment with lithium might ameliorate or prevent not only manic but also depressive recurrences. This was a new and unexpected observation and it called for closer examination.

Baastrup started to give long-term lithium treatment to patients with both mania and depressions and in spite of the geographical distance between Risskov and Glostrup he invited me to cooperate with serum lithium analyses and methodology. We carried out a trial that ran over six and a half years and involved 88 bipolar and unipolar patients. These had been selected for having had two or more episodes within the last year or one or more episodes per year for the last two years. The Archives of General Psychiatry published our paper (Baastrup and Schou 1967) which revealed several things. Firstly, the start of long-term lithium treatment was associated with a remarked 87% drop in the frequency of both manic and depressive recurrences. Secondly, the recurrences that did occur usually developed after the patients had stopped taking lithium, or in patients with atypical manic-depressive disorder, mostly schizoaffective disorder. Thirdly, the efficacy of lithium did not disappear with time or after interruption and subsequent resumption of the treatment. And finally, the prophylactic effect of lithium was equally good in unipolar and bipolar patients.

The outcome of this trial gave Baastrup and me an intense feeling of fulfillment. For the first time we had come upon a maintenance treatment that could break the almost inexorable development of recurrences and could stabilize the mood of patients who previously had suffered frequent and destructive attacks of mania, depression or both. Our patients were seriously ill; no less than 40% of them had attempted suicide before they were given lithium.

After publication of this study it became customary to talk about prophylactic or recurrence–preventive treatment of mood disorders. The terms mood stabilization and mood stabilizers were not used until after 1990 and the users of these terms did not always specify whether they referred to prevention of manic or depressive recurrences. Lithium prevents both manic and depressive episodes.

Psychiatrists in Denmark and other countries then began to use lithium prophylactically. They confirmed our findings and were gratified with lithium's efficacy. However, psychiatrists from the Maudsley Hospital in London (Blackwell and Shepherd) expressed their skepticism forcibly and they did it in The Lancet, i.e., a journal other than the one in which we had published. They were not skeptical because they failed to confirm our findings, for they never tried to give lithium to patients. Their skepticism was purely speculative.

Blackwell and Shepherd (1968) felt that the evidence did not support our claims of a prophylactic lithium action. They argued that some of the patients had a "fragmented" rather than a recurrent course of illness; that the follow-up period had been too short; that the chosen statistical method weighted the facts in favor of the hypothesis; and, finally, that the non-blind evaluation of the recurrences was biased. This led to somewhat heated discussions between them and us, and the disagreement involved both methodological and personal issues. Lader (1968) argued that the patients selected for having had frequent episodes for some years must be expected to have fewer episodes during the following years. In our refutation (Baastrup and Schou 1968a,b) Baastrup and I went over the first paper's many misunderstandings and erroneous calculations. We also repeated that most of the patients had been discharged after they were given lithium; it was the general practitioners who decided when there had been a recurrence and we had no influence on this. We furthermore pointed out that the frequency of recurrences could not be expected to drop but rather to rise year by year in the way that is characteristic of the course of recurrent affective disorders (Angst and Weis 1969; Angst, Grof and Schou 1969).

The disagreement between us and our critics involved important methodological issues. Shepherd was one of the first psychiatrists in Great Britain to use randomized, placebo-controlled trials and he was convinced that valid evidence could be obtained only with this procedure and that any other evidence must be rejected. Baastrup's and my trial was not randomized and placebo controlled. It had started, more or less, on an exploratory basis and had grown gradually. The marked change in the course of the disease of patients having had a median of nine episodes before the lithium treatment coincided with the start of that treatment and this was unlikely to be fortuitous. Psychiatrists who followed their patients longitudinally found our observations and conclusions convincing. Our critics disregarded the serious long-term prognosis of untreated bipolar disorder.

The controversy created uncertainty among British and American psychiatrists, and they hesitated to start prophylactic lithium treatment. Baastrup and I could not help but feeling responsible for this to some extent. If we had carried out our study with a double-blind design from the beginning, matters might have taken a different turn. However, things being what they were, we had to consider carefully whether we should, after all, supplement our open study with a double-blind one in order to subject the question of prophylactic efficacy to further testing under the strictest precautions.

We presented this and other arguments in a reply in Lancet (Lader 1968), but Blackwell and Shepherd remained skeptical and did not give lithium to their patients. They overlooked, or chose to overlook, the serious long-term prognosis of bipolar disorder not given prophylactic treatment.

Personal issues are more difficult to analyze, but it is worthy of note that when Shepherd in 1967 heard me lecture about prophylactic lithium treatment in Germany and express gratification with the results, he immediately perceived me as a naïve and biased "believer." The crucial point seems to have been reached when I told how my brother, who for twenty-five years had had depressions every spring, stopped having recurrences when he was given lithium. Shepherd obviously found that this was the final testimony of my folly and subjectivity. He referred to me as "an enthusiastic advocate." The term "enthusiast" might refer to someone who is strongly engaged in his work, but in the given context the term "advocate" can hardly have been meant as a compliment, an advocate being seen as a person who supports only one side of a case. A scientist, on the other hand, is someone who gathers all relevant evidence and then weighs it carefully before drawing a conclusion. This is usually in the form of a hypothesis that may later be rejected, by the scientist himself or by others. I learned later (Baastrup and Schou 1968) that at Maudsley there were people who explained my position by hinting that I myself was manic-depressive and on lithium. That is not so.

Reporting here what may appear to be a personal grudge involves a question of principle. If a reader pays attention to an author's assumed motives and mental state, this may sharpen his critical sense. But if the reader rejects the data, arguments and conclusions of an author because he does not find his motives acceptable or does not deem his mental state sufficiently sane, science and patients might be deprived of valuable information.

The idea of putting prophylactic efficacy to further testing under the strictest of precautions was tempting, but difficulties arose. Could Baastrup and I, who found the likelihood of a prophylactic action of lithium very high, justify a trial that meant that half of our patients would be given placebo instead of what we considered an active drug? Could we, who were responsible for the patients' health, expose them to the risk of prolonged suffering or possibly suicide? Was consideration for the interests of manic-depressive patients in other hospitals or other countries sufficiently important to outweigh consideration for our own patients?

I pondered these questions with personal feelings involved since my younger brother had suffered recurrent depressions every spring from the time he was 20-years-old. He had been treated with electroconvulsive therapy and antidepressants that to some extent relieved the current episodes, but the attacks came again and again. Then I started him on lithium and the disease stopped. After years of being disabled he could resume work; he and his family were able to look to the future with new hope. Could Baastrup and I subject him or others like him to a one-to-one risk of being deprived of the treatment that had altered their lives so radically?

But a potentially interminable discussion did not serve any useful purpose. New data were needed and Baastrup and I decided to carry out a double-blind trial, but only after I had designed a trial protocol that took our special ethical problems into consideration.

We selected about a hundred patients with recurrent depressive disorder or manic-depressive disorder who had been in lithium treatment for a year or more were; they were allocated randomly to continue lithium treatment or to be switched to placebo. (At that time the concept of informed consent did not yet exist). The trial was blind to the observers, but non-blind outsiders could transfer a patient who relapsed during the trial back to lithium without telling the observers whether that patient had been on lithium or on placebo. The trial accordingly remained double-blind.

A sequential analysis terminated the trial as soon as a statistically significant difference ($p < 0.01$) had been reached between the placebo-treated and the lithium-treated patients. By using such a procedure, we exposed as few patients as possible for as short a time as possible to placebo and minimized the ethical problem of giving placebo to patients who seemed to benefit from lithium treatment.

The trial lasted less than six months (Baastrup, Poulsen, Schou et al. 1970). In the group of unipolar patients 9 out of 17 on placebo had recurrences and 0 out of 17 on lithium ($p < 0.001$). In the group of bipolar patients 12 out of 22 on placebo had recurrences and 0 out of 28 on lithium ($p < 0.00001$). A trial in which we pooled our data with data from Prague and Zurich confirmed our findings (Angst, Weis, Grof et al. 1970). Michael Shepherd never commented on these studies.

Controlled trials from Ireland, England, Scotland and North America using both open trials, discontinuation trials and prospective trials, led to the same results as our trial. The evidence of a marked prophylactic action of lithium became so strong that under pressure from a few American psychiatrists FDA acknowledged lithium as a prophylactic agent in bipolar disorder. It was taken into use worldwide and lithium became the prophylactic agent of choice. Prophylactic lithium treatment has been most helpful for many seriously ill patients.

Over the years I have studied numerous aspects of the pharmacology, toxicology and clinical use of lithium. One of the studies dealt with the effect of prophylactic lithium treatment on artistic productivity (Schou 1979). Among the 24 artists I interviewed, six found their creativity reduced when they were given lithium, six felt no difference and 12 noted that their creativity had increased in quantity and quality as lithium prevented their barren depressions and their overactive manias that resulted in artistically valueless works.

Other topics were the psychological and social effects of lithium treatment; treatment management and monitoring; treatment regimen; lithium effects on the normal mind; somatic and psychological side effects; the effects of lithium treatment on the function of the kidneys and other organ systems; interaction with other drugs; and acute and late effects of lithium intoxication. These studies involved both experiments on animals and clinical observations.

Since my retirement in 1988 I have published reviews dealing with topics of current interest. The renal lithium clearance is of decisive importance for lithium's safety and Klaus Thomsen and I have worked out measures to prevent lithium intoxications (Thomsen and Schou 1999). It was for some time thought that lithium treatment during pregnancy was teratogenic, but later studies without a biased selection have shown that the risk of fetal changes is minimal (Schou 1998).

I have with particular interest studied and reviewed the literature about the prophylactic effects of other medications (Schou 1998, 2001). Canadian studies from recent years have shown that the efficacy of prophylactic medications depends primarily on the kind of patients treated. In patients with typical bipolar disorder, those with completely symptom-free intervals and in whom there may be bipolar disorder in the family, lithium is clearly the best prophylactic agent. In patients with atypical bipolar disorder, those with residual symptoms during the intervals, with other psychiatric disorders in the family, or with co-morbidity, some of the anticonvulsants and atypical neuroleptics are better. We should not cease to look for better prophylactic drugs, but until the superiority of a new drug over lithium has been unequivocally established, psychiatrists will serve their patients with typical bipolar disorder best by prescribing lithium.

Lithium cannot be patented and consequently has little commercial interest. Occasionally I have been asked whether it would have been an advantage if lithium had been subsidized by the pharmaceutical industry. With such support it might have been as massively promoted as the contending drugs are and that could have been an advantage for the patients. However, the drug companies were not interested and I have had complete scientific freedom. It seems unlikely that a sponsoring pharmaceutical company would have permitted me to study and publish about adverse effects of lithium more extensively than anyone else.

Since there is no commercial support for lithium, I myself have had to collect and disseminate information about it. I have used a database and a reprint library that I started in 1954 and have kept updated since then. I have travelled extensively and lectured to, as well as learned from, general practitioners, practicing psychiatrists, hospital physicians and patient groups around the world. It has also been interesting and rather difficult to write books in non-technical language for patients and relatives, but it has given me many contacts. The books have appeared in 12 languages, some of them in six editions. The importance of that kind of activity, now called "psychoeducation," is being increasingly recognized.

Although lithium is still considered the gold standard against which all newer prophylactic agents are measured, it continues to have a rather limited use. Patients and psychiatrists take it for granted that an old drug must be less efficacious than newer drugs and powerful pharmaceutical companies see inexpensive lithium as a competitor for their more expensive products. There is a dire need to inform patients and physicians about recent advances.

It is of particular importance to inform about the evidence of a marked anti-suicidal effect of long-term lithium treatment. In affectively ill patients the frequency of suicide attempts and of completed suicides is 10-15 times (not per cent) lower in patients on lithium than in patients not on lithium (Müller-Oerlinghausen, Ahrens, Grof et al. 1992; Baldessarini, Tondo and Hennen 2001). It is surprising that lithium is not used more often in patients with severe depressive symptoms, whether they are bipolar, suffer from major depressive disorder or have schizophrenia. One could give lithium prophylactically to patients with suicidal thoughts, to patients with suicide attempts in the past and to patients with suicides in the family. In no other agent with prophylactic action in mood disorders has convincing evidence of an anti-suicidal effect been presented.

The discovery that long-term lithium treatment has a neuroprotective effect has also increased the interest in lithium. Even if these observations have not yet led to diagnostic, prognostic or therapeutic advances, they give new hope to patients and psychiatrists.

I admit to having often felt frustrated on my journey with lithium, but lately I have been encouraged and gratified by the increased research interest in, and use of, lithium, even in the United States.

John Cade and Poul Christian Baastrup have been of special importance to my work and development. Cade and I met on three occasions: when he and his wife visited us in Denmark in 1972 (1970), when he and I shared the International Scientific Kittay Foundation Award in 1974 and when my wife and I visited the Cades in Melbourne the following year. He was a mild-mannered, modest person who once said of himself: "I am not a scientist. I am only an old prospector who happened to pick up a nugget." But prospectors find because they seek. John Cade was characterized by insatiable curiosity, keen observation, willingness to test even absurdly unlikely hypotheses and the courage to run the risk making a fool of himself.

Poul Christian Baastrup was a friend and associate and the role he played in the development of prophylactic lithium treatment was essential. I once characterized Cade, Baastrup and myself as the artistic, the persevering and the systematic scientist, respectively. Baastrup was characterized by unusual consistency of approach and double devotion to scientific truth and the welfare of his patients. In addition to monitoring his lithium-treated patients for the rest of their lives, Baastrup gave them unceasing psychological support and this undoubtedly increased their compliance and adherence.

I have benefited from cooperation and friendship with many other brilliant and conscientious scientists. Paul Grof from Prague, later Ottawa, and Bruno Müller-Oerlinghausen from Berlin are particularly close friends who always have given me inspiration and support. It was together with them that in 1988 I initiated an International Group for the Study of Lithium-treated (IGSLI) patients. It has had participants from Belmont, Berlin, Dresden, Freiburg, Fullerton, Halifax, Hamilton, Lübeck, Ottawa, Poznan, Prague, Risskov, Stockholm, Vienna and Zürich. Members meet once a year, rotating meeting venues, to discuss past and present joint projects.

Bruno Müller-Oerlinghausen suggested that the mortality and suicidal behavior of lithium-treated patients should be one of the first topics to be studied. As noted above, I considered the anti-suicidal effect of lithium one of the most important advantages of prophylactic lithium treatment. Other projects initiated and headed by Paul Grof and Martin Alda, deal with so-called "excellent lithium responders," carefully defined by IGSLI. These studies are yielding important information about the course of the disease, subtyping and prediction of response in the patients themselves and in their children.

Why did I become so involved with mood disorders and lithium? My choice contained an element of luck, but it was not purely accidental. As already mentioned, my father took a special interest in manic-depressive illness and scientific curiosity is contagious. Then lithium came along and turned out to be efficacious - another felicitous juxtaposition of observation, circumstance and a tuned mind. I have not seen any reason to stray from the topic of lithium while there is still so much to find out.

Perhaps more than most scientists I have been granted the privilege of reaping the fruits of my labor. A number of family members have been or are given lithium with marked effect. If prophylactic lithium treatment had not emerged, they might today have been hospitalized or dead.

In Haiti, where voodoo is the prevailing religion, psychotic persons are believed to be "ridden" by a Loa, a spirit. Scientists engaged in their work are likewise possessed. Their Loa never leaves them in peace, rides them day and night, year after year. During my life I have been ridden, but with generosity. It has been a rewarding experience to meet so many kind and generous persons and to work in a field where many scientific interests and insights converge. It has been still more gratifying to participate in the combat of a protracted, devastating and potentially deadly illness.

References:

Angst J, Weis P. Zum Verlauf depressiver Psychosen. In: Schulte W, Mende W, editors. Melancholie in Forschung, Klinik und Behandlung. Stuttgart: Thieme, 1969. pp. 2-9.

Angst J, Grof P, Schou M. Lithium. Lancet 1969; I:1097.

Angst J, Weis P, Grof P, Baastrup PC, Schou M. Lithium prophylaxis in recurrent affective disorders. Br. J. Psychiatr. 1970; 116:604-14.

Baastrup PC, Schou M. Prophylactic lithium. Lancet 1968a; I:1419-22.

Baastrup PC, Schou M. Prophylactic lithium. Lancet 1968b; II:340-50.

Baastrup PC, Poulsen JC, Schou M, Thomsen K, Amdisen A. Prophylactic lithium: Double-blind discontinuation in manic-depressive disorders. Lancet 1970; II: 326-30.

Baastrup PC, Schou M. Lithium as a prophylactic agent: Its effect against recurrent depressions and manic-depressive psychosis. Arch Gen. Psychiatr. 1967; 16:162-72.

Baastrup PC. The use of lithium in manic-depressive psychosis. Compr. Psychiatr. 1964; 5:396-408.

Baldessarini RJ, Tondo L, Hennen J. Treating the suicidal patient with bipolar disorder. Reducing suicide risk with lithium. Ann. NY Acad. Sci. 2001; 932:24-38.

Blackwell B, Shepherd M. Prophylactic lithium: Another therapeutic myth? An examination of the evidence to date. Lancet 1968; I: 968-71.

Hartigan GP. The use of lithium salts in affective disorders. Br. J. Psychiatr. 1963;109: 810-14.

Lader M. Prophylactic lithium. Lancet 1968; II:103.

Müller-Oerlinghausen B, Ahrens B, Grof E, Grof P, Lenz G, Schou M, Simhandl C, Thau K, Volk J, Wolf R, et al. The effect of long-term lithium treatment on the mortality of patients with manic-depressive and schizoaffective illness. Acta Psychiatr Scand. 1992 Sep;86(3): 218-22.

Schioldann J, Strömgren LS. Erik Robert Volter Strömgren. 28 November 1909 –15 March 1993. A Bio-Bibliography. Acta Psychiatr. Scand. 1996; 94:283-302.

Schou M, Juel-Nielsen N, Strömgren E, Voldby H. The treatment of manic psychoses by the administration of lithium salts. J. Neurol. Neurosurg. Psychiatr. 1954; 17:250-60.

Schou M. Lithium ved mani: Praktiske retningslinier. Nord. Med. 1956; 55:790-4.

Schou M.: Artistic productivity and lithium prophylaxis in manic-depressive illness. Br. J. Psychiatr. 1979; 135:97-103.

Schou M. Has the time come to abandon prophylactic lithium treatment? A review for clinicians. Pharmacopsychiatry 1998; 31:210-15.

Schou M. Lithium treatment at 52. J Affect Disorders 2001; 67:21-32.

Schou M. Treating recurrent affective disorders during and after pregnancy: What can be taken safely? Drug Saf. 1998; 18:143-152Thomsen K, Schou M. Avoidance of lithium intoxications: Advice based on knowledge about the renal lithium clearance under various circumstances. Pharmacopsychiatr. 1999; 32:83-6.

*Printed in: J. Schioldann. History of the Introduction of Lithium into Medicine and Psychiatry. Birth of Modern Psychopharmacology 1949, Appendix III (pp. 312-320). Adelaide Academic Press, 2009. Danish edition: Mogens Schou: Min rejse med lithium. Selvbiografiske noter.

Bibibliotek for Læger September 2005:217-228, "introduced" by J. Schioldann: [The lithium pioneer Mogens Schou – half a century with lithium]. Ibid. pp. 209-216, accompanied by a reprint of the Danish edition of Schou's et al.'s original lithium paper, 1955 (Ugeskrift for Læger 1955;117:93-101). – Coincidentally, Mogens Schou died on 29 September 2005. - J. Schioldann. Obituary: Mogens Abelin Schou (1918-2005) – half a century with lithium. History of Psychiatry 2006;17(2):247-52.

August 30, 2018

PAUL GROF'S COMMENT

Thank you for reprinting Mogens Schou's "My Journey." Although Mogens wrote it a number of years ago, it has gained relevance as, for several reasons, lithium is regaining popularity and interest: a kind of "Lithium Renaissance."

One issue seems new. Since the publication of Johann Schioldann's English translation of Lange's Periodic depressions and of his observations on lithium in those conditions, several people have recently raised a sensible question: Was Mogens Schou and Christian Baastrup 's discovery of the stabilizing effects of lithium an original idea or, did Schou merely extend Lange's work to manic-depressive patients? As in this report, My Journey, Mogens Schou mentions that his father knew about Lange, this question now adds on intensity.

Verification

I am convinced that, until late in his life, Mogens did not know that Lange successfully used lithium in the long-term treatment of his "periodic depressions." When the extraordinary efficacy of lithium was confirmed in manic-depressive illness around 1970, some psychiatrists and historians went back and brought to light many previously unknown historical facts. That, of course, was all the usual wisdom of hindsight.

First of all, during the initial battle for the recognition of lithium's efficacy, had Mogens known about Lange's earlier findings, he would have quoted them as support and with great joy. At that time, whenever he could find any indication that lithium was useful, he would immediately quote it.

Second, Mogens was unusually meticulous about searching his sources. One of the things that I hugely admired and try to emulate was that any research report, even seemingly utterly insignificant, in Mogens' mind deserved a prudent consideration and analysis. Initially, I thought that he was perhaps too obsessive. He would carefully analyze even reports that to me seemed irrelevant and banal. However, gradually I learned that his attention to details and minutia was well justified. This meticulousness was reflected in several ways: for example, he insisted that he pronounce the name of any foreign author in the way it is pronounced in the author's language.

Third, throughout the 50 years Mogens and I had close contact, regular correspondence and frequent discussions it was crystal-clear that his primary motivation for research was to improve the life of patients. One can see particularly in his early publications in the 1970s how comprehensive he was in entirely covering literature about all the various uses of lithium. That the prophylactic work with lithium is recognized as his own had relatively little importance for him, if any. His joy came primarily from the patients reporting how well they became.

I think Lange's observation about lithium may have some effect on Mogens' thinking when it was published during his final years. The last investigation he actually designed was a study of the stabilizing effect of lithium specifically in recurrent depressions.

January 10, 2019

JANUSZ K. RYBAKOWSKI'S COMMENT

My comment on the Mogens Schou autobiography, written by Johann Schioldann, is based on the speech I delivered in Copenhagen, November 23, 2018, when we celebrated the 100th anniversary of Mogens Schou's birthday.

Mogens Schou was a great clinician and scientist - a true giant of lithium research and treatment. For the establishment of contemporary lithium therapy, Mogens Schou probably achieved more than anybody in the world. There was more than a half century of his indefatigable lithium activity which he performed with great and exceptional scientific scrutiny. Among lithium researchers, Mogens Schou can be named Primus Inter Pares as he, together with his Danish colleagues, were the first to perform pivotal studies and to make important clinical observations on lithium therapy. Concomitant with this, Mogens Schou was also extremely engaged in the care of patients receiving lithium.

The year Mogens Schou began his lithium studies, 1952, coincides with the year of the death of his father Hans Jacob Schou, a prominent Danish psychiatrist. From him, Mogens inherited a dedication to patients and to neurobiological studies of psychiatric disorders. The initial fruit of his clinical studies on lithium took place two years later, with the publication of the first controlled study on lithium's effectiveness among patients in a manic state (Schou, Juel-Nielsen, Strömgren and Voldby 1954). When it was performed over half a century ago, the study was kind of unusual because the researchers used a neutral preparation (placebo) for comparative purposes to show the "real" effect of lithium. The study included 38 patients in a manic state, among whom 30 had "clear" affective symptoms - a spectacular improvement was noted in 12, improvement in 15 and a lack of effect in three. During therapy, measurements of the concentration of the drug in blood serum were systematically made and in six of them in cerebrospinal fluid. It was found that concentrations of lithium ion in the serum remained within 0.5 to 2 mmol/l, which was an important element for further research on relations between the concentration of lithium in serum and its clinical effectiveness and toxic symptoms. Three years later Mogens Schou summed up in his extensive article published in the Pharmacological Reviews the whole contemporary knowledge concerning pharmacology, biochemistry and clinical effects of lithium (Schou 1957).

The real breakthrough for the understanding of lithium's therapeutic action in mood disorders occurred in the early 1960s when the first reports pointing to a possible prophylactic effect of lithium therapy on manic and depressive recurrences appeared. They came from England (Geoffrey Hartigan 2014) and Denmark (Paul Christian Baastrup 1964). In connection with this, Mogens Schou, together with Paul Baastrup, performed a mirror-image study of lithium prophylaxis on 88 patients with unipolar and bipolar affective disorder in Denmark's Glostrup hospital. The trial lasted six and half years and the main finding was that the average duration of disordered mood (mania or depression) within a year before lithium was 13 weeks, while during a year on lithium it was shortened to the average of two weeks. The results were published in the Archives of General Psychiatry (Baastrup and Schou 1967).

The next year, 1968, was marked by Mogens Schou's important

clinical observations and studies. For the first time, the adverse effect of lithium on thyroid function (goiter) was described, based on findings in a big group of 330 lithium-treated patients (Schou, Amdisen, Eskjaer et al. 1968a). Also, a study on renal handling of lithium elucidated the mechanism of renal lithium reabsorption (occurring in the proximal tubule) and its relationship to sodium reabsorption. This discovery provided a plausible explanation of lithium toxicity with sometimes fatal outcome in subjects receiving lithium as a salt substitute which occurred in turn of 1940/1950s (Thomsen and Schou 1968). And, based on eight cases, the first comprehensive description of lithium poisoning was published, with a characterization of prodromes, clinical picture and outcomes, as well as suggested management (Schou, Amdisen and Trap-Jensen 1968b). However, in the same year, a strong backlash against lithium prophylaxis provided by the British psychiatrists Barry Blackwell and Michael Shepherd appeared in Lancet, titled "Prophylactic lithium. Another therapeutic myth?" The article was questioned the validity of the findings on lithium effectiveness and requested double-blind trials on this issue (Blackwell and Shepherd 1968). Fifty years after this publication, Barry Blackwell, who initiated INHN discussion on the topic with "The Lithium Controversy. A Historical Autopsy" (2014) seemed to be confident that lithium remains the best first choice for mood stabilization in bipolar disorder.

Eight placebo-controlled trials in which Mogens Schou exercised a significant initiative were performed in Europe (in Denmark and the UK) and the USA in 1970-1973. In these studies patients were to have had at least two recurrences of illness in the two years preceding lithium treatment. Most of these studies employed a method comparing the course of illness in a group in which lithium was discontinued and replaced with a placebo with a group which continued to receive lithium (discontinuation design). Recurrence of illness was defined as a deterioration that would require psychiatric hospitalization or commencing regular antidepressive or antimanic treatment. Analysis of all research showed that the percentage of patients in whom recurrences of depression or mania occurred was significantly lower while receiving lithium (on average 30%) than while receiving placebo (on average 70%) (Schou and Thomson 1976).

Because lithium therapy can be administered during pregnancy, Mogens Schou in 1968 helped initiate the "Register of Lithium Babies" (Schou, Goldfield, Weinstein and Villeneuve 1973). The clinical observations to-date have shown that lithium use during pregnancy by women with a mood disorder, especially by those previously treated with this drug, makes a favorable risk/benefit ratio in favor of lithium (Poels, Bijma, Galbally and Bergink 2018).

In his promulgation of lithium therapy, Mogens Schou was very interested in how such therapy influences the various aspects of the patient's life. As bipolar disorder is overrepresented among artists, he was the first to examine the issue of the effect of lithium prophylaxis on artistic creativity. From 24 artists treated with lithium due to bipolar disorder, 12 reported an increase in their artistic productivity, six a slight decrease and six noted no change at all (Schou 1979).

Schou was extremely dedicated to the best clinical practice of lithium therapy. Since 1980 there have appeared successive issues of Mogens Schou's book Lithium Treatment of Manic-Depressive Illness, a practical guide to lithium therapy for doctors, patients and their families. Successive revised editions appeared in 1983, 1986, 1988 and 1993. The 6th edition was titled Lithium Treatment of Mood Disorders (Schou 2004).

Mogens Schou, together with Bruno Müller-Oerlinghausen from Berlin, and Paul Grof from Ottawa were the Founding Fathers of the International Group for the Study of Lithium-Treated Patients (IGSLI), created in 1988. In the 1990s the group published seminal papers showing a favorable influence of lithium on the decrease of mortality and prevention of suicidal behaviors (Müller-Oerlinghausen, Ahrens, Volk et al. 1991; Müller-Oerlinghausen, Wolf, Ahrens 1994; Müller-Oerlinghausen, Wolf, Ahrens et al. 1996). Recently, the IGSLI publication confirmed the neuroprotective effect of lithium (Hajek, Bauer, Simhandl et al. 2014). Since its conception, the group has had yearly meetings; the most recent, the 32nd IGSLI conference, took place in Santiago, Chile. There participants could visit the Acatama Dessert, the world's largest and purest active source of lithium.

In the years 1990-1994 the journal Lithium was published. Mogens Schou was on the editorial board and became the author of the first scientific article in the journal; it was on lithium and treatment-resistant depression (Schou 1990). After many years, lithium augmentation of antidepressants is the best evidenced pharmacological strategy in treatment-resistant depression (Bauer, Adli, Ricken et al. 2014). By some researchers, it is even regarded as the second main indication for lithium use (after preventing mood recurrences) in mood disorders. With the foundation in 1999 of the International Society of Bipolar Disorders (ISBD), Mogens Schou was nominated as its honorable president. Since 2001, during the society's annual international conferences, Mogens Schou's awards have been given for exceptional achievements in the field of research, educational activity and organizational and media activity concerning the bipolar affective disorder.

On September 23 25, 2005, Mogens Schou participated in the 19th IGSLI conference that took place in Poznań, Poland. In spite of limitations connected with his advanced age, he was very glad that he could actively participate in this conference; during it, he presented one of his new research proposals. It concerned the issue of lithium for prophylaxis of unipolar depression where he suspected a significant efficacy, especially among so-called "hidden bipolars." Over the years, a growing number of controlled studies have been published confirming that lithium has prophylactic effectiveness in unipolar depression. Recently, it was reported from Finland, on the basis of an observational study, that lithium monotherapy is the pharmacological treatment associated with the lowest risk of psychiatric hospitalization in patients with severe unipolar depression (Tiihonen, Tanskanen, Hoti et al., 2017). There was no sign then that several days after the Poznan IGSLI conference Mogens Schou would finish his busy lithium-oriented life.

Verification

My account of Mogens Schou spanned from 1971, when I wrote the letter to him about my interest in lithium treatment, until the IGSLI conference in Poznan in 2005 when Mogens brought me the copy of this letter as a token of our long-term acquaintance. This was a very emotional event for both of us. In the meantime, I was a Mogens's student, visiting him on several occasions in Risskov, Denmark. Gradually, I became his partner in lithium research. The crowning achievement of this relationship was the Mogens Schou Research award I received during the International Society of Bipolar Disorder conference in Mexico City held in March 2018.

References:

Baastrup PC, Schou M. Lithium as a prophylactic agents. Its effect against recurrent depressions and manic-depressive psychosis. Arch Gen Psychiatry 1967;16:162-72.

Baastrup P.C. The use of lithium in manic-depressive psychoses. Compr Psychiatry 1964; 5:396-408.

Blackwell B, Shepherd M. Prophylactic lithium: another therapeutic myth? An examination of the evidence to date. Lancet 1968;7549:968-71.

Blackwell B. The Lithium Controversy. A Historical Autopsy. inhn.org.controversies. June 19, 2014.

Hajek T, Bauer M, Simhandl C, Rybakowski J, O'Donovan C, Pfennig A, König B, Suwalska A, Yucel K, Uher R, Young LT, MacQueen G, Alda M. Neuroprotective effect of lithium on hippocampal volumes in bipolar disorder independent of long-term treatment response. Psychol Med 2014;44:507-17.

Hartigan G.P. The use of lithium salts in affective disorders. Br J Psychiatry 1963; 109:810-814.Bauer M, Adli M, Ricken R, Severus E, Pilhatsch M. Role of lithium augmentation in the management of major depressive disorder. CNS Drugs 2014;28:331-42.

Müller-Oerlinghausen B, Ahrens B, Volk J, Grof P, Grof E, Schou M, Vestergåard P, Lenz G, Simhandl C, Thau K, et al. Reduced mortality of manic-depressive patients in long-term lithium treatment: an international collaborative study by IGSLI. Psychiatry Res 1991;36:329-31.

Müller-Oerlinghausen B, Wolf T, Ahrens B, Schou M, Grof E, Grof P, Lenz G, Simhandl C, Thau K, Wolf R. Mortality during initial and during later lithium treatment. A collaborative study by the International Group for the Study of Lithium-treated Patients. Acta Psychiatr Scand 1994;90:295-7.

Müller-Oerlinghausen B, Wolf T, Ahrens B, Glaenz T, Schou M, Grof E, Grof P, Lenz G, Simhandl C, Thau K, Vestergåard P, Wolf R. Mortality of patients who dropped out from regular lithium prophylaxis: a collaborative study by the International Group for the Study of Lithium-treated patients (IGSLI). Acta Psychiatr Scand 1996;94:344-7.

Poels EMP, Bijma HH, Galbally M, Bergink V. Lithium during pregnancy and after delivery: a review. Int J Bipolar Disord 2018;6:26.

Schou M, Amdisen A, Eskjaer Jensen S, Olsen T. Occurrence of goitre during lithium treatment. Br Med J. 1968a;3:710-13.

Schou M, Amdisen A, Trap-Jensen J. Lithium poisoning Am J Psychiatry 1968b;125:520-7.

Schou M, Goldfield MD, Weinstein MR, Villeneuve A. Lithium and pregnancy. I. Report from the Register of Lithium Babies. Br Med J 1973;2:135-6.

Schou M, Thompsen K. Lithium prophylaxis of recurrent endogenous affective disorders. In: Lithium Research and Therapy, Johnson FN, editor. London: Academic Press 1976. pp. 63-84.

Schou M. Artistic productivity and lithium prophylaxis in manic-depressive illness. Br J Psychiatry 1979;135:97-103.

Schou M. Biology and pharmacology of the lithium ion. Pharmacol Rev 1957;9:17-58.

Schou M. Lithium and treatment-resistant depression. A review. Lithium 1990;1:3-8.

Schou M. Lithium Treatment of Mood Disorders. A Practical Guide. Basel: Karger; 2004.

Schou M, Juel-Nielsen N, Strömgren E, Voldby H. The treatment of manic psychoses by the administration of lithium salts. J Neurol Neurosurg Psychiatry. 1954;17:250-60.

Thomsen K, Schou M. Renal lithium excretion in man. Am J Physiol 1968;215:823-7.

Tiihonen J, Tanskanen A, Hoti F, Vattulainen P, Taipale H, Mehtälä J, Lähteenvuo M. Pharmacological treatments and risk of readmission to hospital for unipolar depression in Finland: a nationwide cohort study. Lancet Psychiatry 2017;4:547-53.

October 24, 2019

CHAPTER 4.

CONTROVERSY

BARRY BLACKWELL: THE LITHIUM CONTROVERSY: A HISTORICAL AUTOPSY

I am delighted Larry Stein has joined Jose de Leon in expressing interest and concern about aspects of an ancient controversy that may have contemporary relevance. Perhaps it is time to engage in a more detailed and complete analysis of the issues raised, many of which are dealt with in my memoir, *"Bits and Pieces of a Psychiatrist's Life,"* and will be cited in this essay (Blackwell, 2012).

It is now almost half a century since Michael Shepherd and I published our article "Prophylactic Lithium; *Another Therapeutic Myth?"* in the Lancet, which commented on and critiqued a previously published study by Mogens Schou and his colleague in the Archives of General Psychiatry (Baastrup and Schou, 1967), making the claim that lithium had a unique effect in preventing future episodes of manic depressive disorder. Their riposte to our critique appeared later the following year (Baastrup and Schou, 1968).

If history has anything to offer today, then such past events deserve to be dissected. As possibly the sole remaining protagonist in the fierce debate these two papers generated, I offer this autopsy, personally performed, and invite INHN members to comment.

This essay will be in three parts; reciting the facts themselves; an analysis and interpretation of the scientific zeitgeist prevailing at the time, commenting on the emotions aroused; and, finally, the possible relevance of such matters today.

I completed five years of psychiatric training at the London University Institute of Psychiatry and Maudsley Hospital, including a two-year fellowship in animal research leading to my doctoral degree in Pharmacology from Cambridge University. Following this, I completed a two-year research fellowship with Michael Shepherd. At his suggestion, I undertook to analyze and critique Schou's data claiming that continuous administration of lithium prevented future episodes of manic depression. There was no control substance since other "mood stabilizers" were far in the future and Schou rejected placebo as unethical based on his clinical experience and convictions of efficacy. So, there was no double-blind procedure to protect against potential observer bias, although a placebo control was included in the definitive studies that confirmed his beliefs many years in the future (see later). The possibility of bias existed both due to the study design and because Schou was quite open to admitting enthusiasm for his hypothesis, derived from a family member's benefit after all else had failed to stifle recurrences. At this time, prophylaxis was such a unique and unexpected claim it might have evoked a "too good to be true" skepticism, which heightened our concern about potential bias in an uncontrolled study.

There was no established method, at this time, with which to evaluate such a unique claim; Schou's series included a heterogeneous collection of subjects broadly interpreted as suffering from manic depressive disorders but with varying affective manifestations, of differing duration, frequency and severity. This created concerns about the specificity of the claim as well as statistical issues, primarily concerned with regression to the mean – spontaneous remission from a high baseline in a fluctuating disorder. Other statistical concerns were displayed and discussed in sophisticated terms in a paper read to a NIMH/VA study group and subsequently published in Frank Ayd's newsletter (Blackwell, 1969). Similar statistical and methodological criticisms were made by Malcolm Lader in the Lancet (1968). The essence of these concerns focused on the impossibility of distinguishing dependency on a medication, or spontaneous remission from prophylaxis, a problem I dubbed the "panacea paradigm." The scientific caveats evoked sharp rebuttals from clinicians who knew better, including Nate Kline in America (Kline, 1968) and Sargent in Britain (Sargant, 1968). Sargant's comments are especially illustrative of the tone and angst aroused in this debate. He appealed for the abandonment of "crude statistics" and "valueless double-blind sampling" in favor of "bedside observations for the sake of England's treatment reputation in world psychiatry."

Controversy

Seldom noted or commented on is that in addition to concerns about methodology we applied Schou's statistical technique to a convenience sample of 13 manic-depressive patients from the Maudsley data base treated with imipramine and found results comparable to lithium.

It is important to place these events in their broader historical perspective and consider how this colored the controversy. Until the Flexner revolution in the early twentieth century, medicine was an apprentice profession whose materia medica included many panaceas, nostrums and placebos, the popularity of which depended largely on the status of the apothecaries, physicians or barber surgeons who dispensed and endorsed them. As medicine became more scientific and moved from the community into academic medical centers, its remedies became potentially more effective. Trial methodology and statistical analyses developed to rigorously evaluate therapeutic claims. Eventually, the double-blind controlled study became the gold standard. Psychiatry lagged behind in this regard; chloral hydrate, barbiturates, paraldehyde and amphetamines were synthesized and well established with regard to effectiveness and shortcomings but nothing new or potentially more effective existed to compare them against.

Lithium had a persisting role in this evolution. A naturally occurring metallic ion with no commercial potential or synthetic rivals, it was introduced into medical practice, in 1859, as a bone fide treatment for gout but then increasingly as a panacea with Lithia tablets used for a wide variety of ailments, despite absence of benefit and occurrence of side effects. In the earlier days of scientific medicine, it was used as a salt substitute in cardiac disease until the absence of a method for measuring blood levels led to cases of fatal toxicity. It was withdrawn from medical practice, in 1949, the identical year Cade reported its therapeutic effect in psychotic manic patients.

Many pioneers in psychopharmacology consider the two decades from 1950 to 1970 as the seedbed for all the original treatments in every category of psychiatric disorder. Lithium provides twin bookends for this exciting epoch, beginning with Cade's discovery of lithium for acute mania and ending with Schou's discovery of prophylaxis- both enabled by discovery of a method for measuring lithium levels in the blood. In an account of his own discovery, Cade recognizes Schou as "The person who has done most to achieve this recognition."

The trajectory of lithium's ascendancy as a prophylactic agent during these two decades is best told by Schou himself (Schou, 1998) and Paul Grof, with whom he collaborated (Grof, 1998) and who wrote Schou's obituary at the time of his death in 2005 at age 87 (Grof, 2006). The obituary is an appropriate paean of praise for a colleague who was twice nominated for the Nobel Prize in medicine and physiology. Grof traces Schou's dedication to our field from vivid childhood memories of depressed patients in the asylum where his father was medical director, "wandering in the hospital park with drooping heads and melancholic faces waiting for the depression to pass and fearing future recurrences." This impressed on Mogens the need for a sustained prevention of depression "at the time when maintenance ECT was clearly not the ideal."

When Cade published his findings on lithium, in 1949, it attracted Schou's attention although Cade himself had only demonstrated an acute effect in manic psychosis and found that "in three chronically depressed patients, lithium produced neither aggravation nor alleviation of their symptoms" (Cade, 1971). Despite this fact, Schou's interest was piqued by his concern that since age 25, his brother had experienced "yearly episodes of depression. In spite of ECT, drug treatment and hospitalization the depressive attacks came again and again" (Schou, 1998). During the decade 1950-1960 that Cade vigorously pursued his interest and research on lithium, imipramine was probably not available until towards the end of the decade and it is likely that during this interlude, Schou prescribed his brother lithium, which "changed his life and the lives of his wife and children." This leads me to wonder if, in fact, his brother manifested a Type 2 bipolar disorder, in which mild hypomania went unremarked. Grof notes that late in his career, Schou developed a special interest in "hidden bipolars" – patients with depression who had unrecognized bipolar disorders. Schou's last scientific presentation, shortly before his death, was on this topic and a new study he was proposing (Grof, 2006).

Schou was not a founding member of the CINP but participated in the first Congress in Rome, in 1958, when he contributed to the final session, a "General Discussion." He recalls his comment that "On the chemotherapeutic firmament lithium is one of the smaller stars" (Schou, 1998). Baastrup and Schou's seminal publication in the Lancet (Baastrup and Schou, 1968) had been underway for seven years, begun probably in 1961. The above facts help explain why imipramine was not included as a comparative drug, even though the population included both unipolar and bipolar depressed patients. Later on, as his familiarity with imipramine grew, he used the term "normothymics" to include both lithium and imipramine (Schou, 1963).

These events resonate with the concerns raised in our paper criticizing Baastrup and Schou's methodology and conclusions (Blackwell and Shepherd, 1968) regarding the uncertain specificity of lithium and the absence of a control comparison. To be fair, Schou and Grof draw attention to the problem of using a placebo control based on the high suicide rate in untreated affective disorder. Schou eventually resolved this obstacle with a novel trial design in which sequential analysis of paired placebo and lithium patients was coupled with an immediate switch to open treatment for any recurrence (Schou, 1998).

Because the ad hominem aspects of this debate still linger, I will quote a few laudatory comments made by his friend and colleague Paul Grof in the obituary. Schou was "a caring man with great humility," with a "love and compassion for people" and also a "highly meticulous" researcher who "never left a task undone."

In 1970, two years after I immigrated to America, my mentor Frank Ayd and I conceived the idea to invite all the scientists and clinicians who had discovered the original therapeutic compounds in each disorder to tell their own story at a conference in Baltimore. These first-person accounts were published the following year in our edited book, *"Discoveries in Biological Psychiatry"* (Ayd and Blackwell, 1971). They included Albert Hoffman (*Hallucinogens*), Frank Berger (*Meprobamate*), Irv Cohen (*Benzodiazepines*), Pierre Deniker (*Neuroleptics*), Nate Kline (*MAO inhibitors*), Roland Kuhn (*Imipramine*), John Cade (*Lithium*), Paul Janssen (*butyrophenones*) and Jorgen Ravn (*Thioxanthines*). I contributed a chapter on The Process of Discovery using the interaction of cheese and the MAOI as a template and Frank Ayd concluded with a summary on *The Impact of Biological Psychiatry*.

Noteworthy now, but not discussed at the time, was that Frank did not include Schou. Perhaps, speculatively, this might have been for two reasons. First, Schou's contribution was derivative to Cade's and more adaptive than original; secondly, because the benefits of all these "serendipitous" discoveries had all been confirmed in well controlled clinical studies. The methodological difficulty of proving prophylaxis and the specificity of lithium in doing so, would linger experimentally (but not in practice) for almost twenty years, until the definitive studies, in 1984, by the Medical Research Council in Britain (Glen et al., 1984) and the NIMH study group in the USA (Prien et al., 1984). This latter study, larger of the two, involved a two-year follow up of 117 bipolar and 150 unipolar patients given lithium, imipramine, both drugs or placebo. It reached three major conclusions:

1. Imipramine is preferable to lithium for long term prevention following recovery from an acute episode of unipolar depression.
2. For both bipolar and unipolar disorders, the preventative effects of both lithium and imipramine parallel their effects in acute episodes.
3. Even when lithium and imipramine are effective, they are not panaceas. Only a quarter to a third of patients with either bipolar or unipolar disease were treatment successes.

Eighteen years after Schou's original study, the issues of diagnostic specificity, comparative and specific benefits for lithium or imipramine and their magnitude were scientifically defined in the absence of potential observer bias and statistical flaws.

Controversy

In retrospect, some of the angst directed to Shepherd and I might have emanated from various attributions; methodological puritanism, unjust allegations of bias or of potential therapeutic nihilism- for which the Maudsley was rather unjustly credited. Nevertheless, it was a contemporary and colleague of mine from the Maudsley who, in comments on events in the 1960's, made the satirical observation that, "Writing from the Olympian heights of the Institute of Psychiatry Barry Blackwell and Michael Shepherd airily dismissed Schou's evidence" (Silverstone, 1998). But we were all scientific babes in the wood when it came to prophylaxis, bias must always be assumed unless it is eliminated and, while the atmosphere at the Institute was decidedly empirical, it was also benevolent to developments in psychopharmacology. The 1998 book, *"The Rise of Psychopharmacology and the Story of the CINP,"* lists the 33 Founders of the organization. 27 were clinicians but only three were from Britain. Sir Aubrey Lewis, Michael Shepherd and Lindford Rees. Sir Aubrey was an active participant in the first CINP Congress.

My first rotation at the Maudsley as a resident, in 1962, was under Lindford Rees, a dedicated psychopharmacologist who carried out early studies on imipramine; my second rotation was on the Professorial Unit, where Aubrey Lewis took me under his wing and, once he was sure I was not interested in psychoanalysis, arranged and endorsed my psychopharmacology training. True, Michael Shepherd was a skeptic and scientific purist but, lest he be blamed for any perceived disrespect towards Schou, I must make clear that I was first author on our Lancet paper, chose its title and was responsible for the data analysis and conclusions reached.

Nor were either of us wedded uncritically to double blind methodology. We were well aware of its shortcomings. Immediately before our paper on lithium, Shepherd and I worked on a drug study for a pharmaceutical company which went nowhere because of rigid, impractical and unrepresentative criteria for recruiting subjects. We published our conclusions on contemporary trial methodology in the Lancet (Blackwell and Shepherd, 1967). During my psychopharmacology research in animals, I collaborated with a colleague evaluating and recording the outpatient use of MAO inhibitors by all the consultants and residents at the Maudsley. This must have been among the first "effectiveness" studies to look beyond the boundaries of conventional controlled clinical trials at what happens in real life (Blackwell and Taylor, 1967). The results were unusual and revealing. One intriguing finding was how the interaction between prescriber and drug influenced outcome, precisely what the double-blind study is designed to stifle or eliminate. The most powerful effect on outcome, above diagnostic and demographic variables, was prescriber behavior. Those who used MAOI's a lot, as "first choice" drugs," had better outcomes than those who used them more reluctantly, as "second choice" drugs. The reasons appear self-evident. First choice prescribers reaped the benefits of their enthusiasm, the placebo response, spontaneous remission and perhaps a willingness to tolerate side effects. The "second choice" population contained more treatment resistant and side-effect sensitive patients alert to the physician's skepticism. Needless to say, these outcomes were likely to reinforce physician attitudes and behaviors. Pharmaceutical reps soon learned to capitalize on this phenomenon by offering physicians a stipend in return for using their new drug in "the next few patients you see."

Another finding was the intriguing comment one enthusiastic prescriber made in the chart, "Although this patient never looked depressed before, she looks less depressed now." Perhaps drug outcomes sometimes influence diagnostic habits. So, in retrospect, one wonders if Schou's late-life interest in "hidden bipolars" was evoked by his extensive experience and enthusiasm for lithium. Perhaps he was curious to find if there were subtle and covert clinical indicators of hypomania in some recurrent unipolar patients who, like his brother, unexpectedly benefited from lithium.

Also relevant to the prophylaxis debate was our finding that 18% of that population remained on an MAOI for three years after recovering from an initial episode of "atypical" depression and relapsing on attempts at withdrawal, a finding we attributed to "dependence" but identical to the 11 out of 60 patients (18%) who took lithium for three years and where "prophylaxis" was the explanation (Baastrup and Schou, 1967). Further complexity is added by noting that, independent of diagnosis or treatment method, about 80% of all outpatients at the Maudsley stopped treatment within three months, while the remaining 20% remained, sometimes for years. What then is the difference between "dependency" and "prophylaxis?" This raises semantic, philosophical and clinical issues and attempts to discriminate by stopping treatment introduce an ethical dimension of potential harm. Perhaps this introduces an "eye of the beholder" component concerning which semantic meaning one applies and is this, in turn, partly based on the physician's temperament?

I am ambivalent; my heart tells me one thing and my head another. Am I a neutral researcher, seeker after truth, or a benevolent healer following the Hippocratic ideal of "first do no harm"? Is what I see "prophylaxis" or "dependence," perhaps some of each?

The issue of potential clinical bias is nuanced; an intimate interaction between clinician and patient, particularly a friend or relative, can sow the seed of a new idea, worthy of further investigation or testing as a hypothesis. The problem arises in how to remove this bias towards the new idea from the outcome of an investigation. Sometimes it is more difficult than others and in my own initiation into research I was fortunate.

As a first-year resident, I became involved in the interaction of MAOI and tyramine containing foods. The first clue to the possible cause of a sometimes-fatal hypertensive crisis came when a hospital pharmacist (GEF Rowe) read a letter I wrote to the Lancet describing the syndrome and its symptoms – predominantly a sudden severe pounding headache. He recognized and described this process in his wife on two consecutive occasions after she ate cheese; "Could there be something in the cheese?" So, a fellow resident and I took an MAOI for two weeks before eating cheese from the hospital cafeteria. Nothing happened. Nevertheless, I subsequently obtained data from twelve cases in less than 9 months, some including measures of blood pressure and one produced under experimental conditions (Blackwell, 1963). Nobody suggested my interest and potential bias was artificially elevating a patient's blood pressure or causing a headache. But the research director of the pharmaceutical company making the MAOI did write a letter to the Lancet stating that my conclusions were "unscientific and premature." Within weeks, researchers at another hospital had isolated tyramine in their body fluids after eating cheese. The issue was no longer moot. Physiological and physical parameters are less subject to observer bias than emotional and behavioral outcomes but finding a glib reason to disparage either is easy.

The issue at stake is also a matter of semantics and timing. The word "bias" has a pejorative connotation, especially when applied retrospectively, to allege an investigator's potential faulty judgment in an uncontrolled study. The term then assumes an unpleasant but perhaps unintended ad hominem element. Contrast this with the prospective benign intent of a controlled study- to protect an investigator from his or her laudable compassion and therapeutic enthusiasm.

On which side of this semantic fence one sits, at a given moment or on a specific issue may be influenced by other factors, including the reputation and fame of the investigator and one's acquaintance with them or sympathy with their claims or ideas. There is no better example than Linus Pauling's orthomolecular beliefs and zeal in promulgating them. He was the only scientist to have won two unshared Nobel Prizes; Chemistry, in1954, and the Peace Prize, in 1962. No person on the planet had better scientific and humanistic credentials. But following the onset of Bright's disease, he developed a strong belief that physical and mental illness might be alleviated by manipulating vitamin levels. In 1968, he published an article in Science on "Orthomolecular Psychiatry." Pauling, himself, took three grams of Vitamin C daily to prevent the common cold and collaborated with a British cancer surgeon on its use in prolonging life. These claims were not disproved until over ten years later by controlled research at the

Mayo Clinic. A physician critic, in an article in The Atlantic (Offit, 2013) commented that although Pauling was "spectacularly right" in his early scientific career, his late career orthomolecular assertions were "so spectacularly wrong that he was arguably the world's greatest quack." Putting this cautionary tale aside, it is only just to remark that Schou was certainly right, while Pauling was unequivocally wrong.

By the time Schou was attempting to demonstrate the prophylactic potential of lithium in Scandinavia, the Congress in the United States had enacted the Harris-Kefauver legislation mandating that drug manufacturers prove their products were effective as well as safe. In 1968, I immigrated to America to become the Director of Psychotropic Drug Research for the Merrell Company, in Cincinnati. The company was just recovering from the stigma of having marketed thalidomide for insomnia and the marketplace was cluttered with compounds in search of a credible rationale or proof they were more effective than a placebo. Merrell had two such products in the psychotropic domain and I had the daunting task of proving they could pass muster. One was "Alertonic" a cunningly named reddish-brown liquid popular in nursing homes for the elderly that contained small amounts of alcohol, B vitamins and an amphetamine like stimulant. A substantial placebo response made the task of proving efficacy impossible.

A still more dubious drug was Frenquel with the marketing claim that it stifled hallucinations whatever the diagnosis and the odd characteristic that the intravenous dose was higher than the oral one. Since no other drug had a similar claim, this was a niche product and the threat of withdrawal produced a flood of protests from patients and clinicians who "could not live without it." The FDA was unimpressed and impervious to testimonials, but I decided to visit one of the more credible supplicants to better define what was going on. The following account appears in my memoir in the piece on "The Pharmaceutical Industry" as a Bit titled "Snake Oil" (Blackwell, 2012).

"I had a trip planned for New York and decided to call on one of the Frenquel seekers. The office where the cab let me off in Greenwich

Village was next to a homeless drop in center. The doorbell was answered by a polite, casually dressed, older physician who greeted me and ushered me into a room in the basement furnished more like a family doctor's office than a psychiatrist's den. In the center of the room stood an examining table rather than a reclining couch with an attached shiny aluminum tray on which lay a large syringe containing a colorless liquid I assumed was Frenquel. Sitting on the table, legs dangling and wearing a brightly colored, mildly revealing dress was an attractive young woman. Almost before I could take in the scene, she leapt to the floor, faced me and began to shout, 'So you're the f----ing drug company man that's going to ruin my life!'"

The doctor moved quickly to take her arm, guided her back to the table, and did his best to calm her. She settled down and lay back, still eyeing me furiously, pulling up the sleeve of her dress to expose the veins in the hollow of her arm. This was obviously a well-practiced routine, which the doctor performed often. He inserted the needle and gently pushed the plunger as the patient closed her eyes and appeared to drift into a light sleep. Visibly relieved the doctor removed the needle, lay down the syringe and leaned towards her. "It's all right, Martha, you can get up now." Her eyes opened, she smiled at us, and thanked me for coming so far out if my way to help her.

Another surprise awaited me; the doctor suggested the three of us have lunch together. We walked to a nearby bistro, and over a meal paid for by Merrell I spent an hour in the company of two friendly, apparently normal people. Over lunch the doctor explained to me that the alcohol and drug detox clinic adjoining the homeless center used Frenquel often to help "bring down" people in drug withdrawal.

On the flight back to Cincinnati, I wrote up my "trip report" explaining I had found two "off-label" novel uses for Frenquel: to calm someone who, most likely, had a borderline personality, and to facilitate drug or alcohol withdrawal. I didn't suggest Merrell pursue research into these potential new indications, but perhaps I was wrong. New uses for old drugs are often discovered by chance; looking for one thing and finding another. It's called serendipity. On the other hand, it seemed more likely that everything attributed to Frenquel might be due to suggestion, the placebo response, or spontaneous remission."

I did not state the obvious – that Frenquel clearly had mild sedative and calming properties but certainly not sufficient to justify the rigors of a controlled study in a market already including meprobamate and the first benzodiazepines. Nor were Alertonic and Frenquel a worthy match for lithium in the effort it would take to prove they were effective remedies for a specific problem.

Finally, we come to the saddest part of this tale – the extent to which scientific disagreements can degenerate into strident squabbles. Almost twenty years after our Lancet article, Michael Shepherd asked me to review the book, "The History of Lithium Therapy" (F.N. Johnson, Macmillan Press: 1984). It was published in Psychological Medicine the following year. The author, an academic psychologist, had authored three previous texts on lithium and claimed Schou and Cade as his friends. In unrestrained hyperbole, verging on the ludicrous, he endorses the enthusiasts who see lithium as "the King of drugs" responsible for the "third revolution in psychiatry." The following quotations illustrate the polemical nature of the book. Lithium is being taken by "one person in every two thousand in most civilized countries" because "depression (sic) is a crippling condition." Lithium alone triggered the chemical revolution in psychiatry; "At a stroke, the elusive ethereal Freudian psyche was replaced as the primary object of attention in psychiatry by the polyphasic, physic-chemical system called the brain." Lithium, "like no other single event, led to psychiatry becoming truly interdisciplinary." Its ubiquitous use "suggests a new basis for classification of psychopathological states." And it is so cheap and easy to administer it will "transform health care in underdeveloped countries."

These absurd claims provoked me to satire and to ending my review by suggesting that those who might buy the book would be those who shared the author's view that lithium was the "Cinderella of psychopharmacology" and who wished to have an unabridged version of the fairy tale at their fingertips. These comments were, in part, a reprise of a lively debate between Nate Kline and me in the correspondence columns of the American Journal of Psychiatry.

The final irony is that this book was published shortly before the two definitive controlled studies (referred to previously) finally arrived at an accurate scientific demonstration of the specific and fairly modest benefits of lithium and imipramine in preventing recurrences of bipolar and unipolar disorders, respectively.

Some reservations about the impact of unbridled enthusiasm for prophylactic treatment have been expressed from the scientific sector. Paul Grof notes that the use of prophylactic treatment for "nearly everyone with recurrent affective disorders has led to the point that the natural history of affective disorder the illness is not known anymore. He also notes that with the extensive use of lithium "the concept of affective disorders has dramatically broadened and mood symptoms, rather than comprehensively assessed psychopathology have become the center of psychiatry assessment." (Grof, 1998).It is worth adding that the parsimony of the DSM system has colluded in this outcome.

What can we make of all this today? To begin with, the testing of new psychotropic drugs has passed almost entirely out of the hands of academic clinicians and federally funded projects and into the realm of the pharmaceutical industry and subcontracted commercial companies who, while they adhere to FDA minimal requirements for controlled studies, have adopted other dubious ways to degrade the process and bias the outcomes. We have also learned that even the best of controlled double-blind studies may not mirror or predict what happens in real world effectiveness. I would gladly return to the time when experienced dedicated clinicians like Mogens Schou did the very best they could, however imperfectly, to show us what works in real practice. After all, their original study was really an "effectiveness" one and not a controlled scientific evaluation. And Schou was, after all, correct. But perhaps Mogens Schou's legacy is better served by the recognition that his truly innovative contribution was the concept of "prophylaxis" itself and not the agents used to accomplish it. This was the very fact that relentlessly recurrent episodes of affective disorder could be checked by continuous, rather than episodic treatment, a technique that also suppressed the phenomenon of kindling.

Now we come to the most tantalizing question raised by this autopsy. Suppose that each of us, Schou, Shepherd, Blackwell and Grof are double blind neuroscientists groping the same elephant. That prophylaxis of recurrent affective disorders is Schou's reality-the body, but that lithium is not a panacea for all its forms (Blackwell and Shepherd)-the tail, and that more scrupulous analysis of the phenomenology, genetics and neurochemistry might reveal which subtypes respond specifically to lithium, imipramine or valproic acid (Grof)-the head. This is a puzzle beyond the capacity of DSM-5 or contemporary trial methodology to solve; worse still, all three compounds are orphan drugs – either un-patentable or generic, so that support for research is unlikely unless the national or federal funding agencies in Britain and America reverse course and revive clinical psychopharmacology research.

At the same time, claims that exceed the level of proof available in efficacy or effectiveness studies should always be challenged and those who exaggerate them beyond belief are free game for Anglo Saxon satire. Mea culpa!

References:

Ayd F, Blackwell B, editors. Discoveries in Biological Psychiatry 1971, reprinted Ayd Medical Communications, Baltimore, 1984.

Baastrup PC, Schou, M. Lithium as a Prophylactic Agent: Its Effect Against Recurrent Depressions and Manic-Depressive Psychosis. Arch. Gen. Psychiat. 1967;16:162.

Blackwell B, Shepherd, M. Early Evaluation of Psychotropic Drugs in Man. Lancet 1967;2:819-22.

Blackwell B, Taylor, D. An Operational Evaluation of MAOI. Proceedings Royal Soc. Med., 1967.

Blackwell B. Hypertensive Crisis Due to MAOI. Lancet 1963;2:849-51.

Blackwell B, Shepherd M. Prophylactic Lithium: Another Therapeutic Myth? Lancet 1968;1:968.

Blackwell B. Lithium: Prophylactic or Panacea? Medical Counterpoint: 1969;52-59.

Blackwell B. Bits and Pieces of a Psychiatrist's Life. Xlibris, 2012.

Glen AIM, Johnson AL, Shepherd M. Continuation Therapy with Lithium and Amitriptyline in Unipolar Depressive Illness; a Randomized, Double-Blind Controlled Trial. Psychological Medicine 1984;14:37-50.

Grof P. Fighting the Recurrence of Affective Disorders. In: The Rise of Psychopharmacology and the Story of the ACNP, Ban TA, Healy D, Shorter E, editors. CINP 1998;101-4.

Grof P. Obituary: Mogens Schou (1918-2005). Neuropsychopharmacology 2006;31:891-2.

Kline NS. Prophylactic Lithium? Amer. J. Psychiat. 1968;125:558.

Lader M. Prophylactic Lithium? Lancet 1968;2:103.

Prien RF, Kupfer DJ, Mansky PA, Small JG, Tuason VB, Voss CB, Johnson WE. Drug Therapy in the Prevention of Recurrences of Unipolar and Bipolar Affective Disorders. Report of the NIMH Collaborative Study Group. Arch. Gen. Psychiat. 1984;41:1096-104.

Sargant W. Prophylactic Lithium? Lancet 1968;2:216.

Schou M. Normothymotics, "Mood Normalizers". Are Lithium and Imipramine Drugs Specific for Affective Disorders? Brit. J. Psychiat. 1963;109:803.

Silverstone T. Psychopharmacology in the 1960's. In: The Rise of Psychopharmacology and The Story of the CINP, Ban TA, Healey D, Shorter E, editors. CINP 1998;285-8.

June 19, 2014

PAUL GROF'S COMMENTS
SOMEWHAT DIFFERENT HINDSIGHT

For quite a while, lithium treatment had fallen out of favor in the mainstream. Non- patentable and inexpensive, lithium could not compete with the skillful marketing of new profitable neuroleptics and antiepileptics and could not withstand other pressures exerted by the pharmaceutical industry. The finest example was the clever advertising of divalproex which, despite the absence of evidence for stabilizing patients, quickly became the best-selling drug for bipolar disorder in the United States. But recently, a renaissance of interest in the use of lithium treatment has unexpectedly emerged.

Several motives may be converging here. Lithium's rather unique antisuicidal properties, proven for some time (Müller-Oerlinghausen, Ahrens, Volk et al. 1991) have recently been widely publicized. In neuroscience laboratories lithium has turned out neuroprotective (Hajek, Cullis, Novak et al. 2012) and it might even become helpful in the management of several obstinate neurological and geriatric disorders (Quiroz, Drevets, Henter and Manji 2012). More important clinically, the re-evaluation of atypical neuroleptics in the treatment of bipolar disorders has lately curved sour. Furthermore, voices have now arisen suggesting that lithium may actually be the only true mood stabilizer, as it demonstrably acts against both polarities of manic-depressive disorder (Grof and Müller-Oerlinghausen 2009).

Perhaps it was this resurgence of interest that led colleagues to ask independently Barry Blackwell and myself to address again the history of the lithium controversy. And as Barry Blackwell completed his interesting reminiscences (Blackwell 2014) and invites comments on his version of the autopsy, I happily oblige.

It is in this context that I think it is useful to dissect the lithium controversy. I concur with Blackwell that we can learn from the past. In psychiatry we now live in an era of conceptual turmoil and absorbing lessons from our history has become critical. Each story has at least two ways of interpreting. With the passage of time our differences have softened, and I agree with most of what Barry Blackwell says in general but still part with him on the weighing of the usefulness of long-term lithium treatment.

Preceding events

What was the controversy actually about? Let me first briefly sum up, from my perspective, the events that preceded the disagreement. In the 1950s the maintenance treatment offered to manic-depressive patients used to be psychoanalysis and maintenance ECT (Geoghegan 1949). The former was unfortunately not helpful and the latter effective but not favored by patients. Lithium was initially used only for the management of acute mania.

Since 1956 however anecdotal observations started emerging about other possible benefits of lithium. Schou (1956) reported an observation of a manic patient who subsequently stopped having both manic and depressive recurrences when he maintained lithium during the free intervals. Beneficial action against depressions was also mentioned by Vojtechovsky (1957). Hartigan (1963) and Baastrup (1964) similarly noted that patients maintained on lithium had a marked reduction of both types of recurrence.

Baastrup and Schou (1967) then carried out a longitudinal study of patients with many previous episodes of illness. Patients with both bipolar and unipolar disorder were involved. The analyses indicated that recurrences occurred in patients significantly less frequently during lithium treatment than before such treatment, or even disappeared completely. Schou, Angst and I then decided to collaborate and to use a "mirror-image" design, utilizing the ample information we had about the previous course of illness of these manic-depressive patients. Against marked editorial resistance, our joined prospective observations on 250 lithium-treated patients were eventually published in the British Journal of Psychiatry. Together with clinical reports published earlier, an ample body of similar observations was emerging and demonstrating lithium as a useful drug in the treatment of manic-depressive illness.

Opposition against such interpretation emerged quickly however and, among experts, views about the issue became sharply divided. Some psychiatrists expressed strong support for lithium prophylaxis, based on their own clinical experience. Others disagreed. On methodological grounds, Blackwell and Shepherd (1968) concluded that the claims for prophylactic efficacy were just a myth, supported by faulty evidence. They raised several critical points; their main objections were, first, a bias due to the open, non-blind evaluation of the recurrences and, second, a statistical approach which in their opinion weighted the facts in favor of the hypothesis.

But the objections could be effectively counteracted only by a tightly designed double-blind evaluation.

Barry Blackwell's invaluable contribution

Before commenting on these methodological disagreements, I want to express my gratefulness to Barry Blackwell. Even though his objections were incorrect, it was an invaluable service to moving ahead. Had it not been for his widely quoted procedural condemnation, I really wonder if lithium would now be in clinical practice, all over the world. The national regulatory bodies insist on double-blind tests. It was Blackwell's somewhat sarcastic, sharp, articulate arguments that made a strong impression and eventually forced the randomized double-blind trial. My feelings of gratefulness may not have been quite the same then but in hindsight they are strong, and I have expressed them repeatedly publicly.

When Mogens Schou, Jules Angst and I completed the replication study published in the British Journal of Psychiatry (1970), the last thing on our minds was to switch any of these patients to placebo. Many of them had suffered from severe, frequently recurrent mood disorder, had been hospitalized numerous times and badly incapacitated by their illness. On lithium they were stable for the first time and it seemed not only unethical but also unimaginable to ask them to stop it, in order to participate in a clinical trial with placebo.

Before they went on lithium, I followed my patients for up to six years, failing to stop their depressions and manias. I could not imagine putting them and their families through the same misery again. In addition, in most of these patients the effect of lithium stabilization was so convincing, so different from the previous course of illness, that to use placebo just to prove that they again relapse appeared unethical and redundant. Furthermore, the Swiss and Czech findings were already an independent replication of the earlier Danish findings.

Finally, our analysis also indicated that the criticism aimed at our methodology was not correct. Barry Blackwell and Michael Shepherd raised two main methodological objections against the findings: that the marked recurrence reduction the patients experienced was to be expected naturally – that it was the result of a "regression to the mean" - and that the observations were not made blindly and thus biased by enthusiasm.

As for the duo's first protestation, the patients experienced frequent episodes qualifying them to enter the trial. Blackwell and Shepherd felt that the less frequent episodes that followed were the result of the recurrence frequency regressing back to a mean of lower value. To demonstrate their point, they quoted Saran's (1968) data of 13 patients who entered the follow-up with frequent episodes but lost that frequency with the passage of time.

But the problem was that, because of the small number of patients, Saran's example was neither representative nor applicable to the problem. Issakson and Ottosson (1969) and Laurel and Ottosson (1968) showed that the "mirror image" design is justified. In a sufficiently large sample of patients not receiving maintenance treatment the mean frequency of recurrences in the past becomes replicated in the future.

In essence, the individual clinical course of manic-depressive illness is capricious, overall seemingly random. Given this capriciousness, in a small group of patients the future frequency of recurrences will vary in any direction. It may decrease - as it did for Saran's 13 patients, it may increase, or it may remain about the same. But to obtain a predictable, anticipated mean frequency, one requires a sufficiently sizable cohort, as was the case in our open trials with a "mirror" design (1994).

As for the Blackwell and Shepherd's second objection – biased open assessment – blind evaluation is often very important but not a panacea. As Schou later demonstrated (1992), the results from long-term clinical trials of lithium were well comparable, regardless of whether the evaluations were carried out blindly or openly. Obviously, if one were evaluating the effects of an anxiolytic in neurotic patients, the placebo effect and bias would usually play a huge role. Double-blind arrangement would be indispensable. Blackwell illustrated clearly the relationship between observer enthusiasm and treatment outcome earlier with MAOI inhibitors (Blackwell and Taylor 1967).

But in a maintenance treatment of manic-depressive patients the task is markedly different: to assess if a patient who was previously symptom-free, develops in a free interval an acute manic or depressive episode. If in this task there would be large, systematic discrepancies between different psychiatrists with a similar training, we could forget psychiatry altogether.

Parenthetically, the biases of the involved investigators were actually markedly different, and not all positive. Schou and Baastrup were openly enthusiastic, because of their previous promising observations. Jules Angst appeared curious but neutral as to the expected outcome. And my previous 6attempts to prevent the recurrences of manic-depressive illness were so dismal (Grof and Vinao 1996, 1969), that I did not believe anything could work preventatively. As I wrote earlier, I was hoping to prove Schou wrong. Yet despite our different preconceptions, our results with long-term lithium treatment were comparable.

Lithium's efficacy was subsequently proven in a trial (Baastrup, Poulsen and Schou 1970) that employed the design with blind evaluation and randomization. As to the ethical concerns, using sequential analysis minimized the number of patients receiving placebo. Using sequential analysis can markedly reduce the number of patients needed to reach a statistically significant difference by utilizing, in addition, the probability hidden in the sequence in which the observations come in.

In this manner it became possible to complete the double-blind trial within six months and with a minimum of patients having been given placebo. All of the patients who became ill again were those switched to placebo, none of the lithium patients experienced recurrences during the same time.

Methodology in diapers

I fully concur with Barry Blackwell that one of the main reasons for our disagreements was the fact that the methodology of maintenance trials in bipolar disorders was in diapers then. In fact, we were developing the methodology while proceeding with the studies (Grof

1970).

As I read Barry Blackwell's "autopsy," I felt there were good reasons why we could not and cannot see lithium treatment in quite the same light. Our background, professional careers, experience and interests were different. As I understand it, his central interests were clinical trials, psychopharmacology and pharmacology. He was frustrated by many methodologically inadequate studies in the past and did not want to see another shabby study confusing psychiatrists. And, after his critique of lithium, he moved on to the industry and then academic and clinical practice. He seemed more interested in anxiety states than in following manic-depressive patients (Blackwell, 2014).

We, on the other hand, prior to lithium studied the natural course of manic-depressive illness in hundreds of patients (Angst 1969; Angst, Dittrich and Grof 1969). Since the heated lithium debate, I have treated more than thousand patients with lithium, some of them up to 40 years and researched who does respond. With experience being so different, even now Barry Blackwell and mine evaluation of lithium cannot be the same.

The efficacy of lithium is neither a myth nor imipramine-like

Barry Blackwell feels that, after the initial trials, uncertainty about Lithium's efficacy lingered until later studies published in 1984. He singles out Prien, Kupfer, Mansky et al. (1984), a double-blind trial carried out mainly in the US VA hospitals. The results are interpreted as indicating that in bipolar patients imipramine is better in cases of mild depressions and lithium in more severe cases. To claim that the efficacy of lithium is comparable to imipramine requires disregarding fully the rest of the published evidence. Such assertion seems to me idiosyncratic, neglecting the existing regulatory decisions, numerous clinical trials and expert consensus.

There is a body of double-blind clinical investigations together demonstrating prophylactic efficacy of lithium both against manias and depressions (Schou 1994; Coppen, Peet, Bailey et al. 1973); trials that have dealt well with Blackwell's methodological objections. On this basis, by the early 1970s, lithium was approved for long-term treatment in most Western countries, by regulatory agencies requiring solid double-blind evidence. Expert committees that have produced more than 25 guidelines for the treatment of bipolar disorder now quote lithium trials as the best (class I) evidence for efficacy. Despite Prien's study, imipramine is nowhere recommended for long-term treatment of bipolar disorders.

Prien's findings only can be interpreted if they are placed in the context of what had happened between 1968 and 1984 with diagnosing mood disorders. Manic-depressive illness was transforming into a much larger and more heterogeneous "bipolar spectrum disorders." As lithium treatment had a striking success in patients with typical manic-depressive illness, the diagnostic fashion for mood disorders broadened (Baldessarini 1970; Grof and Fox 1987), and in "bipolar spectrum" disorders many patients with mood-incongruent symptoms and multiple comorbidities were included. In addition to manic-depressive illness the experimenting with lithium also expanded to other indications: schizoaffective conditions, cycloid psychoses, aggressive states, alcoholism, potentiation of antidepressants, and several other situations.

But lithium prophylaxis is the treatment of choice only for what used to be "manic-depressive illness": in essence, remitting, episodically recurring bipolar and unipolar disorders. It may also be of partial help in other conditions, but the effect is quantitatively and qualitatively different: for example, one will see low efficacy and intense rebound after discontinuation. The diagnosis of manic-depressive illness used to require, among others, the exclusion of mood incongruent psychotic symptoms, the exclusion of other psychiatric diagnoses (i.e. exclusion of comorbidity) and the presence of episodic course.

This development created a very interesting situation. Recent studies have shown that bipolar disorder is now often underdiagnosed, particularly in recurrent depression. At the same time, as bipolar diagnosis is now given simply on the basis of a symptom set, without further analysis and exclusions, it is also grossly overused instead of other diagnoses. As a result, the bipolar spectrum disorder has become very fashionable and highly prevalent, but the classical lithium responsive manic-depressive patients are only a minority subgroup.

For whatever it's worth, while the Prien, Kupfer, Mansky et al. study was going on, two experienced American colleagues who knew my interest in lithium and participated in the study contacted me. They were very critical of the patient selection, partly due to the population of VA hospitals, and warned me not to believe the findings once the study is completed. In hindsight, the Prien, Kupfer, Mansky et al. study can hardly be considered the main pillar for the evaluation of lithium's usefulness.

Wide Acceptance and Narrow Opposition

Lithium treatment for bipolar disorder has gradually been accepted in most countries of the world, including the Third World countries. Lithium is now available as an effective mood stabilizer worldwide, but its use is geographically uneven. It should help in the Third World that lithium is inexpensive, particularly in comparison with new putative stabilizers.

But repeated questioning lithium's efficacy does happen and comes particularly from those who had been using lithium outside of the established evidence and in naturalistic studies with looser diagnosing and monitoring. But careful analyses have shown that lithium remains effective for patients with clinical profile for which it was proven effective in the first place (Berghöfer, Alda, Adli et al. 2013).

Despite overwhelming evidence of the efficacy in typical manic-depressive cases, continuing debates about lithium are likely to occur between opponents who incorrectly believe that they are discussing the same issue but have used lithium in other bipolar types. Unfortunately, the correct evaluation of the outcome of stabilizing treatment in recurrent mood disorders is much more challenging than one would assume. Capricious course, fluctuating compliance with medication, and a varying speed of stabilization all make it difficult to evaluate the relationship between the medication and a changed course of illness in any individual patient. Bipolar disorders have distinct subtypes responding preferentially to different mood stabilizers, and lithium offers a variety of markedly different benefits to patients outside the classical manic-depressive illness (Grof 1998, 2003).

Squall

I do not know if Barry Blackwell really believes - as he seems to indicate in his writing – that the effect of lithium treatment on bipolar disorders is indeed comparable to the effect of imipramine, or whether this is just another expression of his mastery of hyperbole. But we certainly do approach this issue from different angles.

When I think of lithium stabilization, my thinking is unavoidably colored by my experience of treating many bipolar patients for more than five decades. Before lithium treatment we lost every year several patients to suicide and the life of those who continued living was marred by their illness: the impact of frequent episodes of manias, depressions and hospitalizations and the influence on their families and professional life. Since we have been using lithium, the situation changed dramatically and these problems have been minimized, and often completely eradicated.

For Mogens Schou the initial heated debates were stressful. He was a very compassionate physician and switching stabilized patients from lithium to placebo troubled him greatly. He was also an extremely meticulous researcher. The possibility raised by Blackwell and Shepherd that he may have overlooked something important in methodology bothered him very much. He was extremely careful, as he kept moving between his laboratory and his clinical investigations.

The accusation of biased observation was not easy for him to swallow. There was some irony in blaming him for not having carried out the observations double-blind as he, in fact, performed the first double-blind study in psychopharmacology fifteen years earlier. Particularly unfortunate was, I thought, Michael Shepherd's criticism ad hominem: he repeatedly stressed that Mogens Schou was a biased enthusiast because Mogens' brother's depressions responded well to lithium and, replying to questions, he never publicly conceded that lithium works.

From what Barry Blackwell has written about his professional life (Blackwell 2014), his professional interests have been different than ours and he worked more along different lines. His critique of lithium was an important but a relatively short-lived involvement and reflected more his interest in methodology and history of clinical trials than in the treatment of bipolar patients. Thus, I may be biased in favor of lithium but from his text I tend to conclude that he underestimates the helpfulness of lithium treatment and oversimplifies its use in bipolar disorders. Nevertheless, as I mentioned, in hindsight I see enormous value of his critique during the early days of lithium's clinical trials.

Impact of Lithium Treatment on Psychiatry

Up until 1967 no medication had seemed capable of averting recurrences of affective disorders; therefore, only acute episodes had been treated. The introduction of long-term lithium treatment, lithium prophylaxis, changed things radically. From a practical point of view, it was primarily lithium's ability to prevent recurrences that made an impression. For research the introduction of lithium was a major stimulus for neurobiology, demonstrating that a simple element can produce major neurobiological changes. Lithium became the focus of attention of pharmacologists, biochemists, physiologists, psychiatrists, psychologists, and many others. It was probably the advent of lithium therapy that made psychiatric research truly interdisciplinary. Research on all aspects of the affective disorders has been greatly stimulated by the demonstration of the effectiveness of lithium in the treatment of these conditions.

For academic psychiatry the acceptance of lithium treatment led to the important recognition that mood disorders are much more common than previously presumed, and that the existing classification systems must be reconsidered. As the history of the past four decades has shown, lithium therapy has made a significant contribution to modern psychiatry, both in relation to its specific uses in alleviating recurrent endogenous affective disorders, and in stimulating psychiatric research and conceptual thinking.

References:

Angst J, Weis P, Grof P, Baastrup PC, Schou M. Lithium prophylaxis in recurrent affective disorders. Br J Psychiatry. 1970;116:604-14.

Angst J BP, Grof P, Hippius H, Poeldinger W, Weiss P. Clinical course of affective disorders. Psychiatry. 1969;76:489-500.

Angst J, Dittrich A, Grof P. Course of endogenous affective psychoses and its modification by prophylactic administration of imipramine and lithium. Int Pharmacopsychiat. 1969;2:1-11.

Baastrup PC. The use of lithium in manic-depressive psychosis. Compr Psychiatry. 1964;5:396-408.

Baastrup PC, Schou M. Lithium as a prophylactic agent: its effect against recurrent depressions and manic-depressive psychosis. Arch Gen Psychiatry. 1967;16(2):162-72.

Baastrup PC, Poulsen JC, Schou M. Prophylactic lithium: Double blind discontinuation in manic-depressive and recurrent-depressive disorders. The Lancet. 1970;2:326.

Baldessarini RJ. Frequency of diagnoses of schizophrenia versus affective disorders from 1944 to 1968. American Journal of Psychiatry. 1970;127:59-63.

Berghöfer A, Alda M, Adli M, Baethge C, Bauer M, Bschor T, Grof P, Müller-Oerlinghausen B, Rybakowski JK, Suwalska A, Pfennig A. Stability of lithium treatment in bipolar disorder - long-term follow-up of 346 patients. Int J Bipolar Disord. 2013;1:11.

Blackwell B. The Lithium Controversy: An Historical Autopsy. inhn.org.controversies. June 19, 2014.

Blackwell B, Shepherd M. Prophylactic lithium: Another therapeutic myth? An examination of the evidence to date. The Lancet. 1968;I:968-971.

Blackwell B, Taylor D. An Operational Evaluation of MAOI. Proceedings Royal soc. Med. 1967.

Coppen A, Peet M, Bailey J, Noguera R, Burns BH, Swani MS, Maggs R, Gardner R. Double-blind and open studies of lithium prophylaxis in affective disorders. Psychiatr Neurol Neurosurg. 1973;76:501-10.

Geoghegan JS, Stevenson GH. Prophylactic electroshock. Am J Psychiatry. 1949;105:494-6.

Grof P, Müller-Oerlinghausen B. A critical appraisal of lithium's efficacy and effectiveness: the last 60 years. Bipolar Disorders. 2009;11:10-19.

Grof P. Designing long-term clinical trials in affective disorders. J Affect Disord. 1994;30:243-55.

Grof P, Vinao O. Maintenance and prophylactic imipramine doses in recurrent depressions. Activitas Nervosa Superior. 1966;8:384-5.

Grof P, Vinao O. Comparison of various prophylactic procedures in affective psychoses. In: Das Depressive Syndrom, Hippius H, Selbach H, editors. Berlin 1969. pp. 101-4.

Grof P, Schou M, Angst J, Baastrup PC, Weis P. Methodological problems of prophylactic trials in recurrent affective disorders. Br J

Psychiatry. 1970;116:599-603.

Grof P, Fox D. Admission rates and lithium therapy (letter to the editor). British Journal of Psychiatry. 1987;150:264-265.

Grof P. Has the effectiveness of lithium changed? Impact of the variety of lithium's effects. Neuropsychopharmacology. 1998;19:183-8.

Grof P. Selecting effective long-term treatment for bipolar patients: monotherapy and combinations. J Clin Psychiatry. 2003;64 Suppl. 5:53-61.

Hajek T, Cullis J, Novak T, Kopecek M, Hoschl C, Blagdon R, O'Donovan C, Bauer M, Young LT, Macqueen G, Alda M. Hippocampal volumes in bipolar disorders: opposing effects of illness burden and lithium treatment. Bipolar Disord. 2012;14:261-70.

Hartigan GP. The use of lithium salts in affective disorders. Brit J Psychiat. 1963;109:810-814.

Isaksson A, Ottosson JO, Perris C: Methodologische Aspekte der forschung uber prophylaktische Behandlung bei affektiven Psychosen. In: Das Depressive Syndrom Hippius H, Selbach H, editors. Berlin. 1969, pp. 561-574.

Laurell B, Ottosson JO. Prophylactic Lithium? The Lancet. 1968;2:1245.

Müller-Oerlinghausen B, Ahrens B, Volk J, Grof P, Grof E, Schou M, Vestergård P, Lenz G, Simhandl C, Thau K, et al. Reduced mortality of manic-depressive patients in long-term lithium treatment: an international collaborative study by IGSLI. Psychiatry Res. 1991;36:329-31.

Prien R, Kupfer DJ, Mansky PA, Small JG, Tuason VB, Voss CB, Johnson WE. Drug therapy in the prevention of recurrences in unipolar and bipolar affective disorders: report of the NIMH collaborative study group comparing lithium carbonate, imipramine, and a lithium carbonate-imipramine combination. Archives of General Psychiatry. 1984;41:1096-1104.

Quiroz J.A.C.; Drevets, W.C.; Henter, I.D.; Manji, H.K.: Mood Disorders (Chapter 3). In: Translational Neuroscience, Barrett JEC, Williams M, editors. Cambridge University Press; 2012. pp. 27-69.

Schou M. Litiumterapi ved mani: Praktiske retningslinier. Nord Med. 1956;55:790-4.

Saran BM. Prophylactic lithium? Lancet 1968 Aug 3; 2(7562):284-5.

Schou M: Phases in the development of lithium treatment in psychiatry. In: The Neurosciences: Paths of Discovery II, Samson FAG, editor. Birkhäuser: Boston, Basel, Berlin. 1992. pp. 148-66.

Vojtechovsky M: Zkusenosti s lecbou solemi lithia. Problemy Psychiatrie v Praxi a ve Vyzkumu. Prague, Czechoslovak Medical Press 1957. pp. 216-24.

January 22, 2015

Thomas A. Ban

JULES ANGST'S COMMENTS
STUDIES ON THE LONG-TERM NATURAL
HISTORY OF MOOD DISORDERS

Knowledge of the course of mood disorders is essential when deciding whether long-term prophylactic medication is justified. This is especially the case if the natural history of a disorder shows not spontaneous improvement but rather persistent recurrence or even an increase of episodes, reflected by shortening cycle lengths. A cycle is defined as an episode plus the subsequent interval, i.e. the time between the onset of two subsequent episodes.

In 1967 Angst and Weis (1967), investigating a group of 375 subsequent hospital admissions of patients with mood disorders in Zurich (Switzerland), found a log-normal distribution of episode and cycle lengths in four subgroups (125 recurrent depression, 117 involutional melancholia, 45 bipolar and 85 schizo-affective psychoses). This signified that studies should no longer base on arithmetic means. More important, however, was that the longitudinal analysis of cycle lengths showed a clear acceleration of recurrences with an increasing number of episodes. This was most marked in patients with bipolar disorder, followed by schizo-affective disorder and was lowest in patients with depressive disorders.

These findings were reproduced in 386 patients from a further three centers (Basle, Berlin, Landeck) by Angst, Grof, Hippius and Weis in 1968. In 701 patients with bipolar disorder and 988 patients with recurrent major depression a progressive shortening of cycles correlated with age at onset, age, and number of episodes over 20 years (the subsequent cycle was about 10% shorter than the previous one. Despite the clear finding of an increasing recurrence risk by shortening of cycles, in our statistical testing of the long-term effect of prophylactic treatment we applied the very conservative mirror model, which assumes, as the zero hypothesis, merely an equal occurrence of the number of episodes before and under treatment during identical, individual observation periods.

Studies on prophylactic treatment of mood disorders with imipramine and lithium

A first study by Angst, Dittrich and Grof in 1969 dealt with patients treated with imipramine (N=63) or lithium (N=91) in Prague and Zurich. Statistically the mirror model was applied with Wilcoxon signed rank tests. Under imipramine there was a significant deterioration in the course of depression during the second intra-individual period, whereas lithium showed a positive effect in bipolar disorders (p<.025) and a trend to an effect in recurrent depression or involutional melancholia (p<.07). The negative and positive effects of the two drugs were comparable and significant in both samples (Prague and Zurich). This was the first statistically based demonstration of the efficacy of lithium in treating mood disorders.

In a larger analysis of lithium data undertaken in Glostrup (DK), Prague and Zurich (Angst, Weis, Grof, Baastrup and Schou 1970) equal observation periods (before and under treatment) were again compared with regard to hospital admissions and number of episodes before and during lithium prophylaxis. In all three centers there was a reproducible significant decrease in the number of episodes (p<.001) during the lithium period. Taking all 244 patients together, there were significantly fewer hospital admissions for patients with manic-depressive disorders (p<.001), recurrent depression (p<.002) and schizo-affective disorders (p<.01). The average observation periods of the three groups compared were 2x38.5 months for bipolar disorder, 2x26.7 months for recurrent depression and 2x28.1 months for schizo-affective psychoses.

Thus, in contrast to the repeatedly confirmed deterioration of the spontaneous course of mood disorders, a significant improvement was achieved with lithium but not so with imipramine.

Personal reminiscences

Ervin Varga from Budapest and I worked under Michael Shepherd for a few months, researching 981 records of patients treated for depression in the Maudsley Hospital. At that time my monograph showing the differences between unipolar depression, bipolar disorder and schizo-affective disorder (published in 1966) had already been accepted for print. Bleuler, Strömgren and Aubrey Lewis agreed that the results could not be true, but fortunately Eliot Slater believed in the correctness of the findings. Strömgren and Bleuler changed their minds after Perris published similar results. Michael Shepherd had by self-admission never treated a patient with lithium and I would be interested to know whether Blackwell himself had done so at the time of their joint article in the Lancet.

During these years we held annual meetings of the IGSAD (International group of studies of affective disorders, founded by Ottosson, Perris, Winokur and Angst). I invited Michael Shepherd to join the group. Some members (Christian Baastrup, Mogens Schou, Max Hamilton, Martin Roth, Paul Grof, Jules Angst, etc.) discussed the ethical and feasibility problems of a placebo-controlled study on lithium and decided finally on the design of a cessation study carried out in Glostrup (Baastrup, Poulsen, Schou et al., 1970).

The positive results of this study were first presented to an IGSAD meeting and were the subject of intense debate. Michael Shepherd remained silent during the discussion and when asked for his opinion, replied "no comment." At the end of that year, I asked him to retire from the group, which he did; we remained on very friendly terms for the rest of his life.

References:

Angst J, Weis P. Periodicity of depressive psychoses. In: Brill H, Cole JO, Deniker P, Hippius H, Bradley PB, editors. Neuropsychopharmacology. Proceedings of the Fifth International Congress of the Collegium Internationale Neuropsychopharmacologicum. Washington D.C. 1966, 28-31 March 1966. International Congress Series No.129. Excerpta Medica Foundation 1967, pp 703-10.

Angst J, Grof P, Hippius H, Poeldinger W, Weis P. La psychose maniaco-dépressive est-elle périodique ou intermittente? In: Cycles biologiques et psychiatrie, De Ajuriaguerra J, editor. Paris, Masson, 1968, pp 339-51.

Angst J, Dittrich A, Grof P. Course of endogenous affective psychoses and its modification by prophylactic administration of Imipramine and Lithium. Int Pharmacopsychiat 1969;2:1-11.

Angst J, Weis P, Grof P, Baastrup PC, Schou M. Lithium prophylaxis in recurrent affective disorders. Br J Psychiatry 1970;116:604-14.

Baastrup PC, Poulsen JC, Schou M, Thomsen K, Amdisen A. Prophylactic lithium: Double-blind discontinuation in manic-depressive and recurrent-depressive disorders. Lancet 1970;2:326-30.

January 22, 2015

BARRY BLACKWELL'S REPLY TO PAUL GROF'S AND JULES ANGST'S COMMENTS

I thank Paul Grof for the kindness and generosity of his comments and must confirm what both he and Jules Angst suggest was my youthful inexperience at the time of the controversial "Prophylactic Lithium" article in the Lancet co-authored with Michael Shepherd. Much of my residency training (1962-1967) was preoccupied with human and pharmacology research on the interaction of MAO inhibitors and tyramine containing foods so I had virtually no practical experience with lithium.

It is also accurate that different career patterns have colored our opinions of the research and its practical implications. Both Drs. Grof and Angst have devoted significant portions of their careers to sophisticated research on the natural history and drug treatment of the bipolar affective disorders in large populations of patients. My own career trajectory has been entirely different, devoted to a wide spectrum of interests in pharmacology, psychosomatic medicine, medical education and specific topics such as patient compliance, homelessness, chronic pain, physician career development and administration of two academic departments. As a result, my continuing interest and knowledge in the arena of bipolar disorder became that of a journeyman (albeit academic) psychiatrist with only a modest involvement in everyday clinical practice and a patchy knowledge of the evolving literature.

From my personal experience and those of colleagues I did learn how the depressive component of bipolar disorders often persists in subdued form despite lithium and is difficult to treat with imipramine (or anything else) without the risk of aggravating manic symptoms. So, this debate in enlivened by the question of how much a body of academic research knowledge can be reliably and usefully transferred as relevant to everyday clinical practice.

How much of value I may have missed in this search is problematic. Paul Grof's bibliography confirms his comment on the lengthy lapse in general interest and research on lithium's effects in bipolar disorder. His list of references covers over seven decades (1940-2015) and of his 64 citations exactly half (32) appeared during the single decade (1961-1970) when this debate erupted. No other decade has more than three citations until 2010, since when five new publications appear of which Paul is a co-author on three.

Review of this and Jules Angst's literature suggests that although our differences are largely reconciled lingering issues are worthy of debate.

It is a fact that one methodological concern raised by Shepherd and me related to potential bias due to lack of a double blind and also true that we underestimated the understandable concerns about safety and suicide that later resulted in imaginative alternative research designs. A second was the possibility of statistical regression to the mean. A third, and perhaps major concern, was the heterogeneity of the patient sample. Both of these latter two concerns were elegantly displayed by the article's graphic portrayal of episodes of illness and remission including recurrent manic, depressive and mixed forms. At a time when imipramine had established its efficacy as an antidepressant in single episodes of unipolar depression we questioned if it also might have a prophylactic effect. We tested this hypothesis using Baastrup and Schou's statistical model in a sample of recurrent unipolar depressed patients treated with imipramine from the Maudsley Hospital data base and found it to be confirmed. This colored our conclusion that lithium was unlikely to be prophylactic for the entire spectrum of bipolar disorders. In retrospect our overboard response to this finding might belong in the category known as "throwing out the baby with the bathwater."

Much of Paul Grof's and Jules Angst's ongoing research has been devoted to a more specific clarification of what types of bipolar spectrum disorder respond in which manner to lithium, imipramine and other mood stabilizers. Grof notes (p.24) that, "recent studies have shown that bipolar disorder is now often undiagnosed, particularly in recurrent depression." This conclusion may have been embedded in Baastrup and Schou's original study and unkindly labeled by us as "bias." My current assumption based on Paul Grof's information is that Schou's brother failed both ECT and imipramine before responding dramatically and persistently to lithium despite being previously considered to suffer from recurrent unipolar depression. Perhaps this conviction was reflected in their diverse patient population and claim for ubiquitous benefit across the spectrum of disorders. Schou's late life interest in this topic suggests he might have been seeking for subtle manifestations of hypomania between episodes of severe depression that would indicate a lithium responsive diathesis. Experienced clinician that Schou was, perhaps he was correct in this also.

Dr. Grof is dismissive of the Prien, Kupfer, Mansky et al. (1984) study and the weight it accords in support of imipramine's potential benefit in recurrent depressive disorder. He cites an impressive body of contradictory evidence which includes personal phone communications from two experienced American colleagues working with Prien who were, "very critical of the patient selection, partly due to the population of V.A. hospitals, and warned me not to believe the findings once the study was completed." The precise scientific basis for this conclusion is not revealed but the allegation is sadly reminiscent of the "ad hominem" feelings evoked by us in Schou's sensitive response to our better articulated concerns. I regret this.

Overall, I strongly agree with Grof and Angst that this kind of historical dissection can be beneficial to contemporary understanding of the evolution of neuropsychopharmacology. We all make mistakes and owning them may benefit posterity. Perhaps the lithium controversy belongs in the larger context pervading our entire field. The first two decades of clinical psychopharmacology were filled with expectations that we would "discover the right drug for the right patient." The story of lithium, the first of our truly psychotropic drugs, so well portrayed by Paul and Jules, shows how far we have come but have yet to go in achieving that end. As Dr. Grof notes, expert committees around the world have produced 25 guidelines for the treatment of bipolar disorder despite which he notes the lax diagnostic practices, overuse and unrealistic expectations for lithium.

Despite the best efforts of dedicated researchers to define therapeutic specificity the general practitioners in our field (of which I was one) continue to operate on a "trial and error basis" when selecting drug treatment for an individual patient. This is contributed to by our still incomplete knowledge of the natural history, genetic origins and phenotypic presentations of the disorders, an unhelpful DSM system of diagnosis, complicated by side effect sensitivity, drug interactions, differing drug profiles, variable compliance and misleading commercial mythologies regarding drug specificity.

Controversy

If this sounds like, "masterful hyperbole" (of which Paul Grof accuses me) please read our essay, "Sir Aubrey Lewis" (Goldberg, Blackwell and Taylor 2015) to better understand the differences between hyperbole (OED: deliberate exaggeration, not to be taken literally) and empiricism (OED: knowledge based on observation and experiment). The latter philosophy of science was the model in which I was trained, a style for which the Maudsley was both renowned and denigrated and of which our article, "Prophylactic Lithium: a Therapeutic Myth" remains, for all its faults, a paradigm.

This deconstruction of the lithium controversy brings to mind a final concern. At their inception over half a century ago both the ACNP and the CINP established policies and memberships dedicated to translational research and dialog. This had dual implications; that basic science might illuminate clinical research while clinical research of the caliber conducted by Grof and Angst would translate to improved everyday diagnosis and treatment by practitioners in the general fields of psychiatry and medicine.

During my own residency training "Descriptive Psychiatry" was the prevailing idiom in European psychiatry – a dedicated interest in the nosology and natural history of mental disorders, illuminated by biological, psychological and social influences and insights although treatment options were sparse. As the new drugs appeared this interest survived initially but began to wane as the connection between clinical features and outcomes was influenced by discoveries, speculations and false hopes involving neurotransmitters, receptors, neural pathways, hormonal and genetic influences. The membership and interests of the ACNP began to tilt unevenly in the direction of neuroscientists (often with dual doctorates), the number of talented clinicians dwindled by attrition while clinical research and data analyses were increasingly usurped by industry. At the same time the NIMH withdrew from new drug research. The well-intentioned DSM nosology is capable, if scrupulously used, of sustaining interest in descriptive psychiatry and sophisticated biopsychosocial formulations but its multi-axial potential has been degraded to become primarily an Axis 1 diagnosis for insurance purposes and ubiquitous use of the Not Otherwise Specified (NOS) categories.

I hope that this renaissance of interest in natural history, nosology and treatment outcomes in bipolar spectrum disorders, sparked by Grof and Angst's research will have a wider influence on the future direction of our field.

Reference:

Goldberg D, Blackwell B, Taylor D. Sir Aubrey Lewis. Professor Sir Aubrey Lewis, the Maudsley Hospital & the Institute of Psychiatry. inhn.org.biographies. February 19, 2015.

February 5, 2015

CHAPTER 5.

RE-EVALUATION

Thomas A. Ban

PAUL GROF: MORE HINDSIGHT THOUGHTS

Barry Blackwell's two sets of comments (2019a,b) on Mogens Schou: My journey with lithium revisit events that happened five decades ago. It's helpful to look at the happenings, in hindsight, to see what we can still learn.

While incorrect, Blackwell and Shepherd's 1968 critique of lithium studies (Blackwell and Shepherd 1968) was beneficial and served a crucial function. I had stated that repeatedly. At that time, Mogens Schou, Jules Angst and I wavered to proceed to a placebo test of our findings. Without Blackwell and Shepherd's article, a strict placebo test and the subsequent introduction of lithium into stabilizing bipolar treatment may have been delayed for a long time. Many bipolar patients would have missed stability.

As Leonardo Tondo correctly stresses (Tondo 2019) our intense hesitation to conduct a double-blind discontinuation trial was based on concerns about patient well-being. Patients included in our open studies were not like patients who nowadays start taking lithium after a brief illness. The several hundred patients included in the open evaluation (Baastrup and Schou 1967; Angst, Grof and Schou 1970) had often been sick for countless years before starting lithium; many had also attempted suicide. While on lithium, they remained in remission for the first time in their life.

Convincing such patients to enter a discontinuation trial with placebo was important for science, but for patients the participation was dangerous or possibly disastrous. This dilemma was much greater than in the usual double-blind studies. In particular, Mogens Schou's compassion for manic depressive patients was profound. As I wrote earlier: "Upon receiving one of many awards, he said: 'For me, every single patient whose life was changed radically by lithium outweighs honors and awards. I trust that you understand and agree. . .'" (Grof 2006).

Had it not been for the biting criticism of the 1968 "Myth" article, the double-blind discontinuation (Baastrup, Poulsen, Schou et al.

1970) may not have been initiated. Yet, it was the strongly positive result of the blind discontinuation study that started altering the previously negative view of lithium. It has triggered the official approvals. Moreover, the use of sequential analysis made it possible to terminate the experiment after a mere six recurrences on placebo.

As I understand Barry Blackwell's comments, their concern about the absence of double-blind studies was prompted by many uncritical clinical reports that afterwards failed the double-blind tests. Blackwell and Shepherd concluded that the only way to eliminate bias, false optimism and unfounded enthusiasm was via a placebo-controlled double-blind study.

One also needs to appreciate the context: The 1960s was a golden era of introducing double-blind studies into psychiatry en masse. For instance, in our psychopharmacological department, Psychiatric Research Institute in Prague, the enthusiasm went so far that all psychotropic medications had only experimental numbers; none had an identifying label.

As researchers, we all are bound to make mistakes, but we react to them differently. I remember vividly that when I met Barry for the first time, much to his credit, he without hesitation conceded that their conclusions were unjustified. What a sharp contrast with Michael Shepherd who was later asked on various occasions about their 1968 article. I never heard him admit that he made a mistake.

In hindsight, I feel that I have learned two relevant, methodological lessons. First one was pointed out in several explorations. If one investigates changes in the bipolar course using mirror image method, and wants to arrive at interpretable, replicable findings, the patient sample must exceed about 100. The size must make up for the large individual variability of the course (Grof 1994).

Missing this point led Blackwell and Shepherd to one wrong conclusion that unfortunately Barry reiterates in his comments here: "Seldom acknowledged in the ensuing debate was the fact that we demonstrated equivalent efficacy for imipramine using the same statistical methodology on a small sample of bipolar patients from the

Maudsley database." I believe Barry is referring here to a report on13 Maudsley patients published by Saran (1968). On the other hand, our cohorts included more than 250 patients.

Second, double-blind placebo-controlled trials are vital but not a panacea. Such trials are necessary for most of the problems in psychopharmacology, but at times they are not essential or feasible. Schou, for example, compared the results of open and double-blind trials carried out with lithium stabilization and the findings were indistinguishable. Presumably, it depends on the severity and type of pathology one assesses.

Similarly, when dealing with issues such as pregnancy or mortality, one cannot use a double-blind methodology yet must answer vital clinical questions by compiling relevant observations. In addition, the double-blind method does not always provide the correct answers. Misapplied, for example, to very heterogeneous samples, it may offer misleading conclusions.

References:

Angst J, Weis P, Grof P, Baastrup PC, Schou M. Lithium prophylaxis in recurrent affective disorders. Br. J. Psychiatr. 1970;116:604-14.

Baastrup PC, Schou M. Lithium as a prophylactic agent. Arch. Gen. Psychiat. 1967;16:162-72.

Baastrup PC, Poulsen JC, Schou M, Thomsen K, Amdisen A. Prophylactic lithium: Double-blind discontinuation in manic-depressive disorders. Lancet 1970;II:326-30.

Blackwell B, Shepherd M. Prophylactic lithium: Another therapeutic myth? An examination of the evidence to date. Lancet 1968;I:968-71.

Blackwell B. The lithium controversy: a historical autopsy. inhn.org.controversies. June 19, 2004.

Blackwell B. Barry Blackwell's comment (Mogens Schou: My journey with lithium). inhn.org.biographies. March 21, 2019a.

Blackwell B. Barry Blackwell's additional comments (Mogens Schou: My journey with lithium). inhn.org.biographies. June 6, 2019b.

Grof P. Mogens Schou (1918-2005): Obituary. Neuropsychopharmacology 2006;31:891-2.

Grof P. Designing long-term clinical trials in affective disorders. J Affect Disord. 1994;30(4):243-55.

Saran, BM. Prophylactic lithium? Lancet. 1968;2(7562):284-5.

Tondo L. Leonardo Tondo Comment. (Mogens Schou: My journey with lithium). inhn.org.biographies. February 7, 2019

October 31, 2019

BARRY BLACKWELL'S REVIEW OF JOHAN SCHIOLDANN: HISTORY OF THE INTRODUCTION OF LITHIUM INTO MEDICINE AND PSYCHIATRY: BIRTH OF MODERN PSYCHOPHARMACOLOGY 1949

I am grateful to Tom Ban and Sam Gershon for drawing my attention to, and inviting me to review, this remarkable book, eight years after its publication. Its provenance is as unique and gratifying as its contents. The author is a Norwegian psychiatrist educated at the

University of Copenhagen, interested in medical historical biography, married to an Australian wife, living in Australia since 1984 and now Emeritus Professor of Psychiatry at the University of Adelaide.

What better progenitor to explore the historical enigma surrounding the Australian, John Cade, who reported the effectiveness of lithium as treatment for acute mania in 1949, a compound with a long prior history of use in gout and its associated psychiatric manifestations, beginning 90 years earlier in Norway.

To grasp the premises, scope, nature and validity of this historiographical enterprise, first read the Preface by German Berrios, Chair of Epistemology in Psychiatry at the University of Cambridge, England. Among his observations is a cogent comment that priority questions often raise issues of a nationalistic nature: "The Lange brothers and Schou in Denmark fulfill the same social function as Cade does in Australia. All that a good historian can (and should) do is try and understand why it is so important for countries to have heroes, and why some official stories, however mythological they may be, cannot be changed or replaced."

This should be enough to whet any reader's curiosity as they are about to enter a dense forest of fact, inference and conjecture. The volume opens with a prescient quotation, "All knowledge is cumulative, and dependent on previous discoveries that have been made available to the scientist and to his fellow man" (Keys 1944). An introduction lays out the scope and skeleton of a 390-page volume that aspires to weave, "as far as the source material allows, an in depth, comprehensive and scholarly fabric that extricates, even if not fully possible, the actual events and sequence of the intricate, checkered and quixotic story of lithium."

The Historiographic Method

An amateur historian at best, this is my first exposure to the pleasures and pitfalls of this method. Google informs me it was developed to make history a respected academic discipline and exists in many different forms applied to a wide variety of topics, both cultural and scientific.

In this instance, the author is concerned with identifying the entire world literature encompassing The History of the Introduction of Lithium into Medicine Psychiatry: Birth of Modern Psychopharmacology 1949.

To this end, 1,245 references are cited in many different languages, as far back as the mid-19th century. This unique and massive bibliography is a generous gift to any reader desirous of knowing the breadth and depth of available information on this sometimes-controversial topic.

The subsidiary issue alluded to in the title is to display John Cade's place in modern psychopharmacology and discern which relevant literature might have influenced Cade's thoughts and behavior in his 1949 discovery of lithium's benefit in mania.

A problem arises when Cade himself makes no mention of historical material the author considers relevant. Is this neglect due to ignorance of the source, disregard for its relevance, or did this unmentioned and perhaps long forgotten material influence Cade at a pre-conscious level?

The author's opinion in this latter regard is entirely subjective for which there is no definable objective threshold. This reviewer and the reader might disagree with the author's assumption on common sense grounds, skepticism about pre-conscious attributions, or covert bias derived from collateral sources related to Cade's persona, nationality, scientific credibility or some unknown issues. To this end the reviewer will comment later, but the readers must decide for themselves.

The Text

Each of 30 chapters is scrupulously referenced; there are photographs of the principal protagonists and copious indexes of persons and subjects. The 390-page text is divided into two parts: **Part I**: Birth of Lithium Therapy, 1859, and **Part II**: Renaissance of Lithium Therapy. Birth of Modern Psychopharmacology 1949. An **Epilogue** consists of three appendices: **Appendix I** Carl Lange: On Periodical

Depressions and their Pathogenesis; **Appendix II** The many faces of John Cade, by Ann Westmore; and **Appendix III** My journey with Lithium, by Mogens Schou.

Part I: The Birth of Lithium Therapy

Gout is one of the earliest diseases described in the literature, from the time of Sydenham who suffered from and wrote about the condition (Sydenham 1683); it was considered an affection of the nervous system, with melancholia an inseparable companion (Roose 1888). Neurosis was also considered an etiologic factor (Duckworth 1880). Uric acid was discovered in calculi in 1775 (Scheele 1776) and identified as an etiologic contributor to uric acid diathesis, linked to diet (Parkinson 1805). Mania was also reported to be a manifestation alone (Whytte 1765) or in conjunction with melancholia (Lorry 1789).

The belief that gout, melancholia and mania were co-morbid was widely held throughout the 19th century in America and Europe, endorsed by many of the leading mental health physicians, discussed at international conferences and articles about the subject were published in leading psychiatric journals of the day (Pinel 1809; Esquirol 1838; Trousseau 1868; Reynolds 1877; Rayner 1881).

Naturally enough, treatments proliferated, some from antiquity and others directed mainly towards the presumed uric acid diathesis. Early in the second century AD Soranus of Ephesus recommended alkaline waters for "manic excitement" while Colchicine dated from the sixth century AD (Alexander of Tralles). Deterred by its drastic purgative effects, a spectrum of other remedies flourished, including cautery, moxibustion, acupuncture, bloodletting, non-protein diets and abstemious lifestyles.

Towards the end of the 19th century, a review of the evidence found the author "completely baffled" and doubtful about etiologic assumptions concerning uric acid that were "more acceptable to charity than likely to be accepted by psychologists," but it might be satisfactory and agreeable to "lay some of human frailty to the charge of uric acid" (Fothergill 1872).

Lithium in Gout

Lithium enters the stage with its discovery in 1800 by the Brazilian Jose Bonifacio de Andrada e Silva who found it in a pile of rocks in an iron ore mine (Johnson 1985). It was not chemically identified as a metallic ion and named lithium, Greek for stone, until later (Vaquelin 1817). It was first mentioned as a potential therapeutic agent when lithium carbonate was found to be four times better than sodium carbonate as a solvent for uric acid (Lipowitz 1841). Clinical utility was suggested two years later when lithium carbonate was shown to dissolve a human kidney stone in vitro (Ure 1844), then first used in vivo by Binswanger in 1847 (Sollman 1942).

Lithium's widespread use in gout and addition to Materia medica is attributed to Garrod, who also noted a therapeutic effect on co-morbid affective symptoms, "occasionally maniacal symptoms arise which I have myself witnessed." Garrod's work, including therapeutic dosage levels, was disseminated in the English, German and French literature (Garrod 1863). Lithium was first listed in the British Pharmacopeia in 1864 and in Merck's Index, from its first edition in 1889 until its fifth edition in 1940, after which its use was banned by the FDA due to lethal toxicity in cardiac patients when used as a salt substitute.

During almost a century, between its first use and until its lethal side effect was recognized, lithium was used in various formulations for a variety of conditions in addition to gout. These included lithium bromide in epilepsy (Locock 1857), as a mild tonic (Gibb 1864), as a sedative (Levy 1874) and in America for epilepsy and "general nervousness" (Mitchell 1870).

Lithium in Affective Disorders

The first systematic use of lithium in affective disorders alone occurred at the Bellevue Hospital in New York (Hammond 1871) for "acute mania with exaltation or acute mania with depression" although the compound used was lithium bromide and its effect was attributed to an alleged ability to "diminish the amount of blood in the cerebral vessels causing cerebral congestion." However, Hammond's later publications, from 1882 till 1890, make no further mention of this use which the author speculates might have been due to lithium toxicity because of the "tremendously high doses he administered."

In 19th century America the rationale and sequence of indications for lithium use were reversed. Hammond made no mention of gout or co-morbidity but in New York Leale took on where Hammond left off. At a conference in London, England (Leale 1881) he resurrected the concept of co-morbidity. "When these gouty functional disturbances are ridiculed or neglected by the physician and the sufferer permitted to long continue in this irritable nervous condition under the pleas that he is hypochondriac and permanent changes are allowed to occur in the cerebral meninges then he may have acute mania, ending in incurable insanity, with the remainder of life spent in a lunatic asylum."

Others followed Leale's lead in what became known as "American Gout" (Da Costa 1881) or "Metabolic Narcoses" (Dana 1886). In such cases the orthopedic manifestations were sometimes minimal ("half gout") and while the mental symptoms were also occasionally mild there were clearly recognizable depressive or manic manifestations of affective disorder, often attributed to "lithaemia, lithiasis or uric acid diathesis." Of interest is the work of John Aulde in Philadelphia who was greatly frustrated by the "unwillingness" of some of his patients "to pursue a course of treatment" and who were only willing "to seek the doctor when trouble overtakes them" (Aulde 1887). An interesting comment on poor compliance, a problem that would not be widely noted or named until more than 90 years later (Blackwell 1997).

Lithium in Denmark

In Denmark, lithium would finally emerge as a treatment for specific mental disorders. Pride of place is accorded the Lange brothers during the last quarter of the 19th century and the first decade of the 20th, (1874-1907), after which its popularity dwindled and was eventually extinguished. Carl Lange (1834-1900) was an academic neuropathologist in private neurology practice and his younger brother, Fritz Lange (1842-1907), was an asylum psychiatrist at Middlefart Lunatic Asylum.

Carl propounded his thesis on "periodic depression" and its response to lithium treatment (Lange 1886). His description of this disorder was later categorized as recurrent unipolar depression (Felber 1987) which Carl Lange distinguished from bipolar disorder because "lack of spirits and joie de vivre is their constant complaint" and also from melancholia due to an absence of delusions and hallucinations. In Carl Lange's experience episodes of "periodic depression" never developed states of mania. If they had occurred, he would have classified them as "cyclical forms of insanity." His theory of etiology included both heritability of "decisive significance," as well as "a constant tendency of the urine to deposit uric acid sediment." About the latter he was ambivalent, "in no way is it certain that uric acid is the cause of periodic depression." Nevertheless, he posited that rational treatment to counteract the underlying diathesis required the "alkaline treatment method," which included lithium salts that had been entered into the Danish Materia medica in 1863 (Gazette de Hospitaux 1863), as well as dietary restriction to eliminate sources of uric acid. Significantly, Lange stressed that both of these measures be undertaken, not only during acute episodes of depression but long term and, if possible, lifelong, although this required in both patient and prescriber, "not insignificant amounts of energy." One of his patients (case vignette No, 5) was non-compliant and refused lithium treatment because she did not believe she was ill, but attributed her malaise to existential calamity, "all sin and disaster."

Carl's efforts were devoted more to the nosology of periodic depression and Fritz's more to the etiological theory of "autointoxication" due to the uric acid diathesis. Towards the end of the 19th century criticism came on both fronts from leading contemporary colleagues (Levinson 1893; Pontoppidan 1895; Christiansen 1904). Unfortunately, Carl died in 1900 and Fritz in 1907, three weeks before his attempted rebuttal, "Uratic Insanity," was published (Lange 1908).

With the death of both brothers, interest dwindled, and opposition grew until "in a meeting of the Medial Society of Copenhagen in 1911 the Lange's theory of periodic depression was dealt its death blow" (Faber 1911). The proceedings gave short shrift to the alleged disorder and its treatment: "The dilapidated ruins of uric acid diathesis should be removed, partly because it is a hindrance to newer and more correct understandings, partly because it also results in useless or even harmful therapy."

Lithium around the World

Not surprisingly, however, the Lange's theories and practice spread to other countries around the turn of the century where they gained criticism and little support from psychiatrists as documented by authors in Great Britain, America, France and Germany. In the last edition of his book, Henry Maudsley touched on the occasional co-morbidity of gout and mental disorders, downplayed the significance of uric acid and mentioned neither Carl Lange nor lithium (Maudsley 1895).

American views were reflected in the popular opinion that Lithia springs and water were beneficial for a broad spectrum of maladies assumed to be due to uric acid diathesis, a belief endorsed by a long line of Presidents but eventually debunked in the popular press: "The time is now to overthrow the Lithia water fetish the only use of which is to extract annually many thousands of dollars from the pockets of real and imagined sufferers" (Leffmann 1910).

A more scientific source in America noted that "The uric-acid hypothesis is a scrap basket for all improperly diagnosed cases" (Futcher 1903).

In Europe, Kraepelin's final verdict was to dismiss Carl Lange's beliefs about periodic depression; it had not been confirmed by clinical observations and was not consistent with his own experience that only a few patients had co-occurring gout. He viewed the diagnosis as more likely being manic depressive disorder in which the manic phase had been missed, but did not mention lithium in its treatment, although he did use it for epilepsy (Kraepelin 1927).

The author notes that preceding Lange's work a relationship between gout and symptoms of affective disorder, including mania, had been "the darling of French medicine" including authorities such as Pinel, Esquirol, Trousseau and Charcot, but did not include the use of lithium.

The author also adds a more contemporary note by citing a study which showed a correlation between cyclic changes in manic-depressive illness and changes in daily uric acid excretion, particularly in the early stages of remission - whether natural or lithium induced. The authors speculated that lithium interferes with the active transport of organic acids in the kidney and the brain (Anumonye, Reading, Knight and Ashcroft 1968).

Back to Norway

In 1927, the same year that Kraepelin issued Europe's dismissive coup de grace to Carl Lange's concept of "periodical depression," Hans Jacob Schou, father of Mogens Schou, published a vehement defense of what he described as "one of the most beautiful descriptions, absolutely classical, which can still enrich and instruct readers of our time" (Schou 1927).

Appropriately he delivered this endorsement with caveats: Lange had made the mistake of separating periodic depression from melancholia and periodical mania when, in fact, the mental and physical symptoms he described were "completely analogous to those of melancholy, differing by degree only," coupled with the fact that both mild and severe forms "occur in manic-depressive families" and had a similar natural history. Schou also speculated that Lange had missed many manic episodes because "his patients were exclusively non-hospitalized, and they would consult him when depressed but not in their exalted periods." Later in life he modified this view to speculate that what would become unipolar depression might be separate from manic-depressive forms (Schou 1940). He recommended treatments ranging from psychotherapy, opium and barbiturates to "the modern shock treatment" (Schou 1946).

Schou also considered that Lange's etiologic theory of uric acid diathesis was refuted by his own research. He disapproved of Lange's suggestion that work and exercise were prime remedies but did not mention the Lange brother's interest in alkaline medicinal remedies (including lithium) or any investigations of his own involving lithium (Schou 1938). Since the uric acid diathesis did not exist there was no reason to mention any medicinal remedies for it.

This logical assumption was later mistakenly characterized as the deliberate abandonment of prophylactic lithium treatment by the father of Mogens Schou, (Amdisen 1985) creating a mythical father-son disagreement (Schou 2005).

While Mogens Schou's denial that his father was the indirect source of any knowledge of lithium's potential therapeutic efficacy is definitive the potential role of the Lange's own work is equivocal. In one publication (Schou 1996), he conceded the brothers treated many hundreds of patients "with dosages large enough to lead to serum concentrations of the same magnitude as those used today," but two years later (Healy 1998) he dismissed their work for lack of convincing case histories, lacking statistics or double blind technique.

Nevertheless, the author considers that Schou senior missed the rediscovery of lithium's effect in manic-depressive disorder "by a whisker." Interestingly, he noted the use of "nerve mixtures" in the disorder's treatment, many of which, listed in the Danish Pharmacopoeia in 1907, contained various salts of lithium (Schou 1946). If the Lange brother's ingenious observations had been followed up, that discovery might have come even earlier (Schioldann 2000).

In a helpful synthesis of the massive amount of preceding information the author provides a prologue to Cade's discovery in 1949. The lithium story began with the fallacious uric acid diathesis which invited alkaline remedies as a treatment repertoire for its allegedly protean manifestations, including psychiatric symptoms.

Equally fallacious was the premise that because lithium was a preferred remedy based on its superior solvent properties in vitro this would transfer to in vivo use, an assumption never clinically confirmed. In addition, the earliest use was with lithium bromide- bromide itself having sedative properties.

The first to use lithium in the acute phase of manic-depressive illness was possibly Hammond (1871), while Da Costa (1881) suggested prophylaxis using lithium citrate. In using lithium prophylactically, both Aulde and Fritz Lange were frustrated by patients' unwillingness to commit to systematic treatment. Both Lange brothers were the first to use lithium carbonate for acute treatment and prophylaxis of periodical depression, finding it superior to the bromide salt. Carl's findings were based entirely on outpatients, while Fritz's included some inpatients suffering from bipolar mood swings. Indisputably, the Lange brothers were the "founding fathers of the systematic use of lithium in psychiatry."

In the first decades of the 1900s, the uric acid diathesis was discarded as an erroneous concept by leading Danish psychiatrists (Faber 1911) and lithium was ushered out with it. The Lange's theories experienced a brief renaissance two decades later with regard to the nosology of manic-depressive disorders, but the "old Danish lithium treatment" was ignored, "only to fall into oblivion" half a century before Cade "rediscovered" its use in acute mania.

Part II: Renaissance of Lithium Therapy. Birth of Modern Psychopharmacology 1949

Appropriately, the author begins with a historiographical analysis of whether Cade's discovery was spontaneous or influenced by what had historically preceded it. In doing so, he cites seven sources beginning with Johnson and Amdisen (1983) whose conclusions are both ambivalent and equivocal. First, they state there had been others "unknown to Cade who had already done so, and indeed, for exactly the same purpose – the control of manic excitement." Later, in the same paper they state: "It hardly seems likely that the various claims which had been put forward for over a hundred years for the therapeutic benefits of lithium in a wide range of disorders, including mental affections, were either totally unknown to Cade or failed to influence his thought, at least in a general way." In another publication, a year later (Johnson, 1984), the author states: "The evidence is difficult to establish, often equivocal and almost always circumstantial." A year later (Amdisen 1984) concurred: "It had escaped Cade's historical research that for as long as 80-90 years before he published his results a presumably not seldom used treatment for mania existed."

Frank Ayd, in a volume on the Early History of Psychopharmacology (Ayd 1991) notes that "In his original report on lithium (1949), Cade reviewed the history of lithium as he knew it then, but in time, it became evident that he had, in fact 'rediscovered' the use of lithium… when Cade learned more of the early history of lithium he acknowledged its earlier uses in mania."

But in 1970, when Cade, along with all the other pioneers in the field, presented his story of lithium at a conference on "Discoveries in Biological Psychiatry" neither in the text nor the references is any mention made of an earlier use by others of lithium in psychiatric disorders (Cade 1970).

Having reviewed the early history of lithium treatment Vestergåard (2001) concluded Carl Lange's observations and writings "were probably known to Cade, but there was nothing to indicate he had been influenced by them." Himmelhoch (2001) concluded, "I would guess (sic) that Cade himself was well aware of Lange's ideas."

Finally, Callahan and Berrios (2005), in a brief book chapter on The Story of Lithium state: "Unknown to him, Cade was retracing the steps of a Danish neurologist, Carl Lange, who had reached the same conclusions 50 years earlier and who had successfully given lithium to patients with affective disorders. However, locked in the Danish language Lange's work was not available to Cade."

The author's conclusion, based on these citations and "a great array of additional source materials," is that it may not be possible to tell the full story to "support an attempt at unravelling the elusive puzzle that is Cade's discovery of lithium." Nevertheless, the chapter ends with a paean of praise for initiating the third revolution in psychiatry. the biochemical revolution in 1949, three years before the discovery of chlorpromazine (Fieve 1997).

This story of Cade's discovery predates the publication of a more detailed analysis of the origins of his ideas about the etiology of the major mental disorders (de Moore and Westmore 2016). Essentially, in addition to a childhood living on the grounds of mental hospitals where his father was a psychiatrist and with a demonstrated interest and involvement in research as a medical student and postgraduate, Cade's views were influenced by his experiences as an officer and general medical practitioner in a Japanese prisoner of war camp during World War II. These experiences shaped a conviction about the organic etiology of severe mental illness, coupled with the simplistic idea, derived from thyroid disease that depression might be due to the absence of a centrally mediated metabolite and mania due to an excess akin to myxedema and thyrotoxicosis (Cade 1947). He communicated these ideas to his wife in a letter en route home from captivity and remained loyal to them in his final publication (Cade 1979) where, not for the first time, he expressed his negative views about Freud and psychoanalysis.

Lithium in Guinea Pigs

Cade's search for a toxic substance began logically in collecting fresh, concentrated morning urine from manic patients and controls with other diagnoses. In a primitive laboratory in the pantry of a chronic ward at the Bandoora Hospital, where he was Superintendent, Cade injected these samples into the peritoneal cavity of guinea pigs and reported his finding that "urine from a manic patient often killed much more readily" (Cade 1947). Identifying urea as the culprit, he described its toxic effects, proceeding from ataxia to quadriplegia, myoclonus, tonic convulsions and eventually status epilepticus leading to death. Interestingly, he discovered that creatinine produced 25% suppression of convulsions and a 50% reduction in mortality, noting the similarity between its structure and that of the anticonvulsant

Dilantin.

Putting aside this distraction, Cade returned to his attempt to find a toxic substance in the urea of manic patients and selected uric acid as a candidate. Confronted by its insolubility in water, he chose the most soluble urate, which happened to be lithium. He now observed the toxicity was far less than expected which he described as the great paradox, "speculating that the lithium ion might be exerting a protective effect" (Cade 1949). Now, using a 0.5% of lithium carbonate, he found this protected all 10 animals injected with an 8% aqueous solution of urea which had previously killed 5 five out of 10 animals. This result of lithium was accompanied by making the animals lethargic and unresponsive for up to two hours before returning to normal. The only extant records of Cade's guinea pig experiments with lithium are in his seminal publication Lithium Salts in the Treatment of Psychotic Excitement (Cade 1949), published in the Medical Journal of Australia, which became the journal's most cited publication. Close inspection of cards (by the author) describing his experiments in guinea pigs deposited by his wife in the Medical History Museum at the University of Melbourne contain none that describe his experiments with lithium (Four Items. Series 22, c.1950).

Cade's observations on guinea pigs when injected with lithium carbonate have been the object of interpretation and controversy among investigators who attempted to replicate the findings. Schou noted that the apathy and slow reaction might be due to intoxication or a direct action on the brain. Experiments in mice and rats also failed to show any comparable effects. Schou's eventual conclusion was critical (Schou 1992): "The reasoning behind his animal experiments was far from clear… and it is my conclusion that the lethargy observed in those guinea was in fact caused by over dosage rather than by a specific tranquilizing action of lithium. I have at least not been able to produce such an effect in guinea pigs or rats with anything but strongly toxic doses." A similar conclusion was expressed (Gershon 1968) with the later caveat that despite a faulty interpretation, the observation provided the incentive to administer lithium to patients with remarkable benefits (Soares and Gershon 2000).

In his 1949 paper, Cade's only reference to earlier medical use of lithium was in gout when he mentions Garrod's text (Garrod 1859). About gout's many "manifestations," he makes no reference to depression or mania mentioned by earlier authors. His conclusion about the historical use lithium was unequivocal: "…the uselessness of lithium in most of the conditions for which it was prescribed, and the fact there was other, more efficacious, treatment in the only disease in which it been shown to be of some value, (and so) it is not surprising that lithium salts have fallen into desuetude." Long after his own discovery he was able to write: "So the introduction of the lithium ion into medicine was all a silly mistake. It was perfectly useless for the conditions for which it was prescribed" (Cade, 1978). He did, however, note that, "The water of certain wells were considered to have special virtue in the treatment of mental illness… it is very likely that their supposed efficacy was a real efficacy and directly proportional to the lithium content of the waters."

Lithium in Patients

Cade's decision to proceed to clinical use was expedited by two factors: first he experimented on himself to determine the safe dose, correctly arriving at 1200 mgs of citrate thrice daily and 600 mgs of the carbonate; and secondly, "I was able to go my own way, unhindered by advice, criticism or caution. I don't think it could happen these days. One would be suffocated by hospital boards, research committees, ethical committees and head of a department. Instead I was answerable only to my own conscience and personal drive" (Cade 1981).

Despite the total lack of evidence in Cade's own writings that he knew of lithium's prior use in affective disorders, the author advances slender evidence that it might have been otherwise. Cade's immediate predecessor in the Victoria Department of Mental Hygiene, W. Ernest Jones, had been Medical Superintendent to an asylum in Wales, UK. His successor, after Jones' move to Australia, discovered a half empty large canister of lithium presumed to date from the early 20th century.

Brian Davies, immigrant from the Maudsley and first Professor of Psychiatry at Melbourne, discussed this hypothesis with Cunningham Dax, Cade's and Jones's superior, who never heard them discuss the possibility of its use in mania, nor did Jones' own research mention it. Another slender thread in the rumor mill was provided by a psychiatrist who worked at Sunbury Mental Hospital from1947 to 1950, the same hospital where Cade's father was Medical Superintendent in 1932 (Ashburner 1950). When Ashburner heard of Cade's discovery and wanted lithium to prescribe, the pharmacist found a big jar of lithium carbonate, a relic from years earlier when the vogue was to use lithium in the treatment of rheumatism. The final piece of tendentious deductive reasoning was derived from the case card of Cade's first patient with mania which records the prescription of lithium with the added comment that he had "an extremely high blood uric acid." The author states, "This case card is highly indicative of the fact, if not proof, that Cade was fully acquainted with the views of his scientific forbears of a presumed connection between mania (gouty mania) and uric acid"; a belief never expressed in any of Cade's writings about his discovery and totally inconsistent with the views about lithium he expressed above.

This issue would remain speculative in the minds of others who wrote about Cade's discovery. Johnson, an ardent and consistent admirer, felt it was "hardly likely" Cade was totally unaware of its use "in a wide range of disorders, including mental affections" (Johnson 1985), but then concluded: "The evidence for this is difficult to establish, often equivocal and almost always circumstantial." An even more remarkable psychoanalytical hypothesis and linguistic analysis was advanced that Cade projected lethargy (a human idiom) onto the guinea pigs while supposedly suppressing prior preconscious knowledge of the historical use of lithium in humans (Reines1991), a tendency ascribed in general to "modern psychopharmacologists (who) either are unaware of or choose to ignore the older clinical literature."

Cade's trial, described in his 1949 paper, included 10 manic patients (three with chronic mania and seven with recurrent episodes), six schizophrenic patients and three with melancholy. Without any control, the results were unequivocal; the manic patients all recovered between a few days and a couple of weeks, relapsing if lithium was discontinued or they were non-compliant. The schizophrenic patients showed a reduction in excitement or restlessness, but no improvement in the core symptoms, although he later reported two patients diagnosed as schizophrenic who did respond (Cade 1969).

The individual case histories of Cade's sample are provided in more detail elsewhere (de Moore and Westmore 2016), but the fate of his first patient (W.B.) is spelled out in detail in the chapter: "Cade's first lithium patient: a paradigm of lithium therapy." According to the original medical record (Davies 1983), which extends from February 24, 1946 (a synopsis of the disorder prior to treatment) and continues until March 3, 1949: "The patient continued well with occasional biliousness." This, however, was not the end of the matter. Johnson (1984) gives a more complete account leading up to the patient's death from lithium toxicity. On March 8, 1950, W.B. was readmitted with lithium toxicity and the drug was discontinued when Cade commented: "Under all circumstances it seems that he would be better off as a care-free restless case of mania rather than the dyspeptic, frail little man he looks on adequate lithium." Two days later, on May 12, 1950, lithium was reinstituted because his manic state worsened. "This state seems as much a menace to life as any possible side effects of lithium." Within a week, by May 19, 1950, lithium was ceased again when he was semi-comatose and had three fits; three days later, on May 22, W.B. was in extremis and died the next day. Cade recorded the death as "toxemia due to lithium salts, therapeutically administered," a verdict accepted by the coroner in October 1950.

Cade never publicly admitted the cause of death and, years later, in four publications he portrayed the final outcome as successful (Cade 1967; Cade 1970; Cade 1978; Cade 1979). Mogens Schou and Cade began corresponding in 1963. Subsequently, Cade learned of lithium's potential as a prophylactic agent in recurrent manic-depressive disorders and Schou accurately predicted it would become far more widely used worldwide. Meanwhile, routine plasma monitoring had made it a far safer drug to use by work done in his own backyard (Noack and Trautner 1951), something Cade also never publicly acknowledged. Sam Gershon, a psychiatric resident under Cade, later reported his statement that, "If you are a good clinician you don't need the machine" (Gershon 2007).

Another unexplained mystery is that in 1950 Cade banned the use of lithium at his own hospital. The author notes that based on his own experience Cade was fully aware of lithium's toxic effects and warned his colleagues of precautions to take in its use (Cade 1949). In February and March 1949 JAMA published reports of fatal toxicity in cardiac patients given lithium as a salt substitute in America. This was published in the Medical Journal of Australia in July, two months before Cade's paper was published on September 3rd. In March, lithium had been banned from all uses in America by the FDA. Nine months later, Cade's first patient, W.B., died of lithium toxicity. This might certainly have been what triggered Cade's decision to ban its use, although this is something to which he never alluded.

Lithium around the Globe

The question arises as to how quickly the use of lithium spread around the globe. A first unpublished account of its use by a British psychiatrist in 1949 was reported as a personal communication years later (Johnson 1984). The first published account after Cade was in Australia (Roberts 1950) of just two cases, one of which, a female with chronic mania, was fatal. The timing of this might well have contributed to Cade's concern even though that might have been ameliorated by a letter to the journal in which Roberts (1950) claimed to have treated more than 50 patients without toxicity at another Australian mental hospital, safety he attributed to use of lithium carbonate, far safer than the chlorate or citrate Roberts was using.

Measurement of Lithium Levels

Re-Evaluation

Also, in 1950, a world authority on gout and uric acid published a paper on lithium as a salt substitute (Talbott 1950) suggesting that monitoring serum levels might stave off toxicity. The idea was picked by a psychiatrist at Mount Park Hospital in Melbourne and a faculty member in the Department of Physiology at Melbourne University (Noack and Trautner 1951). Using a flame photometer, they decided to study Cade's findings in detail, including three fatalities since they were published. They studied more than 100 patients suffering from mental disorders and confirmed Cade's findings without any serious intoxication (Noack and Trautner 1951). By 2004 their paper, like Cade's, was among the 10 most cited articles in the Medical Journal of Australia. In a letter written in 1974, Schou congratulated them on a method of primary importance in the development of lithium as a safe and efficient procedure (Goodwin and Ghaemi 1999). Cade, for the reason given above, remained silent (Gershon and Daverson 2006).

Mogens Schou and Prophylaxis

In 1951, Strömgren in Denmark learned of Noack and Trautner's work at a conference in Paris and drew the attention of "his brilliant research assistant, Mogens Schou" to Noack and Trautner's paper (Strömgren 1951). In 1952 and 1953, Schou collaborated with colleagues in Denmark on the use of lithium in 38 manic patients in a double-blind placebo-controlled study, (Schou et. al., 1954) confirming the work of Cade. This might be the point at which lithium could be considered a scientifically based safe and effective treatment of acute mania.

According to the author, both Strömgren and Schou disavowed any influence of the Lange brothers in their decision to study lithium; Schou also denied hearing his father speak of it. Schou gave the credit entirely to Cade and they soon became close friends, exchanging approximately 40 letters between 1963 and 1970, by which time the scope of lithium began to be vastly inflated by Schou's discovery of its prophylactic effect.

Following his presentation at the 1970 Baltimore Conference on

Discoveries in Biological Psychiatry, Cade (1970) visited Schou in Denmark where Schou heaped praise on him in a lecture as "the man who introduced lithium into psychiatry and described its anti-manic effect." Cade reciprocated as follows: "I feel rather like woman who as a girl had an illegitimate child and had adopted it out. And now, 20 years later, I am visiting the adoptive parents and finding out what a fine big boy he has grown into but knowing far less about him than his adoptive parents" (Schou 1983). This apt and colorful quotation coveys a strong and synergistic relationship between the two men and a somewhat humble contribution made by Cade. It was described by Schou as, "The nicest compliment we have ever received" (Schou 1983).

Serendipity or Not?

The author spends 13 pages addressing this somewhat controversial and provocative topic which plays a recurrent theme throughout the discovery of all the earliest treatments in psychopharmacology (Ban 2006). While it is a term sometimes used by the discoverers themselves, others have viewed it as dismissive or even derogatory. The author notes that Cade "was very annoyed that his discovery was considered by many as serendipitous… he never ceased to point out that it was based on a specific hypothesis and experimental observations." And later, "that he was emphatic that the discovery was the result of a continuous and consistent chain of reasoning."

Among the many citations relevant to this issue, ranging over more than half a century and many countries, a pattern emerges. In the earlier years, while Cade was still alive, there are no less than 16 authors worldwide, alone or together, who use the term "serendipitous." In his book, Serendipity: Accidental Discoveries in Science, Roberts (1989) singles out lithium's discovery as "the most improbable of all." Rejection of this attribution occurs much later and from fewer sources, often linked to memorial occasions celebrating the discovery and Cade himself in Australia. Two individuals stand out in defense of Cade's own position. Johnson, a psychologist and long-time author and advocate for Cade who, in his obituary (Johnson 1981) notes: "He always strenuously denied that his work with lithium contained any element of serendipity." His most vehement advocate was Mogens Schou who consistently attributed his own knowledge of lithium's anti-manic effect to his friend John Cade. In 1977, he addressed the topic at the 43rd Beattie Smith Lecture in Melbourne and in 1982, during the First John Cade Memorial Lecture, he expressed his distaste for the way in which serendipity was used "in a derogatory sense; arbitrary success, random discovery, sheer luck." Interestingly, Schou's overall views of Cade's work were quite nuanced. He noted: "The hypothesis which started his work was crude. His experimental design was not particularly clear. And his interpretation of the animal data may have been wrong. Those guinea pigs probably did not just show altered behavior, they were presumably quite ill." Nevertheless, placing more emphasis on the revolutionary consequences of the discovery for sufferers of manic-depressive illness, Schou added: "...and this is the marvel of the thing – a spark jumped in John Cade's questing mind and he performed the therapeutic trial which eventually changed life for manic-depressive patient all over the world" (Schou, 1996a). Perhaps understandably, Schou conflates Cade's discovery by integrating it with his own.

The author offers no reconciliation or adjudication between these conflicting views of the role or not played by serendipity in Cade's discovery of the effect of lithium in mania.

Cade's Legacy and Role in the Birth of Modern Psychopharmacology

This penultimate chapter begins, appropriately, by singling out America as most tardy in the recognition of lithium for mania. "The magnitude of this discovery is not yet realized in this country (Williamson 1966). This was undoubtedly due to the complete ban placed on lithium in 1949 by the FDA, the year of Cade's discovery, triggered by its lethal toxicity in cardiac patients when used as a salt substitute. This ban stubbornly persisted until 1970 due largely to the failure of academic psychiatry and the FDA to recognize the fact that toxicity could be avoided by blood monitoring (Noack and Trautner 1951). Paradoxically, the ban on use in mania, but still not for prophylaxis, was lifted in 1970 at exactly the time Cade was invited to present his work for the first time in America (Ayd and Blackwell 1970). Doubtless the ban was also not vigorously opposed because lithium was a basic ion, not a patented or marketed drug, backed by the large pharmaceutical companies busy developing and eventually selling expensive, less effective, "mood stabilizers" with more side effects.

Ironically, in 1949, Sweden had awarded the Nobel Prize to Egaz Monez for frontal lobotomy while lithium, discovered in the same year, went largely unnoticed, although it was "difficult to find a specific drug that is as efficacious in a high percentage of patients of a specific nosological category" (Lindheimer and Schafer 1966).

It was not until after Schou and his colleagues reported lithium's prophylactic effect in recurrent manic-depressive disorder, a far broader indication with wider usage, that in the mid to late 1960s Cade's earlier contribution in mania began to gather widespread recognition with vastly magnified claims to its significance in the entire field and history of psychopharmacology. In America, Nathan Kline's article, "Lithium Comes into its Own" (Kline 1968), gave rise to exuberant correspondence in the American Journal of Psychiatry triggered by his description of lithium as "The 20 year old Cinderella of Psychiatry." Hyperbole spread round the globe like the Plague. In an editorial, the Medical Journal of Australia (1999) eulogized lithium and the man: "John Cade was among the highest order of scientists whose work on lithium in patients with mania revolutionized their management and facilitated return to society." Another American psychiatrist, in a book for lay public, declared: "Cade's discovery initiated the third revolution in psychiatry" (the first two were Pinel and Freud) (Fieve 1997). In a commemorative article, a lay journalist in Australia described Cade's original paper as, "one of the most revolutionary in medical history" (Haigh 2004). A trio of psychiatrist's expressed the view that "lithium not only had profound effects for patients with affective disorder, but has also launched the pharmaceutical revolution (Watson, Young and Hunter 2001). Others felt that the introduction of lithium by Cade in 1949 can be "considered to have heralded the modern era of psychopharmacology" (Baldessarini, Tondo and Viguera 2002). Last, but certainly not least, was Johnson (1975) in an early edition of his book, The History of Lithium Therapy: "Cade's discovery is considered by many working in the field of psychiatric research to have been one of the most significant in pharmacology."

Appendix I: Carl Lange; on Periodical Depressions.

This is a verbatim translation from Danish into English by the book's author of Lange's speech to the Medical Society of Copenhagen in 1886, the essence of which is discussed in the text.

Appendix II: The Many Faces of John Cade by Ann Westmore

Ann Westmore (2016) is the co-author of the book, Finding Sanity: John Cade, Lithium and the Taming of Bipolar Disorder.

She gives a brief synopsis of John Cade's youth and character traits, including his interest in collecting, classifying and experimenting as well as his strange hobby of studying animal footprints and fecal patterns. He also shared an interest in literary skills with a younger brother and journalist although his scientific articles tended toward brevity and had been criticized for that.

After medical training, Cade undertook a post graduate doctoral degree (without thesis), a mirror of the British practice preparing for an academic or research career, and also an approach he urged his colleagues to pursue following his discovery of lithium. In his first Beattie-Smith lecture, Cade said: "Let us never rest content with the present bounds of knowledge, it is up to us to initiate a particular approach to a psychiatric problem and if we have not the necessary knowledge to seek it."

During the span of his career, he fulfilled many teaching

assignments, helping to train as many as 300 psychiatric residents, as well as medical students, between 1952 and his retirement in 1977. Like Frank Ayd, he wrote a column for thousands of fellow Catholics on a whole range of medical, psychiatric, ethical and social issues. But he was "equally capable of undermining doctrine," including a witty paper on Masturbational Madness (Cade 1973).

Westmore comes to a modest conclusion: "By teaching curiosity with crude research techniques and the freedom to pursue ideas, John Cade helped to generate an Australian presence in the modern psychopharmacology revolution."

Appendix III: My Journey with Lithium; Mogens Schou

In addition to a synopsis of his own career, Schou provides a profile of his relationship with John Cade. In addition to a long correspondence, they met on three occasions between 1972 and 1975. "He was a mild- mannered modest person who once said of himself 'I am not a scientist – I am only an old prospector who happened to pick up a nugget.'" But, Schou comments: "Prospectors find because the seek." John Cade was characterized by an insatiable curiosity, keen observation, a willingness to test even absurdly unlikely hypotheses and the courage to risk making a fool of himself." Schou characterized Cade as an "artist" compared to "myself as the systematic scientist."

This Reviewer's Comments

Because I have played a personal and significant role in the controversies swirling around lithium (Blackwell 2014) and this is the second book I have reviewed on the topic (Blackwell 2017), I have shunned commenting as far as possible in my review of the book itself and have chosen to address five important aspects that play central roles in the enigmatic story of Cade and lithium.

A Histiographic Fallacy?

In my untutored opinion, there seems to be a strong implication that a long-ago historical archive would almost inevitably be known to an enlightened investigator even when it was not acknowledged in that person's publications or evident in collateral information. I will challenge this assumption both with regard to Cade's biography and personal experience.

Cade's passage to becoming a psychiatrist was unusual by today's standards. He did not start out wanting to be one. From 1929 till 1935 he was a medical student and in his final year he attended 12 psychiatric lectures. Following graduation, he spent a year as an intern in medicine and pediatrics ending with a near fatal episode of pneumonia in pre-antibiotic days. After recovering, he decided to follow his father and become a psychiatrist.

In November 1936, he was appointed as a Medical Officer at Beechwood Mental Hospital "having spent a few months studying psychiatry" (de Moore and Westmore 2016). For the next two years he experienced on the job training in a rich clinical environment and also studied for a post graduate degree in general medicine (M.D.) which he obtained in 1938. Also, during this time, he became involved in research and had two publications.

In September 1939, Australia joined Britain in declaring World War II against Germany and later, Japan. John Cade enlisted in December 1939 and joined up fulltime in July 1940 to begin training as an army general medical officer; he shipped to Burma in January 1941. What followed was four years as a POW of the Japanese in Changi, a time during which he was bereft of medical journals and literature.

Driven by a strong sense of urgency and creative ideas incubated at Changi, Cade returned to Bandoora Repatriation Hospital in 1946 and almost immediately supplemented his demanding work as Superintendent with his intense solitary search in guinea pigs for a toxic cause of mania. "He was a man in a hurry." (de Moore and Westmore, 2016).

To Cade's credit, we know that, despite fragmented and distracting formal training at the start of his career, he was a voracious reader of medical texts who annotated them meticulously. After studying this archive, previous reviewers noted: "John Cade, it seems, was completely unaware of these previous endeavors to use lithium in psychiatric illness." By the late 1940s, notions of lithium's supposed curative properties in all diseases had lost favor and it seems to be included in reference books, almost apologetically, as a testament of past faulty reasoning (de Moore and Westmore 2016).

It is equally unlikely that lithium or uric acid diathesis were mentioned in the curriculum of medical school or postgraduate medical studies.

Even supposing, however unlikely, that Cade did know of the early Danish work decades earlier, why would he fail to acknowledge that in his own work? Most scientists bolster the credibility of novel findings by citing prior work that corroborates their own.

The extent to which early and long-buried knowledge may be overlooked in the discovery process is the subject of an essay on Adumbration (Blackwell 2014). This tells the story of the tardy discovery of the sometimes-fatal interaction between MAO inhibitors and tyramine containing foods five years after these drugs were introduced for the treatment of tuberculosis and depression. A compelling archive of information in prominent journals that might have predicted this toxic interaction was unknown to basic scientists and clinicians working for several pharmaceutical companies, as well as academic and journeyman physicians in various disciplines who treated thousands of patients.

Serendipity

In preparing my thoughts on this matter, I consulted the Oxford English Dictionary (OED) and was delighted to find that serendipity might be considered a portmanteau word that carries the burden of more than one meaning (The example given is brunch, for breakfast and lunch).

A second discovery was an excellent article, the best and most comprehensive I have come across, on the history and role of the word (Ban 2006). Tom traces its origins to a 16th century fairy tale The Three Princes of Serendip, a text translated from Persian to Italian and then French over the centuries until Horace Walpole (1717-1797), an

Re-Evaluation

English literary genius, in a letter to a friend in June 1754, coins the term "serendipity" which describes the three princes who were "always making discoveries by accident and sagacity of things they were not in search of." In my opening lecture on The Process of Discovery (Blackwell 1970), at the Conference where Cade received the Taylor Manor Award for this discovery, I related the example which Walpole gives in the letter to his friend, drawn from the original story. One of the princes "deduces a mule is blind in the right eye because the grass was eaten only on the left side of the path." This is clearly an example of deductive reasoning reflective of the prince's sagacity. Note no experimentation was required which might have demanded a scientist's inductive skills.

More than three centuries of usage in three languages have blurred the precise definition of the word serendipity. Ban cites three dictionaries with differing definitions.

1. "Making happy and unexpected discoveries by accident" (OED).
2. "Finding valuable and agreeable things not sought after" (Webster).
3. "Finding one thing while looking for something else" (Stedman).

The essence common to all three is a search in which the outcome is unexpected. In none of them is there any hint that the word might or can be used in a derogatory way which both Schou and Cade assumed to be the case.

Ban systematically and rigorously applies these definitions to nine different psychotropic medications and divides them into four categories: 1) in four drugs, LSD, meprobamate, chlorpromazine and imipramine, "one thing is found while looking for another"; 2) in three drugs, potassium bromide, chloral hydrate and lithium carbonate, the discovery was serendipitous because, "an utterly false rationale led to correct empirical results"; 3) in one drug, iproniazid, "a valuable indication was found that was not initially sought"; and 4) only with chlordiazepoxide was discovery due to "sheer luck."

In conclusion Ban notes, "Serendipity is one of the many contributing factors in the discovery of most of the psychotropic drugs." Also included is the potential of findings based on knowledge or past experience and he cites Goethe's aphorism, "Discovery needs luck, invention, intellect – none can do without the other" (Kuhn 1970). He also mentions Pasteur's well known, "Chance favors the prepared mind"– cited in the original French.

Tom Ban's conclusions about Cade's discovery concur with the significant majority of the independent opinions cited by the author of this volume. It does not explain the rationale for Cade and Schou's opinions that the use of the term serendipity was dismissive or derogatory.

Cognitive Style

In a previous review of another book about Cade (Blackwell 2017), I raised the issue of Cade's cognitive style based on a brief book by Michael Shepherd (1985) who claimed both Sigmund Freud and Sherlock Holmes used deductive reasoning to arrive at untenable conclusions, contrasting it with the kind of systematic inductive reasoning commonly used in research by scientists. What seemed odd was that Cade castigated Freud's clinical theories but admired and taught medical students and psychiatric trainees using deductive examples. He was also a disciplined clinician well versed in classical nosology and epistemology. Shepherd says nothing about the possibility that the same person might use different methods for separate tasks. I was also struck by the fact that Schou contrasted his friend Cade's "artistic" style with his own as a "systematic scientist." Cade's ventures into etiology seem to be based mainly on deductive reasoning in the case of both schizophrenia, due to absence of "protective foods" (Cade 1956), and mongolism, due to manganese deficiency (Cade 1958). Attempts to decipher the logic and cognitive style of his inquiries into uric acid, lithium and mania have also been frustrating due, at least in part, to lack of data.

Legacy and Primacy

The author's assessment of the importance of Cade's discovery of lithium in 1949 and its impact on the early development of psychopharmacology tilts strongly in a positive direction in a manner not supported by the data. This clearly defines two distinct time periods: from 1949 to 1963 and from then to the present.

Within less than three years of his discovery Cade had banned the use of lithium in the hospital where he was superintendent, a topic about which he remained silent although it coincided with the death of his first patient due to lithium toxicity, followed by the death of another patient at a different hospital and preceded by a total ban on its use in America. During the remainder of this first period Cade's interests shifted dramatically. He was preoccupied with administrative manners dictated partly by the arrival of a new administrator recruited from Britain who supervised his work and implemented innovative changes in mental health care, but also by a shift in Cade's clinical interest to schizophrenia and insulin coma. During this time, he was also sent to Britain for six months to study changing trends in mental health care possibly applicable to Melbourne.

It was during this period, from 1958 to 1963, that the CINP was formed and convened its first three international Conferences, none of which Cade participated in nor did any psychiatrist from Australia. The first to do so was Brian Davies, recruited from the Maudsley in Britain to become Professor of Psychiatry at the University of Melbourne, who joined the CINP in 1961. Lithium was not mentioned in the main program in any of the first three meetings in 1958, 1960 and 1962.

It was in 1963 that Schou first wrote to Cade informing him of an interest in prophylaxis, congratulating him on his discovery and initiating a continuous correspondence. It is from this point on that Cade's interest in lithium was vigorously renewed and from this point forward that comments begin to appear in the literature about the positive influence of events in 1949 on the entire history of the field. The flood of positive attributions stems largely from authors with a special interest in lithium, writing 20-30 years after Cade's discovery and at a time when innovation in the field had slowed to a crawl.

In 1970, when Ayd and I planned and convened the Baltimore

Conference, we invited 16 of the world's leading researchers and clinical pioneers to participate. All agreed and each received the same Taylor Manor Award. Included were Chauncey Leake (Amphetamine), Tracy Putman (anti-convulsants), Alfred Hoffman (LSD), Frank Berger (Meprobamate), Irv Cohen (Benzodiazepines), Hugo Bein (Reserpine), Pierre Deniker (Neuroleptics), Jorgen Ravin (Thioxanthenes), Nathan Kline (Iproniazid), Ronald Kuhn (Imipramine) and John Cade (Lithium).

This meeting provides a different perspective on events in the field. Three drugs were in use before lithium: LSD, amphetamine and diphenylhydantoin. Joel Elkes, regarded by some as the successor to Thudichum, presented on "Beginning in a New Science" during which he described work on neurochemistry at the Department of Pharmacology and Experimental Psychiatry between 1942 and 1950 when he moved to the NIMH at Saint Elizabeth's Hospital in Baltimore (Blackwell 2015). Also included was a paper by Irvine Page on "Neurochemistry as I have known it," describing his work in Germany from 1928, his book on The Chemistry of the Brain in 1938 and at the Cleveland Clinic after 1945, including the discovery of serotonin.

Frank Ayd gave a concluding talk on the Impact of Biological Psychiatry. There was a friendly sense of collegiality among participants and a shared awareness of being part of a group of pioneers in the field. Lithium was considered one compound among many and no speaker was singled out for special credit or leadership of the field of psychopharmacology.

In 1985, Michael Shepherd asked me to review the latest edition of Johnson's History of Lithium Therapy. In doing so I quoted the following paragraph as an expression of concern about how far the book portrayed the biases in the field about lithium: "Lithium is being taken by one person in 2,000 in most civilized countries, possibly more in Denmark. At a stroke the elusive ethereal Freudian psyche was replaced by the polyphasic, physico-chemical system called the brain. Lithium, like no other single event led to psychiatry becoming truly interdisciplinary. Its ubiquitous use suggests a new basis for classification of psychopathological states. It is so cheap and easy to administer that it will transform healthcare in underdeveloped countries whose psychiatric services are otherwise stretched to the limit."

On the 50th anniversary of Cade's discovery, two leading psychiatrists informed the public: "Lithium inaugurated the psychopharmaceutical revolution. Essentially it saved psychiatry as a medical specialty" (Goodwin and Ghaemi 1999).

Plasma Monitoring

This constitutes perhaps the greatest enigma of all: Why did John Cade never speak of the work of Noack, Gershon and Trautner, carried out in Melbourne's own university, when Gershon had been a resident under his care and the biggest obstacle to lithium's safe and wider use would have been plasma monitoring? The only clue we have is that when Gershon asked Cade he commented that a good clinician didn't require laboratory help. This is consistent with a confident self-image of his own skill as a clinician, based perhaps on having experimented on himself and the early experience he had with the 10 patients he was treating. But after his first patient died with a puzzling mixture of medical deterioration and side effects, and soon after that a patient at another hospital died on what appeared to be therapeutic dose, why not change his mind and acknowledge plasma monitoring augmented clinical judgment? One can only imagine pride might enter the equation, especially if he had already decided to ban lithium's use. But this hardly seems consistent with a concern for the many other psychiatrists treating patients with lithium unless he simply did not feel an obligation to be involved now that he had decided to ban lithium use and perhaps believed others would disseminate the information. Added to all this is the fact that 20 years later, when he presented his paper in Baltimore, Cade knew of lithium's increasing and widespread use and openly praised Schou for his discovery of prophylaxis, but still could not bring himself to mention Trautner's work. This suggests a deep-seated personal antipathy he was not able to resolve.

National Heroes

I have left this to last because I suspect it may be the most important factor bearing not just on the interpretation of the book under review, but the enigmas of the entire lithium story. It is also a response to the clue Professor Berrios handed us in his prescient forward to the book and the historiographical method. Berrios noted that "priority questions often raised issues of a nationalistic nature" which Cade and Schou fulfill in Australia and Norway and that however mythological these "official" stories are "they cannot be changed or replaced."

In responding to this assertion, a distinction is made between the first and second parts of the book. The massive database of lithium's pre-1949 history is impressive and valuable to all clinicians and research workers interested in lithium. I have only one caveat to assert that however compelling it might be, there is not a shred of evidence, real or circumstantial, from his own or the writing of others, that John Cade knew anything of that. As a matter of fact, neither apparently, did Mogens Schou, who always asserted he learned of lithium when his mentor Strömgren drew his attention to Cade's work in 1951 or 1952 (Appendix III) and not from either Lange's research or Schou's father. This, apparently, was the bond that created such a powerful synergy between Cade and Schou. There appears to be something of a historiographical bias that if research is well established in the literature, an educated professional must know about it even without evidence to substantiate such an assumption.

In the second part of John Schioldann's book we can see how Cade's Hero status is preserved and protected. The voluminous database is somewhat subjectively and selectively mined to favor Cade and Schou's view that the discovery of lithium was not serendipitous, a word they regard as dismissive or derogatory and not the product of deductive reasoning, although Schou does consider Cade to be "artistic" in contrast to himself as a "systematic scientist." The burden of proof tilts in favor of both serendipity and a deductive cognitive style.

Furthermore, Cade's discovery of lithium's value in mania is combined and conflated with Schou's later discovery of serendipity to claim that this body of work formed a foundation for the whole of psychopharmacology as a discipline, an assumption not supported by close scrutiny of the relevant literature. Other concerns a careful reader might raise are doubts about Cade's ban on lithium; failure to acknowledge Trautner and colleagues work, which made lithium safe to use; and concealment of his first patient's death due to lithium toxicity. It is true that the literature assembled does not cast new light on these blemishes, but failure to mention them does serve the purpose of embellishing a perfect Hero image.

Experience informs me that an unfortunate side effect of commenting on a Hero in anything less than affirmative terms may be perceived as an ad hominem attack on their persona or integrity. I plead for the reader's indulgence to avoid such an attribution and accept my assurance that Cade and Schou, Trautner and Gershon each deserve a place in any lithium pantheon of pioneers; but as colleagues and peers, diverse and without preferred status.

References:

Anumonye A, Reading HW, Knight F, Ashcroft GW. Uric acid metabolism in manic-depressive illness and during lithium therapy. Lancet 1968; 1:1290-3.

Amdisen A. Lithium treatment of mania and depression over one hundred years. In: Corsini GU, editor. Current trends in lithium and rubidium therapy, Lancaster: MTP Press, 1984: 11-26.

Amdisen A. Carl Lange pa fransk visit I psykiatrien. Dan. Medicinhist. Aurb 1985:14; 9-40.

Aulde J. The use of lithium bromide in combination with a solution of sodium citrate. Med. Bull. 1887;39:35-9.

Ayd FJ. The early history of modern psychopharmacology,

Neuropsychopharmacol. 1991; 5: 71-84.

Baldessarini RJ, Tondo L, Hennen J, Viguera AC. Is lithium still worth using? An update of selected recent research. Harvard Rev. Psychiatr. 2002; 10: 59-75.

Ban TA. The role of serendipity in discovery. Dialogues clinical neurosci. 2006; 335-44.

Blackwell B. The Process of Discovery. In: Ayd FJ, Blackwell B, editors. Discoveries in Biological Psychiatry. Philadelphia, Lippincott, 1970; 205-17.

Blackwell B. From compliance to alliance: A quarter century. In: Blackwell B, editor. Treatment Compliance and the Therapeutic Alliance. Harvard Academic Publishers USA, 1997; 1-16.

Blackwell B. The lithium Controversy: A historical autopsy. inh.org.controversies. June 19, 2014.

Blackwell B. Adumbration; A History Lesson inh.org controversies. December 18, 2014.

Blackwell B. Joel Elkes. An Integrative Life. inhn.org.biographies. August 30, 2015.

Blackwell B. Review. de Moore G, Westmore A, editors. Finding Sanity: John Cade, lithium and the Taming of Bipolar Disorder. Melbourne, Allen and Unwin, 2016. inhn.org.biographies. February 2, 2017.

Cade JF. The anticonvulsant properties of creatinine. Med. J. Aust. 1947;2: 621-3.

Cade JF. Lithium salts in the treatment of psychotic excitement. Med. J. Aust. 1949; 2; 349-52.

Cade JF. The aetiology of schizophrenia. Med. J. Aust. 1956; 2: 135-9.

Cade FJ. Manganese and Mongolism. Med. J. Aust. 1958; 2: 848-9.

Cade JF. The use of lithium salts in the treatment of mania. Supplement to the Bulletin of Post-Graduate committee in Medicine. University of Sydney, 1969; 25: 528-33.

Cade JF. The story of Lithium. In: Ayd FJ, Blackwell B, editors. Discoveries in Biological Psychiatry. Philadelphia, Lippincott, 1970; 218-29.

Cade JF. Masturbational Madness: An historical annotation. Aust. N.Z.J. Psychiatr. 1973; 23-6.

Cade JF. Lithium in Medicine In: Burrows GD, Chiu E, editors. Research in Affective Disorders: Proceedings of the Scientific Meeting in Honour of Dr. John Cade. University of Melbourne, 1977; 7-9.

Cade JF. Lithium - past, present and future. In: Johnson FN, Johnson S, editors. Lithium in Medical Practice. Lancaster, MTP Press, 1978; pp 5-16.

Cade JF. Mending the Mind: A Short History of Twentieth Century Psychiatry. Melbourne, Sun Books, 1979.

Cade FJ. Cade to Johnson, personal communication. John F Cade 1912-1980: A Reminiscence. Pharmacopsychiatr. 1981:14: 148-9.

Callahan CM, Berrios GE. The story of Lithium. In: Reinventing Depression: A History of the Treatments of Depression in Primary Care 1940-2004. Oxford University Press, 2005, pp 95-96.

Christiansen V. Dr. F. Lange, overlaege ved Middlefart Sindssygeanstalt: Slaegter, laggagelseren Sindssgeanstalt. Copenhagen, Bibl. Laeg.1904; 96:459-72.

DaCosta JM. The nervous symptoms of lithaemia. Amer. J. Med. Sci. 1881; 144: 313-30.

Dana CL. On the relation of lithaemia, oxaluria and phosphaturia to nervous symptoms. Med. Rec. 1886; 29(3): 57-64.

Davies B. The first patient to receive lithium. Aust. NZ. J. Psychiatr. 1983; 16: 183-209.

de Moore G, Westmore A. Finding Sanity; John Cade, lithium and the taming of bipolar disorder Australia, Allen and Unwin, 2016.

Duckworth D. A plea for the neurotic theory of gout. Brain 1880;3: 1-22.

Editorial. Medical Journal of Australia 1999; 171: 225.

Esquirol E. Des maladies mentale considerees sous les rapports medical, hygienique et medico-legal. Paris, Balliere 1838, Vol 1, p.75.

Faber E. Urinsyrediathesen. Ugesker. Laeg. 1911;73:751-71.

Felber W. Lithium prophylaxis of depression one hundred years ago – an ingenious misconception. Fortsch. Neurol. Psychiat. 1987; 55: 14

Fieve RR. Moodswing New York, Bantam Books, 1997.

Fothergill JM. The Heart and its Diseases. London, H.K. Lewis 1872, pp 398-409.

Futcher TB. The occurrence of gout in the United States. Practitioner 1903; July: 6-16.

Garrod AB. The Nature and Treatment of Gout. London, Walton and Maberly, 1863, 425.

Gazette de Hospitaux, No.43. Therapeutik (Lithium salts) Hospitalstid 1863;6 (20): 78-80.

Gershon S. Personal communication to Schioldann April 25, 2007.

Gershon S, Daverson C. The lithium story; a journey from obscurity to popular use in North America. In: Bauer M, Grof P, Müller-Oerlinghausen B, editors.   Lithium in Neuropsychiatry, the comprehensive guide. Abingdon, Oxon, Informa 2006; 17-24.

Gibb GD. Note on the action of bromides of lithium, zinc and lead. Reports of the 34TH meeting of the British Association of advances in science. Sept 1864.

Goodwin FK, Ghaemi SN. The impact of the discovery of lithium on psychiatric thought and practice in the USA and Europe. In: Mitchell PB, Hadzi-Pavolic D, Marijc HK, editors. Fifty Years of Treatments for Bipolar Disorder: A Celebration of John Cade's Discovery. Aust.NZ J. Psychiatr. 1999; 33 Suppl.; 354-64.

Haigh G. Matter over Mind. The Bulletin (Australia) 2004; 91-5.

Hammond WA. Treatise on Diseases of the Nervous System. New York. Appleton 1871; Mania (358-66) and Treatment (380-1).

Healey D. The Psychopharmacologists II. London, Altman 1998; 259-84.

Himmelhoch JM. Book Review: Schioldann, 2001. Bipolar Disorder 2005; 7: 477-8.

Keys TE. A Stained Glass Window on the History of Medicine. Bulletin Medical Library Association 1944; 32: 488-95.

Johnson FN. Preface in Lithium Research and Therapy. London Academic Press. 1975.

Johnson FN. John FJ Cade, 1912-1980; A reminiscence. Pharmacopsychiatr. 1981; 14: 148-9.

Johnson FN. The early history of lithium therapy. In: Bach RO, editor. Lithium; Current Applications in Science, Medicine and Technology. New York, Wiley 1985 pp. 337-44.

Johnson FN, Amdisen A. The first era of lithium in medicine; An historical note. Pharmacopsychiatr.1983; 16: 61-3.

Kline N. Lithium comes into its own. Amer. J. Psychiatr. 1968; 125: 558-60.

Kraepelin E. Klinische Psychiatrie, Erster Teil, Neunte, vollstandig umgearbertete Auflage. Leipzig: Barth 1927; p.308.

Kuhn R. The Imipramine story. In: Ayd FJ, Blackwell, editors. Discoveries in Biological Psychiatry B. Philadelphia, Lippincott,1970; 14-15.

Lange C. Om Periodiske Depression Stilstande og Deres Patogeneses. Copenhagen: Lunds Forlag, 1886.

Lange F. Den Uratiske Sindssygdom. Hospitalstid 1908; SR, 1(4); 73-81; 97-107; 137-50.

Leale CA. Eczema and albuminuria in relation to gout. In: Transactions of the International Medical Congress, Seventh Session, London, 2-9 August 1881.

Leffmann H. Lithia waters as therapeutic agents. Mth. Cyclop. Med. Bull. Philadelphia 1910; 111: 138-44.

Levinson F. Urinsyre-Diathesen, Gigt og Nyregus. Copenhagen: Philipsen, 1893.

Levy E. Essai sur l'action physiologique et therapeutique du bromure de lithium. These, Paris 1874.

Lindheimer JH, Shafer DW. Lithium Treatment for mania. Dis. Nerv. Syst: 1966: 27; 558-60.

Lipowitz A. Versuche und resultate uber die Loslichkeit der Harnsaure. Annalen der Chemie und Pharmacologie. 6th edn. 1841; 38: 348-55.

Locock C. Discussion of a paper by EH Sievking; Analysis of fifty cases of epilepsy observed by the author. Lancet, 1857;1: 527.

Lorry AL. De praecipuis morborum conversionibus. Paris 1789, p.280.

Maudsley H. The Pathology of the Mind. A study of its distempers, deformities and disorders. London, Macmillan, 1895. pp.112-15.

Mitchell SW. On the use of bromide of lithium. Amer. J. Sci. 1870; 60: 443-5.

Noack CH, Trautner EM. The lithium treatment of maniacal psychosis. Med. J. Aust. 1951; 38: 219-22.

Parkinson J. Observations on the nature and cure of gout; on the nodes of the joints; and on the influence of certain disorders of diet in gout, rheumatism and gravel. London: Symonds, 1805.

Pinel P. Traite medico-philosophique sur l'alienation mentale. 2nd Edn. Paris: Brossen, 1809, p.53.

Pontoppidan K. To psykiatriske Afhandlinger. Hosp. Tid. 1895; 38: 1204-10.

Rayner H. Gouty insanity. In: MacComac, editor. Transactions of the International Medical Congress, Seventh Session. London: Kolckmann, 1881, pp. 640-1.

Reines BP. On the locus of medical discovery. J. Med. Phil. 1941;16:183-209.

Reynolds JR. Some affections of the nervous system dependent on a gouty habit. Br. Med. J. 1887; 2: 842-3.

Roberts EL. A case of chronic mania treated with lithium citrate and terminating fatefully. Med. J. Aust. 1950; 37: 261-262.

Roberts RM. Accidental Discoveries in Science New York, John Wiley, 1989.

Roose R. Gout and its relations to diseases of the liver and kidneys 5th. Edn. London, Lewis, 1888.

Scheele FW. Undersokning om blasetenen. Kongl. Vetenskaps-Acad. Handl. 1776; 37: 327-32.

Schioldann J. Did lithium therapy of affective disorders turn up one hundred years ago or (only) fifty? Aust. NZ. J. Psychiatr. 2000; supp: A 60:34.

Schou HJ. La depression psychique. Quelques remarques historiques et pathogeniques. Acta Psychiatr. Neurol. 1927; 345-53.

Schou HJ. Lette og begyndende Sindssygdomne og I Hjemmer. Ugeskr. Laeg 1938; 100: 215-20.

Schou HJ. De saakaldte neuroser og deres Bdehandling Maanedsskr. Pract. Laegegern Soc. Med. 1940;18:153-68.

Schou HJ. Periodiske Depressioner. In: Jorgensen C Sjaelens, editor. Laegebog Copenhagen: Jespersen og Plos Forlag, 1946; 162-9

Schou M. Remarks at Risskov Mental Hospital. Personal communication to Schioldann June 8, 1970.

Schou M. Phases in the development of lithium treatment in psychiatry. In: Sampson F, Adelman G, editors. The Neurosciences: Paths of Discovery II). Boston, Birkhauser 1992; pp. 149-66.

Schou M. in Felber, 1996a; pp x-xi.

Schou M. The development of lithium treatment in psychiatry, 1996b. Unpublished manuscript placed at Schioldann's disposal.

Schou M. Personal communication to Schioldann, 5.21.2005.

Schou M, Juel-Nielsen N, Strömgren E, Voldby H. The treatment of manic psychoses by the administration of lithium salts. J. Neurol. Neurosurg. 1954; 17: 250-60.

Shepherd M. Sherlock Holmes and the Case of Dr. Freud. London, Tavistock. 1985.

Soares JC, Gershon S. The psychopharmacologic specificity of the lithium ion: origins and trajectory. J. Clin. Psychiatr. 2000; 61 (Supp. 9): 16-22.

Sollman T. A Manual of Pharmacology and its Applications in Therapeutics and Toxicology 6th Edn. Philadelphia: Saunders, 1942, 906-7.

Strömgren E. (Events in psychiatric science 1951). Nord. Psyk. Med. lemsbl. 1952; 71.

Sydenham T. Tractus de Podagra et Hydrope. Londmi: Kethilby, 1683. In the English translation of his works published by the Sydenham Society, 1850; 2: 123-84.

Talbott JH. Use of lithium salts as substitutes for sodium chloride. Arch. Int. Med. 1950; 85:1-10.

Trousseau A. Clinique Medicale de l'Hotel-Dieu. Tome deuxieme, 3rd Edn. Paris, Bailleres, 1868.

Ure A. Einfuhrung des Lithions in die Materia medica. Repert. Pharm. 1844; 84: 259-63.

Vaquelin M. Note sure une nouvelle espece d'alcali mineral. Annals de Chime et de Physique, 1817; 2(7): 284-8.

Vestergåard P. Book Review: Schioldann J: The Lange theory of "periodical depressions" etc. Ugeskr Laeg 2001; 163: 70-83.

Watson S, Young AH, Hunter A. The place of lithium salts in psychiatric practice fifty years on. Curr. Opin. Psychiatr. 2001; 14: 57-63.

Whytte R. Observations on the nature, causes and cure of those disorders which have been commonly called nervous hypochondriac or hysteric to which are preferred some remarks on the sympathy of the nerves. Edinburgh, Balfour 1765, p.166.

Williamson B. Psychiatry since lithium. Dis. Nerv. Syst. 1966:27: 775-82.

September 14, 2017

JOHAN SCHIOLDANN'S COMMENTS ON BARRY BLACKWELL'S REVIEW

I read with interest Barry Blackwell's review of my work (Schioldann 2009) at the invitation of Thomas Ban and Samuel Gershon, eight years after its publication!

Blackwell's opinion with respect to Part II of my work (Note 1) reads like I had made claims which are not supported by the available sources which I had collected. My aim was to provide an in-depth systematic historiography with consideration of metabolic disorder, auto-intoxication, uric acid diathesis, and, moreover, the use of lithium salts in a variety of illnesses, to establish, as far as possible, what John Cade had been, or might have been, inspired and influenced by, when from the mid to the late 1930s to 1947-49 he formulated his hypothesis about the pathogenesis of manic-depressive illness and schizophrenia, not dissimilar to what a considerable number of investigators had held.

In his book on the history of psychiatry, Mending the Mind (Cade

1979), published one year before his death in 1980, Cade recounts that what caused manic-depressive psychosis "was anybody's guess up to the mid-1930, [but] by that time there was a certain amount of presumptive evidence favoring a pathophysiological or medical rather than a psychopathological explanation." And, "certainly, manic-depressive patients appeared to me to be sick in the medical sense." This made Cade wonder "what medical conditions appeared to provide some sort of analogy?" In this respect he was guided by the view that "manic patients behave in many ways as if they were intoxicated – noisy, restless, disinhibited and flamboyant." Therefore, he raised the question could it be "that they were in fact intoxicated, perhaps by a normal product of metabolism circulating in excess?" If that was the case, melancholia could be explained as the opposite of this condition. Therefore, "the parallel between manic-depressive illness and thyreotoxicosis/myxoedema seemed an attractive proposition and a promising jumping off point" – his "explanatory hypothesis", as he later termed it (Cade 1978, 1979). Further, "if this hypothesis is accepted as a working basis for investigation, it is evident that the key to the problem lies in the study of the manic patient, who ex hypothesi is producing the intoxicating agent in excess." In fact, "if indeed this is so it is not unlikely that, as with other substances circulating in excess, it is being excreted in the urine and may be demonstrable therein" (Cade 1947).

Cade was acquainted with the famous work of Garrod (1859) which appeared in several revised editions (Garrod 1863, 1876) and also with a number of mainly British medical and psychiatric textbooks and journal articles, which presented the views held by many investigators of the connection between "gouty conditions," nutrition impurities, the presence of some poison in the blood and affective disorders. He was also aware of their treatment with "alkalies," e.g., lithium salts. Of special interest to him other than Garrod's work, were the contributions of Maudsley (1868, 1879, 1895), Mitchell (1870), Hammond (1871), Da Costa (1881) (Note 2), Gray (1886), Lange (1886), Aulde (1887), Clouston (1887, 1904), Haig (1888a,b, 1891,

1892, 1893, 1894, 1895, 1896 1897, 1898, 2000, 1899,1900, 1901, 1902, 1903, 1904, 1905, 1906, 1907), Hibbard (1898), Luff (1897, 1898, 1903, 1907a,b, 1908, 1909), Good (1903), London (1903), Folin (1904-1905, 1924), Bruce (1906, 1908), Squire (1908, 1916), Craig (1917, 1926), Kraepelin (1921), Devine (1921), Gjessing (1938), Price (1937) and Bollinger (1947).

To test his hypothesis, Cade started by injecting urine from manic patients and, in way of control, urine from normal, schizophrenic and melancholic individuals, into the abdominal cavity of guinea pigs (Cade 1947). All the animals died (Cade 1947, 1967, 1978). To test whether the same "toxic agent" was operant, he proceeded to inject the animals with the "end-products" of protein metabolism, the nitrogenous constituents of urine: creatinine, urea and uric acid, and found that urea was the "guilty substance." He continued his search for the "actual toxic agent," querying what substances might have a modifying effect on the toxicity of urea. To this end he injected the animals with urea, uric acid (and creatinine). Uric acid showed "a slightly enhancing effect," not immediately explainable, as "the specimens were more toxic than could be explained by the concentrations of urea actually present even if it were being enhanced maximally by uric acid;" as he had already stated, one would have to postulate an impossible concentration of 8% to 16% of urea. In his belief that the urine from manic patients was more or less more toxic than that from non-manic patients, but not established quantitatively, he finally postulated a third toxic substance, which he thought might be "operative" in neutralizing a protective effect of creatinine or an enhancement of the toxic effect of urea. It is here that lithium enters Cade's animal experiments. At no later time did Cade make any mention of such a substance.

Cade (1949) first mentioned lithium in his paper, Lithium Salts in the Treatment of Psychotic Excitement, where he recounts that

> "in the course of some investigations by the writer into the toxicity of urea when injected intraperitoneally into guinea pigs, it appeared desirable to ascertain whether uric acid enhanced this toxicity', but 'the great difficulty was the

insolubility of uric acid in water, so the most soluble urate was chosen – lithium salts."

Injecting "an aqueous solution of urea 8%, saturated with lithium urate," Cade observed that "the toxicity was far less than expected, the great paradox" (Cade 1967). This solution of saturated lithium urate killed half of the animals tested, so "it looked as if the lithium ion might have been exerting a protective effect." To test this further, he now injected solutions of lithium carbonate, carbonate substituted for urate. All test animals survived. This, he argued, showed "the lithium ion to have a strong protective effect against toxic, lethal effect of urea" (Cade 1949).

Cade's next step was to test "whether lithium salts per se had any discernible effects on guinea pigs." He now injected the animals "with large doses of 0.5% aqueous solutions of lithium carbonate" (Cade 1949):

> "A noteworthy result was that after a latent period of about two hours the animals although fully conscious became extremely lethargic and unresponsive to stimuli for one to two hours before again becoming normally active and timid."

The 1949 paper appears to be the only extant record of Cade's experiments with lithium salts in guinea pigs.

Cade now swiftly transitioned from these rodent animals to a pilot study, prescribing lithium to a cohort of psychotically excited patients, including manic as well as depressed patients. He observed a striking anti-manic effect. Therefore, in this swift transition had he been guided by a prior knowledge of the use of lithium in affective disorders: gouty mania, maniacal symptoms (Garrod 1859), by the "old authors" presumed caused by, but by 1947-1949 long since discredited, uric acid diathesis, and not revealed by him? Or was he guided by other reasons? Why has Cade's "story of lithium" remained so enigmatic? Can the puzzle be solved? Was it an expected or unexpected discovery, to him, to us historians? Sheer luck? Serendipity? Cade, for his part, maintained that it was the inevitable outcome of the testing of his hypothesis (Cade

1949, 1970, 1975, 1979) whereas, subsequently, first Gershon (1968) and most authors after him have argued that his discovery is serendipitous, among them Blackwell (1972), who now considers it to be both serendipitous and deductive (Blackwell 2017).

The only extant source that can shed sharper light on Cade's swift transitioning and choice of lithium is found in his case card regarding his first lithium patient, W.B. But this opinion does not appear to be shared by Blackwell, who writes:

"The final piece of tendentious deductive reasoning was derived from the case card of Cade's first patient with mania which records the prescription of lithium with the added comment that he had 'an extremely high blood uric acid.' The author states, 'This case card is highly indicative of the fact, if not proof, that Cade was fully acquainted with the views of his scientific forbears [sic] of a presumed connection between mania (gouty mania) and uric acid,' a belief never expressed in any of Cade's writings about his discovery and totally inconsistent with the views about lithium [Cade] expressed before.'"

Blackwell had already presented a brief summary of Cade's papers with which he intends to document that, in fact, Cade had never expressed a belief of a presumed connection between gouty mania and uric acid and, moreover, that this was totally inconsistent with the views Cade had expressed about lithium:

In his 1949 paper, Cade's only reference to earlier medical use of lithium was in gout when he mentions Garrod's text (Garrod, 1859). About gout's many "manifestations," he makes no reference to depression or mania mentioned by earlier authors. His conclusion about the historical use [of] lithium was unequivocal: "…the uselessness of lithium in most of the conditions for which it was prescribed, and the fact there was other, more efficacious, treatment in the only disease in which it [had] been shown to be of some value, [and so] it is not surprising that lithium salts have fallen into desuetude." Long after his own discovery he was able to write: "So the introduction of the lithium ion into medicine was all a silly mistake. It was perfectly useless for the conditions for which it was prescribed" (Cade, 1978) [sic Cade 1977]. He did, however, note that, "The water[s] of certain wells were considered to have special virtue in the treatment of mental illness…it is very likely that their supposed efficacy was a real efficacy and directly proportional to the lithium content of the waters."

In other words, Blackwell accepts Cade's statements at face value as correct and sufficient, at the latest in 1949, but reiterated by Cade, for instance, in his 1977 paper (with some modification in his 1978 paper), finally followed by, as if in way of some concession, but Blackwell failed to provide author, title and when first published: "The water[s] of certain wells […] it is very likely…" etc., etc. Cade had first paraphrased and commented on the wells in his 1949 paper, its provenance: Henderson and Gillespie's Textbook of Psychiatry, published in 1944 and not included in Blackwell's literature list. However, "it is very likely that their supposed efficacy…" etc., etc., was Cade's comment, thus Cade contradicting himself in the same 1949 paper!

My critical analysis of the source materials to which Cade refers in his 1947 and 1949 papers (Schioldann 2009) drew no comment from Blackwell, nor are the authors and/or publications concerning this period of time (nor most of the prior ones) included in his list of references, except Garrod's work, of which he includes the second edition, 1863, not the 1859 edition. Especially, Blackwell does not seem to think that it begs the question why Cade, in his paraphrasing of Garrod (1859), does not mention gouty mania and maniacal symptoms and their association with uric acid diathesis and consequent treatment with lithium salts.

In Sam Gershon's (1968) opinion, "the introduction of lithium […] would seem to have been quite serendipitous, as we do not have any significant basis for its reinvestigation," and with Soares (2000) he noted: "Looking at the origin of this story we find a fortuitous is path is traveled." Further, Gershon (2000, 1971; Gershon and Daversa 2006) argued that one cannot extrapolate from lithium dosages in animal studies to dosages in humans. Mogens Schou (1992, 1996, 1998, 1999, 2001), for his part, found Cade's work "indeed strange – the hypothesis which started his work was crude. His experimental design was not particularly clear. And his interpretation of the animal data may have been wrong." Also, Schou's attempts to replicate them failed. And critically he asked, "why would a compound counteracting the effect of intraperitoneal urea be of psychiatric interest?"

In accordance with these "expert" opinions, I concluded that Cade's observations cannot be considered to be documentation of scientific fact. Did Cade, therefore, have knowledge that he did not reveal, that made his hypothesis and the outcome of his subsequent clinical not so unlikely? – a question also posed by Neil Johnson (1984; Schioldann 2009). In other words, did Cade have knowledge of the claims of, and was he influenced by, the "old authors" as to a possible therapeutic effect of lithium in a variety of conditions comprising mental disorders, e.g., "gouty mania," "maniacal symptoms," to be caused by the uric acid diathesis, as mentioned before? Further, I argued that Cade cannot not have acquired a broad knowledge of the literature on the relevant subjects (Note 3) and that this broad knowledge would have underpinned his work. Furthermore, that rather than based on erroneous, irreproducible observations in guinea pigs, he made an inductive leap in medias res, with prior knowledge into the undertaking of a pilot study of lithium in psychotically excited patients but **precipitated** or **sparked** by his observations recorded in the W.B case card (Schioldann 2009):

> "Date: 6/3/48. – Time: 12.15pm. – Test: Blood uric acid. – Result: 17.5 mg/%. – Mental State: Chronic mania. This extremely high blood uric acid result is suspect. – 18/3/48 – Blood creatinine 2.4 mg/% - 13/4/48. [Blood creatinine] 2.0 mg/% - [Same day, WB] Has been on large doses of lithium citrate for a fortnight."

Re-Evaluation

Knowledge of the relevant literature, presented in my book, can leave no doubt that W.B.'s case card has all the fingerprints of the old, but erroneous and thus long since discarded concept of uric acid diathesis and its treatment with lithium salts in mental disorders, e.g. 'gouty mania', 'maniacal symptoms' (Garrod 1859), erroneously then assumed and consistently with this I concluded:

> "This case card is highly indicative of the fact, if not proof, that Cade was fully acquainted with the views of his scientific forebears of a presumed connection between mania (gouty mania) and uric acid" (Note 4).

The epithet suspect is the pivot that provides the final evidential weight in this "clinical equation" that the card contains, but which, for some reason, escaped proper attention by Blackwell. Not only the fact that he misquotes and misinterprets the card, but on wrong premises he resorts to cast serious blemish on my work – "the final piece of tendentious reasoning"! In fact, I put it that the W. B. card is the centerpiece or master card along Cade's trajectory that holds the key with which to unlock Cade's enigmatic story. Further, I argued that it was between 6th and 29th March that Cade had self-administered (Note 5) lithium in order to ascertain the right dosage to prescribe from various pharmacopoeias and other published sources.

Cade resurrected the uric acid diathesis (Note 7), though only briefly (Note 8). His discovery, or finding, was not accidental, as he himself persistently claimed: "the inevitable though unforeseen product of a hypothesis and of a series of experiments to test that hypothesis," and thus, in his opinion, not serendipitous. I agree with Cade, but for another obvious reason: Cade had traveled a path or overlapping paths, erroneously though, with a paradoxical outcome, but which, for some reason, he did not reveal or acknowledge. Although consistent with this, his premises erroneous, Cade, retracing the "old authors" (some of whom had observed therapeutic effect of lithium in mental disorders), arguably his seminal (re)discovery was not an unexpected, fortuitous, thus serendipitous outcome, as mentioned before and lastly by Blackwell (2017), but perhaps more fittingly describable as pseudoserendipitous, a derivative term of Walpole's. By the same token, I must refute Blackwell's absurd claim that "In the second part of John [sic] Schioldann's book we can see how Cade's Hero status is preserved and protected" in that "the voluminous database [sic] is somewhat subjectively and selectively mined to favor Cade and Schou's view that the discovery of lithium was not serendipitous [...]."

In this respect, Schou's opinion (1977, 1982, 1984) could appear equivocal, but he did hold an extended opinion of Walpole's concept (Note 9). All other things being equal, a couple of months before Schou died, in September 2005, when I was in the final stages of my studies on Cade's "story of lithium," which he read, and due to Cade's curious change of subject: from the background for his discovery in 1949 to strontium – to be presented at a lecture at Risskov in 1970 – I queried with Schou, whom I knew well and became friends with, whether he thought that Cade did know about the past, i.e., the old authors and lithium therapy. He replied (2005):

> "I have now perused all the approx. 40 letters Cade and I exchanged between 1963 and 1978 [and also perused by me] [...] I did not hide my admiration and gratitude for the contribution he made with the 1949 article. At no time have I had any skepticism towards his work. I do not know whether there was something behind Cade's choice of lecture when he was at Risskov. I had exhorted him to give an account of the background for his discovery of lithium's antimanic effect, however, against all expectations he spoke about his investigations with strontium. On the basis of your work it could be that he was concerned that I as biochemically and physiologically more knowledgeable was going to ask him delicate questions. This thought never occurred to me. I believed his [1949] account blindly, although I had difficulty in following his logic."

Schou's reply certainly adds support to my interpretation of Cade's "story."

Blackwell, in no uncertain terms, rules out any influence on Cade by "the early Danish work decades earlier," i.e., that of Carl Lange (1834-1900), namely his work on "periodical depression and uric acid diathesis" and its treatment with lithium (Schioldann 2001, 2009, 2011). It was not well received by contemporary psychiatry, either at home or abroad, due to his apparently rigid distinction between melancholy and depression and the fact that he had not been aware of the hypomanic/manic phases (Note 10) – not to mention his associating depression with the disreputed uric acid diathesis, hence the treatment with lithium salts. It was given its final coup de grace in 1927 by no less than Kraepelin, referred to by Blackwell (Note 11).

Given his research interests into manic-depressive illness and schizophrenia ("dementia praecox"), Cade would have read Kraepelin's work, at least in English: Manic-Depressive Insanity And Paranoia (1921), which describes, in overview, some of the topics of interest and relevance to Cade's own hypothesis about manic–depressive illness, and in addition Kraepelin's dismissive comments on Lange's depression thesis:

> "Lange has arrived at the opinion, that increased formation of uric acid may be regarded as the essential cause of states of depression"; "Lange has assumed as the foundation of periodic depressive states with psychic inhibition, which indubitably belong to the domain of the malady ['manic-depressive insanity'] here described, a gouty mode of development, a view which, however, till now cannot be regarded as proved or even as probable."

Blackwell mentions Kraepelin's dismissal of Lange's work in general, but not in any context with Cade, and he was possibly influenced by the opinion espoused by Callahan and Berrios (2005), who did not refer to Kraepelin:

> "Although unknown to him, Cade was retracing the steps of a Danish [neuropathologist], Carl Lange, who had reached the same conclusions 50 years earlier and who had

successfully given lithium to patients with affective disorders. Locked in the Danish language, Lange's work was not available to Cade. This caused an incorrect history of the 'discovery' of lithium treatment that historians are finding difficult to resolve."

Cade's reading of Kraepelin's 1921 edition would have informed him that Lange's depression thesis (1886) had been translated into German by Kurella (1896). But even if he had been sufficiently proficient in German, it would not have been available to him (it is not contained in "Libraries Australia Database"), so it would have remained "locked" in both Danish and German, but he would surely have become aware of the gist of it from Kraepelin's text and thus also linking him in with the "old authors" on the subject, including, as mentioned before, various hypotheses concerning the pathogenesis of manic-depressive illness:

> "[…] in manic-depressive insanity marked disorders of metabolism must take place"; "the endogenous excretion of uric acid […] remains in depressive patients at the lower limits of the normal, whereas in manics it is reduced", querying "abnormally rapid breaking down of the purin bodies to still lower stages of disintegration"; "periodic neurasthenia which certainly belongs to manic-depressive insanity [with] diminution of uric acid excretion at the time of moodiness"; "intoxication by metabolic products of intestinal bacteria"; "insufficiency of thyroid gland activity"; "the relations between Basedow's disease and manic-depressive morbid phenomena and […] auto-intoxication by glandular products"; "the remarkable changes of state often beginning so suddenly [in the form of] the clinical pictures recalling many intoxications (alcohol, products of fatigue)"; "internal poisons."

Cade might also have been acquainted with Carl Lange's thesis via the work of Haig (1891, 1900), who after Garrod was "a leading authority on uric acid." He not only mentions the work, but they had also corresponded about it. For that matter, the German edition of Lange's thesis was reviewed in "Journal of Mental Science" in 1897.

It is not correct, as Blackwell opines, that according to my work both Strömgren and Schou "disavowed" any influence of the Lange brothers in their decision to study lithium. In his letter to Neil Johnson (Johnson 1984), Strömgren would not rule out

> "the old Danish lithium treatment may have prepared me unconsciously and made me sensitive to any new information concerning lithium." But "to the conscious parts of my brain, however, it looks as if I was convinced by the first report from Australia that here was really a thing to be taken seriously" (Note 12).

In an interview of Strömgren by Schou in 1986 (Schioldann 2002), Schou put it to him: "It was surely Trautner's work you read first, and then later Cade's, and then you showed them to me." "Yes," Strömgren replied. Schou, for his part, denied any knowledge of Lange's work initially, although one would find it hard to believe, had Strömgren not mentioned it to him, and he was adamant that he had never discussed lithium with his father, H. I. Schou, who died in the spring of 1952.

Blackwell again claims, more indirectly though, that in my book "Cade's Hero status is preserved and protected," Blackwell arguing that my failure to mention some blemishes in Cade's story "does serve the purpose of embellishing a perfect Hero image": 1) "why did John Cade never speak of the work of Noack, Gershon and Trautner" (1951), "which made lithium safe to use" – "perhaps the greatest enigma of them all"; 2) "doubts about Cade's ban on lithium"; and 3) "concealment of his first patient's death due to lithium toxicity."

I was not driven by any wish to protect or embellish "a perfect Hero image." Interestingly, several of my Australian colleagues expressed their worry that my writing about Cade's "story of lithium" would dent his reputation. As one of them said, remarkably: "You are cutting down one of our tall poppies." I simply riposted: "I am an historian." The issues raised by Blackwell are recounted in my book, including the

Cade-Trautner-Noack-Gershon question; a complete picture cannot be established on the available sources. However, Gershon recounted that Trautner and himself were never asked to present their data in Australia, "only overseas where there was great interest" (Gershon, 2007). Trautner (1954) wrote to Schou: "We are very glad to see, that you were able to confirm our results, particularly in view of a lot of opposition we meet" and the following year (Trautner, 1955): "During the first trials of lithium quite a few incidents occurred. Clinicians discarded the drug as unpredictable."

In 1974 Schou met up with Gershon in New York and they discussed how it all began, including Trautner's great contribution, reiterated by Schou directly to Trautner (1974):

> "I still remember clearly the correspondence we had in the early fifties […] Much has happened to lithium since then, but we are still taking advantage of your contributions. I hope it gives you pleasure to think back on that work."

But, understandably, Trautner not so pleased, replied (1975):

> "It seems that lithium therapy gets slowly accepted, anyway some doctors [not named by Trautner] who violently opposed its use on humans, now scramble to get a share of the credit of its introduction [sic]."

After the death of W.B. in 1950, Cade banned the use of lithium in his own hospital. However, many Australian psychiatrists continued to prescribe lithium, some of them heeding Noack's and Trautner's 1951 report about serum monitoring of lithium, making the treatment safe, others not, e.g., Ashburner (1981) and Glesinger (1954), who found that serum monitoring was not required, leaving this to the academic departments. Intriguingly, although everybody knew about it, Cade remained uncommunicative about W.B.'s cause of death. I refrained from offering any deliberation of possible underlying personal motives, or for that matter, grudges Cade might have harbored, or regarding his manner, style, cognitive or personality-wise, as Blackwell sees fit to do.

Unfortunately, I could not shed any light on whether Trautner, the physiologist (Johnson 1984, Schioldann 2009), and Cade had met at any stage before or during his lithium experiments on guinea pigs, i.e., 1947-1948, and/or whether Trautner himself might have undertaken such or other studies. According to a personal communication to Johnson from D. Wright (1981), Head of the Howard Florey Institute of Experimental Physiology and Medicine, where Trautner worked, he was carrying out investigations on "nervous tissue metabolism" (Johnson 1984).

Blackwell claims that my "assessment of the importance of Cade's discovery of lithium in 1949 and its impact on the early development of psychopharmacology tilts strongly in a positive direction in a manner not supported by the data":

> "It was in 1963 that Schou first wrote to Cade informing him of an interest in prophylaxis […] It is from this point on that Cade's interest in lithium was vigorously renewed and from this point forward that comments begin to appear in the literature about the positive influence of events in 1949 on the entire history of the field. The flood of positive attributions stems largely from authors with a special interest in lithium, writing 20-30 years after Cade's discovery and at a time when innovation in the field had slowed to a crawl. - Cade's discovery of lithium's value in mania is combined and conflated with Schou's later discovery of serendipity [sic] to claim that this body of work formed a foundation for the whole of psychopharmacology as a discipline, an assumption not supported by close scrutiny of the relevant literature."

I find Blackwell's opinion one-sided and prejudiced, if not polemical, but of course difficult to disentangle, not least for the reason that Blackwell has himself, as he puts it emphatically, "played a personal and significant role in the controversies swirling around lithium."

With Schou's placebo-controlled double-blind trial (together with Strömgren, N. Juel-Nielsen and H. Voldby) in 1954, the anti-manic effect of lithium became evidence-based. It was in 1963 Schou first wrote to Cade that his 1949 publication had "[…] meant a good deal to my professional life." He also wanted to inform him of his attendance at the Third Conference of the Collegium Internationale Neuropsychopharmacologium (CINP) in Munich 1962, where he had emphasized that "the new era of psychopharmacology did not start in 1952 with reserpine and chlorpromazine, but in 1949 with your discovery of the effect of lithium."

During the 1960s Schou indefatigably agitated internationally for the introduction of lithium in the treatment of mania – an uphill battle – assisted in this endeavor by Alec Coppen, Nathan Kline and Sam Gershon. By 1964, independently of one another, Hartigan (1963), Baastrup (1964) and Schou had made sporadic observations which were suggestive of lithium also having prophylactic properties in manic-depressive illness. Subsequently, Baastrup and Schou tested this in a non-blind, systematic lithium trial. Obviously, it was not in 1963, as Blackwell recounted, that Schou first wrote to Cade "informing him of an interest in prophylaxis" (Blackwell's wording); it was three years later, on 19 July 1966, to be exact, that Schou expressed himself in very different, exuberant terms – he had attached a copy of the manuscript to be published the following year (Baastrup and Schou 1967):

> "It is indeed a most interesting drug you have introduced into psychiatry. The more I learn about it, the more am I intrigued by it, and I should not be astonished if studies based on the observations with lithium would eventually lead to a real break-through in the control of manic-depressive psychosis."

Cade replied, two weeks later:

> "What is most impressive is your demonstration that lithium is so effective in preventing relapses of depressive as well as manic phases. This was something about which I had never been sure until I read your paper."

Finally, Cade felt vindicated, attested to by his editorial to the inaugural issue of "The Australian and New Zealand Journal of

Psychiatry," 1967, entitled Lithium in psychiatry: historical origins and present position.

The 1967 paper, a non-blind systematic study by Baastrup and Schou, "Lithium as a prophylactic agent. Its effect against recurrent depressions and manic-depressive psychosis," sparked fierce controversy, the infamous Battle of Lithium (Schioldann, 2006, 2009), waged in the international medical press, 1968-1972, and spearheaded by Shepherd and Blackwell, for and against "the beleaguered Danes." Shepherd and Blackwell (1968), labeled the claims of the prophylactic efficacy "another therapeutic myth" based on "serious methodological shortcomings" and "spurious claims." The ethical issue weighed heavily on Schou and Baastrup, conscious that to deprive their patients of lithium prophylactic therapy would expose those with depression to increased safety risk and thus, in accordance with the Helsinki Declaration, be ethically indefensible (Schioldann 2006). As Schou wrote (Schioldann 2009), "the controversy created uncertainty among British and American psychiatrists, and they hesitated to start prophylactic lithium treatment." However, after painful consideration of the ethical dilemma, in 1970 Baastrup, Schou, Amdisen, Thomsen and Poulsen published a prospective-discontinuation double blind design trial: "Prophylactic lithium: double blind discontinuation in manic-depressive and recurrent depressive disorders." Considered "unparalleled in psychiatry" (Grof 1998), they reaffirmed lithium's prophylactic efficacy; their findings were supported by concurrent works from Ireland, England and North America, using open, discontinuation and prospective trial designs (Schioldann 2009). Thus, not only did prophylactic lithium become evidence-based, lithium was to become the first-choice mood stabilizer in manic-depressive illness.

Shepherd did not comment on the trial directly, whereas Blackwell (1970) opined that it had "methodological inadequacies thus rendering the evidence unreliable"; Shepherd (1970-71), in "A prophylactic myth" even used terms such as unethical and unscientific. Deplorably, the controversy was to assume ad hominem proportions, leaving bad memories, if not scars (Schioldann 1999). It has been recounted by

Johnson (1984) and by David Healy (2008), and in some detail by Schou himself in his My journey with lithium (Schioldann 2009), but not commented on by Blackwell in his review. It was 20 years later that Goodwin and Jamison (1990), world authorities on manic-depressive illness, hailed this trail-blazing discovery of lithium prophylaxis as "one of the most important advances in modern psychiatry."

In the wake of the battle of lithium, in 1984 Felix Post (Wilkinson 1993) related that to Aubrey Lewis and Shepherd lithium was "dangerous nonsense" (Note 13). Further, Strömgren (1992; Schioldann 1999) had queried Shepherd, whom he knew well (Shepherd 1982), why the controversy against lithium prophylaxis had been continued. In the words of Strömgren, Shepherd had "quite openly" replied that it was:

> "simply due to the fact that English psychiatry under the reign of Aubrey Lewis did not distinguish between psychogenic and endogenous depression (Schioldann 2003) (Note 14) and if lithium were to be recommended against depression, all doctors in England would use it against all types of depression, with the result that many patients not in need of it would only suffer damage from it – therefore lithium must be ravaged with fire and sword."

In the interview of Strömgren by Schou in 1986 (Schioldann 2002), Schou asked him this delicate question: "Why do you believe that there was so much hesitation towards lithium both internationally, but also here in this hospital [Risskov]?" Strömgren's reply was unequivocal:

> "Yes, in the course of time, one has seen many drug trials give promising results, only afterwards to show that after all it was nothing. So the general skepticism had to be overcome, and there were also then people, as there always are, who meant that it was never a solution to prescribe medication to the patients. There were several of the influential colleagues who meant that this was not the avenue, and therefore they were not interested in carrying

out such a treatment in systematic manner, and which they probably thought sooner or later might be abandoned and perhaps had some side-effects of which the patients should be spared. So, obviously, it took thumb-thick ["tommetykke"] proofs before it became clear to all and sundry that lithium was an essential plus in our armamentarium."

Indubitably, Strömgren is referring to the Lewis-Shepherd-Blackwell prohibitive edict against prophylactic lithium. However, now 45 years on, with Blackwell's statements included in de Moore's and Westmore's (2016) interesting book on Cade and his discovery in 1949, the controversial prophylactic issue can finally be laid to rest. Blackwell to the authors: "It turned out that we were wrong. Lithium was really the start of a revolution in psychiatry." Blackwell must be lauded for placing this on the historical record!

This historical correction also addresses Blackwell's last concern in his review whether lithium has formed "a foundation for the whole of psychopharmacology as a discipline," an assumption, he emphasizes, that was "not supported by close scrutiny of the relevant literature."

Most succinctly it has been expressed by Gershon (Schioldann, 2009), who has played a leading role in the lithium "travelog" right from the start in the early 1950s until the present day: "The introduction of lithium in 1949 makes it the first agent in the modern era of psychopharmacology, in that it preceded the introduction of chlorpromazine and reserpine" and with Daversa (Gershon and Daversa 2006) he wrote: "Lithium sparked a psychopharmacological revolution in psychiatry, or could be considered to be the breeder core."

Notes:

1. Blackwell: "A distinction is made between the first and second parts of the book. The massive database of lithium's pre-1949 history [Part I] is impressive and valuable to all clinicians and research workers interested in lithium. I have only one caveat to assert that

however compelling it might be, there is not a shred of evidence, real or circumstantial, from his own or the writings of others, that John Cade knew anything about that"; "despite the total lack of evidence in Cade's own writings that he knew of lithium's prior use in affective disorders, the author advances slender evidence that it might have been otherwise"; "another slender thread in the rumor mill was […]"; "the final piece of tendentious deductive reasoning was derived from the case card of Cade's first patient with mania […]."

2. Da Costa (1888) is the first author that I was able to retrieve in the medical literature where a lithium salt (the citrate) other than lithium bromide (Mitchell 1870; Hammond 1871) was used to relieve or "remove" exclusively nervous symptoms. Intriguingly, it would appear that Da Costa thought that the remedies should be taken on a more or less permanent basis, for "until the state is permanently remedied," the nervous symptoms "may appear for years."

3. Detailed reading lists of the requirements in the course of Diploma of Psychological Medicine and for the examination for the degree of Doctor of Medicine: The Melbourne University Calendar 1938 (Schioldann 2009).

4. Neil Johnson (1984): "This observation is interesting in the light of the uric acid diathesis which had held sway in medicine prior to this [1948]."

5. Chiu E. and Hegarty RM. (1999): Cade took "lithium carbonate for 2 weeks to test whether it was toxic or had unpleasant side-effect," and they recounted that his wife, Jean, recalled that "I looked at him the next day, and the weeks that followed and wondered what I would do if he was changed by the lithium."

6. Cade FN. (1970, 1978). "The original therapeutic dose, decided on fortuitously, proved to be the optimum, that is 1.200 mg of the citrate thrice daily or 600 mg of the carbonate."

7. Cade did not use the term or concept of uric acid diathesis in his single-author articles, but in his paper with Neil Johnson (1975), where they made reference to "four papers by [Carl] Lange,

published in 1897, in which the use of lithium salts in the treatment of 'uric acid diathesis' was described: this condition apparently involved both gout and mental depression and some improvement was noted in the latter."

8. A relative of Cade's lithium patient, R.T. had written to him asking whether a poison in the blood could be established as the underlying cause and thus some form of treatment. Cade replied: "Please let me reassure you on several points that [R.T.'s] mental condition is not due to 'poison in the blood' so that no treatment directed to neutralize such a poison would be of the slightest use" (Schioldann 2009).

9. Schou M. Correspondence with G. Kaufmann (1984), who also characterized Cade's discovery as serendipitous. Schou's reply: "It is not quite clear to me what you mean by 'serendipity' […] John Cade himself disliked that word, and I agree with him if it is used with the meaning 'fortuitous' or 'random.' I believe that discoveries often are made if an observation meets the prepared mind, and fortuitous circumstances may decide this, but other factors are at work to decide when a mind is prepared and when the time for the making the relevant observations and drawing the relevant conclusions is ripe."

10. Lange himself was not convinced that "uric acid diathesis" was the cause of periodical depression. In his classic work: Om Sindsbevægelser. Et Psyko-Fysiologisk Studie (1885, On Emotions. A Psycho-Physiological Study, 1922) (cf. The James-Lange theory of emotions), he had virtually formulated alternating periods of mania (as an illness of mood) and depression as a nosological entity, 14 years before Kraepelin (1899) formulated the concept das manisch-depressive Irresein (manic-depressive insanity), Lange commenting that "every psychiatrist knows the strongly developed forms which occur as 'melancholia' or 'mania." He emphasized that "the study of 'the emotional illnesses' becomes particularly important […] once it has become more systematized than hitherto has been the case." It was the following year, in 1886, he presented

just such a study of "the emotional illnesses," namely his depression pamphlet! (Schioldann 2009; Lange and Schioldann 2011).

11. Blackwell (1985): "Much is made of earlier hints that vague mental symptoms associated with uric acid diathesis might benefit from lithium." "Of more compelling interest is that the Danish internist, Carl Lange, published a monograph in 1886 Concerning Periodic Depression and its Pathogenesis which included the use of a lithium-containing mixture for preventative treatment." Blackwell made reference to Schou's father, H. I. Schou, for having denied Lange's claims for lithium (based on Amdi Amdisen's reading of Lange). This is not correct. What he did was to discard the uric acid diathesis as spurious. Had he been as curious, as was Cade, he might have undertaken a pilot study similar to what Cade was to do. Kraepelin had dismissed it in several editions of his work, last in 1927. Co-incidentally, it was the same year that it was resurrected by H. I. Schou due to its nosographical and nosological views. (Schioldann 2001, 2009; Lange and Schioldann 2011).

12. In the same letter, Strömgren wrote that he found it "extremely fascinating if lithium salts which are chemically so simple could have a therapeutic effect in psychiatry, especially so if they were active against just one disease, which could tell us much more about that disease than lots of information concerning the therapeutic effects of complicated compounds which had no clear preference with regard to the different disorders they were used for. This was the reason why I asked my brilliant younger colleague Mogens Schou to devote himself to lithium studies." In Schou's interview of Strömgren in 1986 (Schioldann 2002), he recounted that he had always thought that the biological genesis of the manic-depressive psychosis was relatively simple, and given the illness's ability to swing momentarily, perhaps it was caused by equally simple electrolyte mechanisms, and perhaps analogous to the interaction of electrolyte and hormones, as for instance had been shown by the Zondek brothers (Hermann and Bernhard) and which subject he years earlier had considered for his doctoral thesis. And therefore,

he said: "It came like a revelation to me when I first heard about lithium," this being a simple "chemical element."

13. Felix Post: "[Aubrey Lewis] was a therapeutic nihilist. He didn't believe much in treatment, and it is true, that in those days, treatments were not terribly effective. He was not enamored of ECT and certainly not insulin coma. Lithium he, Shepherd too, thought dangerous nonsense."

14. Since his MD thesis (A clinical and historical survey of depressive states based on the study of sixty-one cases. [ibid. 'Reaction, psychogenesis', pp. 301-316]. University of Adelaide, 1931), Lewis held firm opinions about the dichotomy: endogenous and exogenous (1971), and in 1972, in scathing manner, he advocated for the relegation of the concept 'psychogenic', among whose 'orthodox believers' he grouped Wimmer, Strömgren and Faergeman, thus ultimately Wimmer's concept of psychogenic psychosis (Schioldann 1996, 2003). Lewis died in 1975.

References:

Ashburner JV. Personal communication to Neil Johnson, 15.6.81 (Johnson, 1984, p. 63).

Aulde J. The use of lithium bromide in combination with solution of potassium citrate. Med. Bull. 1887;9:35-39, 69-72.

Baastrup PC. The use of lithium in manic-depressive psychosis. Compr. Psychiatr. 1964;5:396-408.

Baastrup PC, Schou M. Lithium as a prophylactic agent. Its effect against recurrent depression and manic-depressive psychosis. Arch. Gen. Psychiatr. 1967;16:162-72.

Baastrup PC, Poulsen JC, Schou M, Thomsen K, Amdisen A. Schou M. Prophylactic lithium: double-blind discontinuation in manic-depressive and recurrent depressive disorders. Lancet 1970;ii:326-30.

Blackwell B, Shepherd M. Prophylactic lithium: another therapeutic myth? An examination of the evidence to date. Lancet 1968;i:968-71.

Blackwell B. Lithium. Lancet 1970;ii:875.

Blackwell B. Prophylactic lithium: science or science fiction. Am. Heart. J. 1972;83:139-41.

Blackwell B. Book Review: Johnson FN. The History of Lithium Therapy. London. Macmillan Press. 1984. Psychol. Med. 1985;15:695-697.

Blackwell B. Book Review: Schioldan J. 2009. INHN, 2017.

Bollinger A. Recent observations on uric aid. Med. J. Aust. 1947;1:394-5. (B. mentions Otto Folin, vide infra).

Bruce LC. Studies in Clinical Psychiatry. London. Macmillan, 1906, pp. 35-36, 47, 64, 71, 102, 112, 220, 223, 231.

Bruce LC. The symptoms and etiology of mania. The Morrison Lectures 1908. J. Ment. Sci. 1908;54:207-64.

Cade JF. The anticonvulsant properties of creatinine. Med. J. Aust. 1947;2:621-3.

Cade JF. Lithium salts in the treatment of psychotic excitement. Med. J. Aust. 1949;2:349-52.

Cade JF. Lithium in psychiatry: historical origins and present position. Editorial. Aust. NZ. J. Psychiatr. 1967;1:61-2.

Cade JF. The story of lithium. In Discoveries in Biological Psychiatry (eds.) Ayd FJ, Blackwell B. Philadelphia, Lippincott, 1970, pp. 218-229.

Cade JF. Lithium – past, present, future. In: Johnson FN, Johnson S, editors. Lancaster Lithium in Medical Practice. MTP Press, 1978, pp 15-16.

Cade JF. Mending the Mind: A Short History of Twentieth Century

Psychiatry. Melbourne. Sun Books, 1979, pp 65-74.

Chiu E, Hegarty RM. John Cade: the man. Aust. NZ. J. Psychiatr. 1999;33 (Suppl): pp. 24-6.

Clouston TS. Clinical Lectures on Mental Diseases. 2nd Edn. London. Churchill. 1887. pp. 463-5.

Clouston TS. Clinical Lectures on Mental Diseases. 6nd Edn. London. Churchill. 1904. pp. 506-7.

Craig M. Psychological Medicine. London. Churchill, 1917 pp. 28, 87, 110, 328-329.

Craig M, Beaton T. Psychological Medicine. London. Churchill. 1926 (recommended reading for MD candidates at University of Melbourne in 1938).

Da Costa JM. The nervous symptoms of lithiaemia. Am. J. Med. Sci. 1881;144(Oct.):313-30. (p. 325! cf. Schioldann, 2009. pp. 30-3).

de Moore G, Westmore A. Finding Sanity. John Cade

, lithium and the taming of bipolar disorder. Australia. Allen & Unwinn. 2016. p. 256.

Devine H. Recent Advances in Psychiatry. London. Churchill. 1929.

Folin O. Some metabolism studies with special reference to mental disorders. Am. J. Insan. 1904-1905;60:699-732; 61:299-364.

Folin O, Berglund H, Derick C. The uric acid problem. An experimental study on animals and man, including gouty subjects. J. Biol. Chem. 1924;60:361-471. (An extensive review of uric acid is included).

Garrod AB. The Nature and Treatment of Gout. London. Walton & Maberly, 1859, pp. 438, 506, 517, 520-522. (2. ed. 1863; 3. ed. 1876).

Gershon S. The possible thymoleptic effect of the lithium ion. Am. J. Psychiatr. 1968;124:1452-6.

Gershon S. Personal communication. March 13, 2000.

Gershon S. Methodology for drug evaluation in affective disorders: mania. In: Levine J, Schiele BC, Bouthilet L, editors. Principles and problems in establishing the efficacy of psychotropic agents. Am. Coll. Neuropsychopharm. 1971. pp. 123-35.

Gershon S, Daversa C. The lithium story: a journey from obscurity to popular use in North America. In: Bauer M, Grof P, Müller-Oerlinghausen B, editors. Lithium in neuropsychiatry. The comprehensive guide. Abingdon, Oxon. Inform, 2006, pp. 17-24.

Gershon S. Personal communications. May 22 & 29 2007.

Gjessing R. Disturbances of somatic functions in catatonia with a periodic course, and their compensation. J. Ment. Sci. 1938;84:608-25.

Glesinger B. Evaluation of lithium in treatment of psychotic excitement. Med. J. Austr. 1954;1:277-83.

Good CA. An experimental study of lithium. Am. J. Med. Sci. 1903;125:273-84.

Goodwin F, Jamison KJ. Manic-depressive Illness. Oxford University Press. 1990.

Gray LC. The nervous symptoms of so-called lithaemia. N. Y. Med. J. 1886;57-60, 91-95.

Grof P. Has the effectiveness of lithium changed? Neuropsychopharmacol. 1998;19:183-8.

Haig A. Mental depression and the excretion of uric acid. Practitioner 1888;41:342-54.

Haig A. Effects in health and disease of some drugs which cause retention of uric acid, in contrast with the action of salicylates, as shown in a previous paper. Med. Chir. Transact. 1888;71:283-95

Haig A. Uric acid in diseases of the nervous system. Brain 1891;14:63-98. [H. mentions Carl Lange's work, pp. 74, 91].

Haig A. Uric Acid as a Factor in the Causation of Disease. A Contribution to the Pathology of High Arterial Tension, Headache, Epilepsy, Mental Depression, Gout, Rheumatism, Diabetes, Bright's, and other Disorders. Edition 1-6. London. Churchill 1892-1907 (e.g. 1894, p. 146; 1900, p. 287). [H. mentions Carl Lange's work, p. 287].

Haig A. The causation, prevention, and treatment of gout. Practitioner 1903;July:40-60.

Hammond, WA. Treatise on diseases of the nervous system. New York. Appleton. 1871. pp. 358-366 ('mania), pp. 380-381 ('treatment'). (cf. Schioldann, 2009. pp. 29-30).

Hartigan GP. The use of lithium salts in affective disorders. Br. J. Psychiatr. 1963;109:810-14.

Healy D. Mania. A Short History of Bipolar Disorder. John Hopkins University Press. 2008. pp. 115-127.

Henderson Dk, Gillespie RD. A Text-Book of Psychiatry for Students and Practitioners. 6th ed. Oxford University Press, 1944, p. 3.

Hibbard CM. A study of the secretion of urea and uric acid in melancholia and in a case presenting recurrent periods of confusion and depression. Am. J. Insan. 1898;April:503-531.

Johnson FN, Cade JF. The historical background to lithium research and therapy. In (ed.) Johnson FN. Lithium research and therapy. London. Academic Press, 1975, pp. 9-22.

Johnson FN. The History of Lithium Therapy. London. Macmillan Press. 1984, pp. 34-45, 66-78, 154, 160, 183-187.

Kraepelin E. Manic-Depressive Insanity And Paranoia. – From the Eight German Edition of the "Text-Book of Psychiatry", vols. iii and iv [1913]. Edinburgh. Livingstone. 1921 [reprint by Arno Press, 1976]. pp.48-49, 182-3.

Lange C. Om Periodiske Depressionstilstande og deres Patogenese. Copenhagen. Lund. 1886. (cf. Schioldann, 2001, 2009, 2011 (Lange, 2011).

Lange C. On Periodical Depressions and their Pathogenesis. In Schioldann J. History of the Introduction of Lithium into Medicine and Psychiatry. Birth of Modern Psychopharmacology 1949. Preface by German E. Berrios. Adelaide Academic Press. 2009. Appendix I.

Lange C. On Periodical Depressions and their Pathogenesis. Introduction and translation by Johan Schioldann. Classic Text No. 85. History of Psychiatry 2011;22(1):108-130.

Lewis A. 'Endogenous' and 'exogenous': a useful dichotomy? Psychol. Med. 1971;1:191-6.

Lewis A. 'Psychogenic': a word and its mutations. Psychol. Med. 1972;2;209-15.

London B. Literature on gout. Practitioner 1903;337-353 (International bibliography current up until 1902).

Luff AP. The chemistry and pathology of gout. (Gouldstonian Lectures). Lancet 1897:857-63, 942-9.

Luff AP. Gout. Its Pathology and Treatment. London & Melbourne. 1898. pp. 120, 125, 183-184.

Luff AP. The treatment of gout in its various forms. Practitioner 1903;July:91-110.

Luff AP. The treatment of some of the forms of gout. Practitioner 1907;161-75.

Luff AP. Gout. Its Pathology, Forms, Diagnosis and Treatment. New York: William Wood. 1907. Also printed at Oxford, 1907.

Luff AP. In: Squire PW, editor. Squire's Companion to the latest Edition of the British Pharmacopoeia etc. 18th Edn. London. Churchill 1908. Pp. 733-739. (cf. Luff. Lancet 1900;1:931; Luff. Br. Med. J. 1900;1:836).

Luff AP. Treatment of subacute and chronic gout. Ther. Gaz. 1909:798.

Maudsley H. The Physiology and Pathology of Mind. 2nd edition. London. Macmillan, 1868, pp 264-5.

Maudsley H. The Pathology of Mind. 3nd edition etc. London. Macmillan, 1879, 68, pp 111, 120, 196-198.

Maudsley H. The Pathology of Mind. A Study of its Distempers, Deformities, and Disorders. London. Macmillan, 1895, pp 112-115, 546.

Mitchell W. On the use of bromide of lithium. Am. J. Med. Sci. 1870;60:443-5. (cf. Schioldann, 2009. p. 28).

Noack CH, Trautner EM. The lithium treatment of maniacal psychosis. Med. J. Aust. 1951;38:219-22.

Price FW. (ed.) A Textbook of the Practice of Medicine by Various Authors including Sections on Diseases of the Skin & Psychological Medicine by Various Authors [Mapother and Aubrey Lewis]. Oxford University Press, 1937 pp. 436-444, 1298, 1836, 1846). (Recommended reading for MD candidates at the University of Melbourne).

Schioldann J. Erik Strömgren: A biographical portrait. In: Schioldann J, Sand Strömgren L. Erik Strömgren. 1909-1993. A Bio-Bibliography. Acta Psychiatr. Scand. 1996;99:283-302. (pp. 284-290).

Schioldann J. John Cade's seminal lithium paper turns fifty. Invited

Editorial. Acta Psychiatr. Scand. 1999;100:403-5.

Schioldann J. In: Commeration of the Centenary of the Death of Carl Lange [2000]. The Lange Theory of 'Periodical Depression'. A Landmark in the History of Lithium Therapy. Adelaide Academic Press. 2001.

Schioldann J, editor. Erik Strömgren talks about his life with psychiatry. An interview by Mogens Schou. Adelaide Academic Press. 2002.

Schioldann J. Introduction. In: August Wimmer, editor. Psychogenic Psychoses. Adelaide Academic Press. 2003. pp. 56-57, 65-66 (Aubrey Lewis).

Schioldann J. Obituary: Mogens Abelin Schou (1918-2005) – half a century with lithium. History of Psychiatry 2006;17(2):247-52.

Schioldann J. Carl Lange: On Periodical Depressions and their Pathogenesis. In Schioldann J. History of the Introduction of Lithium into Medicine and Psychiatry. Adelaide Academic Press. 2009. Appendix I.

Schioldann J. History of the Introduction of Lithium into Medicine and Psychiatry. Birth of Modern Psychopharmacology 1949. Preface by German Berrios. Adelaide Academic Press. 2009. xxv, 363pp.

Schioldann J. From guinea pigs to manic patients: Cade's 'story of lithium.' Aust. N.Z.J. Psychiatr. 2013;47(5):484-6.

Schou M, Juel-Nielsen N, Strömgren E, Voldby H. The treatment of manic-psychosis by the administration of lithium salts. J. Neurol. Neurosurg. 1954;17:250-60.

Schou M. Letter to J. Cade, 16.3.63 (from Schou).

Schou M. Lithium. Lancet 1970;ii:875-6.

Schou M. Letter to Trautner, November 27, 1974 (from Schou).

Schou M. Lithium in 1977. In honorem John F. J. Cade. The 43rd Beattie-Smith Lecture, University of Melbourne, February 4, 1977. pp. 41-48.

Schou M. Lithium perspectives. Neuropsychobiol. 1983;10:7-12.

Schou M. Correspondence G. Kaufmann, 9.4. 1984 (from Schou).

Schou M. The development of lithium treatment in psychiatry. Unpublished manuscript (of speech delivered at Amsterdam, March 1996) (from Schou).

Schou M. Phases in the development of lithium treatment in psychiatry. In (eds.) Samson F, Adelman G. The neurosciences: paths of discovery II. Boston. Birkhäuser. 1992, 149-166.

Schou M. Lithium treatment for half a century. How did it all start?' Nord. J. Psychiatr. 1999;53:383-4.

Schou M. Lithium treatment at 52. J. Affect. Disord. 2001;67:21-32.

Schou M. Correspondence. July 7, 2005.

Shepherd M. A prophylactic myth. Int. J. Psychiatr. 1970-71;9:423-5.

Shepherd M. Psychiatrists on Psychiatry. Cambridge University Press. 1982.

Soares JC, Gershon S. The pharmacologic specificity of the lithium ion: origins and trajectory. J. Clin. Psychiatr. 2000;61, Suppl. 9:16-22.

Strömgren E. [Internationally famous psychiatrists in an historical perspective]. Lecture delivered at the Psychiatric Hospital, Risskov, 8 May 1992. Unpublished manuscript.

Squire PW. Squire's companion to the latest edition of The British Pharmacopoiea etc. 18th Edn. London. Churchill. 1908. pp. 733-739.

& 19th Edn. 1916. pp. 22, 838-847.

Trautner EM. Letter to Schou, September 15, 1954 (from Schou).

Trautner EM. Letter to Schou, September 28, 1955 (from Schou).

Trautner EM. Letter to Schou, February 9, 1975 (from Schou).

Wilkinson G. (ed.) Talking about psychiatry. (Interview of Felix Post by B. Barraclough, 1984). London. Gaskell. 1993. p. 167.

February 15, 2018

CHAPTER 6.

SAFETY

Thomas A. Ban

JANOS RADÓ: MECHANISM OF LITHIUM INDUCED POLYURIA

ABSTRACT

The present therapy for lithium-induced nephrogenic diabetes insipidus in man is to counter anti-vasopressin action of lithium by administration of thiazide diuretics, antiprostaglandin compounds (indomethacine) combined with large doses of desmopressin. (amiloride supplements the "present therapy" drug group). The "future" treatment seems to be (on the basis of recent animal experiments) to enhance the sensitivity of the kidney to vasopressin action by administering pharmacologic blockade of renal P2Y12 receptor. On theoretical basis it is conceivable that the present therapy of lithium-induced nephrogenic insipidus perhaps could be combined with the "future" pharmacologic blockade.

Introduction

In 1978 we found that in response to indomethacine administered to polyuric patient with familial Bartter syndrome, urine osmolality and free water reabsorption increased simultaneously with the decrease in the excretion of prostaglandin E2 (PGE2) (Radó, Simatupang, Boer and Mees 1978). In 2012 Zhang and his coworkers found that lithium-induced polyuria is due to resistance of the medullary collecting duct to the action of arginine vasopressin, apparently mediated by increased production of PGE2 (Zhang, Pop, Carlson and Kishore 2012). Therefore, PGE2 must be a key factor in the understanding and treatment of lithium polyuria. My early studies on indomethacine and desmopressin in Bartter polyuria, later studies on indomethacine and desmopressin in lithium-induced permanent nephrogenic diabetes insipidus and the results of the new studies of many investigators working in groups with Zhang and with Zhang and Peti-Peterdi ("Zhang and Peti-Peterdi group") are discussed together.

The purpose of this paper is to review the newer literature concerning the

203

relationship between lithium polyuria and chemical (PGE2 and other), as well as genetic (P2Y12 receptor) factors.

Early Studies

In 1978 we investigated the effect of indomethacin and desmopressin on water excretion in a 32-year-old patient with familial Bartter's syndrome in whom urinary concentration was impaired during ad libitum fluid intake without any decrease in maximal concentrating ability (Radó, Simatupang, Boer, Dorhout Mees 1978).

As shown in Figure 1 and Table 1, in response to indomethacin, urine osmolality and free water reabsorption increased simultaneously with the decrease in the excretion of prostaglandin E2. The indomethacin-induced improvement was, however, less than that obtained after desmopressin with or without indomethacin.

Desmopressin (Minirin) was administered in doses of 40 micrograms three times a day intranasally. After a control period (17 days) the effects of daily 200mcg indomethacine was studied during the last 12 days of a month treatment period. One week after discontinuation of indomethacine treatment desmopressin was given again in the same dose as previously.

We compared the urine osmolality findings obtained in healthy subjects and in a polyuric patient with Bartter syndrome without treatment ("no drug") and after administration of desmopressin (DDAVP) or indomethacine, as well as after combined administration of desmopressin and indomethacine during ad libitum fluid intake (Figure 1). Two determinations were done during administration of desmopressin after prolonged water restriction (quadrants).

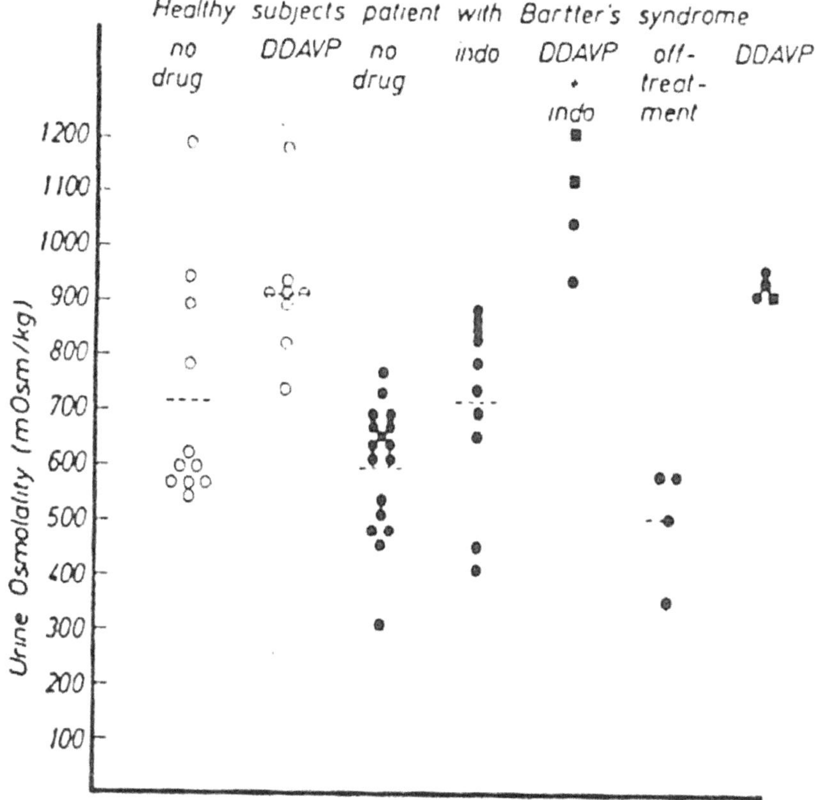

Figure 1. Urine osmolality (U_{osm}) was lower in the untreated patient than in the healthy subjects. After DDAVP this difference disappeared. Indomethacin induced a marked increase in U_{osm} in the patient.

Int. J. clin. Pharmacol. 16 (1978), 22–26 (No. 1)

As shown in Figure 1, in the patient with Bartter syndrome indomethacine potentiated the effect of desmopressin (DDAVP). During prolonged water restriction and desmopressin administration, urine osmolality was 924 mOsm/Kg, increasing to 1169 mOm/Kg in response to indomethacine (quadrant).

Table 1 shows the effects of indomethacine, desmopressin (DDAVP) and indomethacine plus desmopressin on specific renal function. Results of statistical analysis are indicated

Effect of indomethacine on prostaglandins

During indomethacin treatment, excretion of PGE2 was decreased from 138.3 ng/24 hrs to 55 ng/24 hrs (normal range: 9-12 ng/24 hrs). PGA decreased from 205 ng/24 hrs to 97 ng/24 hrs (normal range: 71-144 ng/24 hrs), PGB decreased "from 95 ng/24 hrs to 49 ng/24 hrs (normal range: 36-74 ng/24 hrs) and PGF decreased from 146 ng/24 hrs to 64' ng/24 hrs (normal range: 40-83 ng/24 hrs).

The blood level of PGE1 also decreased from 38.9 pg/ml to 23.2 pg/ml (normal: 5.5 ± 0.8 pg/rnl). PGA changed from 241 pg/ml to 269 pg/ml (normal: 94 ± f 5 pg/rnl), PGB from 129 pg/ml to 107 pg/ml (normal: 1 il9 ± 14 pg/nil) and PGF from 22 pg/ml to 9.4 pg/ml (normal: 17.2 ± 3.3 pg/ml).

(We are greatly indebted to Prof. Dr. A. Hornych, Hôpital Broussais, Paris, who kindly performed the prostaglandin determinations.)

Later Studies on Indomethacine and Desmopressin

In "use of modern antidiuretic agents in the treatment of permanent lithium-induced nephrogenic diabetes insipidus" (Radó 2018a) we found that administration of excessive doses of desmopressin resulted in clinically relevant antidiuresis, enhanced by indomethacine and abolished by calcitonine. A theory was proposed why the presumed antidiuretic drug calcitonine exerted a "diuretic" action by abolishing the effect of desmopressin (Radó, Zdravkova 1991, 1993; Radó 2018b). These results and thoughts were discussed by Gordon Johnson (2018) and Hector Warnes (2019). Renal toxicity of lithium was reviewed in a balanced manner, considering both the renal insufficiency and end-stage renal disease, as well as the prominant tubular abnormality of nephrogenic diabetes insipidus (Radó 2019b). In this review the role of the large doses of desmopressin was analyzed in counteracting polyuria in congenital as well as in lithium-induced nephrogenic diabetes insipidus during combined administration of many different drugs (thiazide diuretics, indomethacine, piroxicam, calcitonine, etc.). Other drugs also having antidiuretic properties but without coadministration with desmopressin were also mentioned (metformin, statins, sildenafil, clopidogrel, prasugral etc.). Finally, antidiuretic drugs which could have been combined with desmopressin, but not promising in the treatment in lithium-induced nephrogenic insipidus, i.e., chlorpropamide, clofibrate and carbamazepine, were also included. From these compounds carbamazepine is an exception: its weak antidiuretic effect, combined with desmopressin, may be advantageous when it is otherwise indicated from psychiatric point of view (Radó 2019a).

New Investigations of the Zhang and Peti-Peterdi Group

Zhang and his coworkers found that lithium-induced polyuria is due to resistance of the medullary collecting duct to the action of arginine vasopressin (AVP), apparently mediated by increased production of PGE2. Genetic deletion of the P2Y2 receptor offered significant resistance to development of lithium polyuria. This change was accompanied by alterations in PGE2 signaling mediated by a marked decrease in the prostanoid EP3 receptor protein abundance thus attenuating the decrease in cAMP, modulator of arginine vasopressin, in the renal medulla (Zhang, Pop, Carlson and Kishore 2012; Zhang, Hansson, Liu, Kishore 2019).

P2Y12 Receptor Localizes in the Renal Collecting Duct

P2Y12 receptor signaling reduces cellular cAMP levels, the central modulator of arginine vasopressin. It was hypothesized that if expressed in the renal collecting duct P2Y12 receptor may play a role in renal handling of water in health and in nephrogenic diabetes insipidus. P2Y12 receptor mRNA expression in rat kidney, and immunolocalized its protein and aquaporin-2 in collecting duct principal cells was found (Zhang, Peti-Peterdi, Müller et al. 2015).

Short-Term Studies in the P2Y12 Receptor Knockout Mice

In the P2Y12 receptor knockout mice, enhanced vasopressin

activity and increased renal sodium conservation was found. These animals were less sensitive not only to the diuresis enhancement induced by lithium, but also to the lithium-induced natriuresis and kaliuresis due to the attenuation of down regulation of the major natrium or kalium transporter/channel proteins in the collecting duct (Zhang, Li, Kohan et al. 2013).

Long-Term Studies in the P2Y12 Receptor Knockout Mice

Age matched wild type and P2Y12 receptor knockout mice were fed regular or lithium-added diet for five months. There was a steady increase in lithium-induced polyuria, nariuresis and kaliuresis in wild type mice, but increases in these parameters were very low in the knockout mice. Lithium-induced collecting duct proliferation was significantly lower in the knockout vs wild type mice. The results demonstrate that genetic deletion of P2Y12 receptor protects against the key structural and functional alterations in lithium-induced nephrogenic diabetes insipidus. Genetic deletion of P2Y12 receptor offers long-term (five months) protection against lithium-induced polyuria, natriuresis, kaliuresis and collecting duct remodeling and cell proliferation (Zhang, Riquier-Brison, Liu et al. 2018)

The most widely studied purinergic receptor in the kidney is ATP-activated P2Y12 receptor which is expressed in the collecting duct. Signaling mediated through P2Y12 receptor antagonizes the vasopressin action by enhancing the production of PGE2 (Kishore, Carlson, Ecelbarger et al. 2015).

The present therapy for lithium-induced nephrogenic diabetes insipidus in man is to counter anti-vasopressin action of lithium. The future treatment is to enhance the sensitivity of the kidney to vasopressin action (Kishore, Carlson, Ecelbarger et al. 2015).

Administration an Irreversible Inhibitor of the P2Y12 Receptor (clopidogrel)

Clopidogrel bisulfate significantly increased urine concentration and aquaporine protein in the kidneys of Sprague–Dawley rats but did not alter urine concentration in Brattleboro rats that lack arginine-vasopressin. Clopidogrel administration also significantly ameliorated lithium-induced polyuria, improved urine concentrating ability and aquaporine protein abundance and reversed the lithium-induced increase in freewater excretion. Selective blockade of P2Y12 receptor by the reversible antagonist PSB-0739 in primary cultures of rat inner medullary collecting duct principal cells potentiated the expression of aquaporine and cAMP production induced by desmopressin (Zhang, Peti-Peterdi, Müller et al. 2015).

Clopidrogel alone increased renal aquaporin 2, Na-K-2Cl cotransporter, Na-Cl cotransporter and the subunits of the epithelial Na channel (ENaC) in renal medulla. When combined with lithium, clopidrogel prevented downregulation of aquaporin, Na-K-ATPase and Na-K-2Cl cotransporter but was less effective against downregulation of cortical sodium channel (α- or γ-ENaC). Thus, clopidrogel primarily attenuated lithium-induced downregulation of proteins involved in AVP-sensitive water conservation (Zhang, Peti-Peterdi, Heiney et al. 2015)

Clopidrogel is an antiplatelet drug of the thienopyridine group extensively used in cardiological clinical medicine. Another such drug is prasugral and both are ADP antagonists acting on the P2Y12 receptor. Administration of prasugral completely suppressed lithium-induced polyiuria and polydipsia in rats (Zhang, Peti-Peterdi, Brandes et al. 2017)

Pharmacologic Blockade of Renal P2Y12 Receptor

Pharmacologic blockade of renal P2Y12 receptor in rodents increases urinary concentrating ability by augmenting the effect of vasopressin on the kidney and ameliorates lithium-induced nephrogenic diabetes insipidus by potentiating the action of vasopressin on the renal collecting duct (Zhang Peti-Peterdi, Müller et al. 2015). This strategy may offer a novel and effective therapy for lithium-induced nephrogenic diabetes insipidus in man.

Conclusion

Pharmacologic blockade of renal P2Y12 receptor may be combined - at least theoretically - with anti-prostaglandin agents (non-steroidal anti-inflammatory compounds) and supplemented with large doses of desmopressin in the treatment of lithium-induced nephrogenic diabetes insipidus. Lithium-induced excessive prostaglandinuria (increased excretion of PGE2) can be prevented by pharmacologic blockade of the renal P2Y12 receptor and antagonized by the administration of indomethacine.

We are all definitely convinced by the enormous work of Ban (2017), Blackwell (2014), Rybakowski (2017), Severus, Taylor, Sauer et al. (2014) and others that millions suffering from bipolar disorder need lithium treatment and making it safer by eliminating (at least partly) its most frequent side effect lithium polyuria, is a decent goal for both the investigators and physicians.

References:

Ban TA. Neuropsychopharmacology in Historical Perspective. Education in the Field in the Post-Neuropsychopharmacology Era. Prologue. inhn.org.education. September 18, 2017.

Johnson G. Comment on Janos Radó's (January 25, 2018) final comment (Barry Blackwell: The Lithium Controversy. A Historical Autopsy). inhn.org.collated. July 5, 2018.

Kishore BK, Carlson NG, Ecelbarger CM, Kohan DE, Müller CE, Nelson RD, Peti-Peterdi J, Zhang Y. Targeting Renal Purinergic Signalling for the Treatment of Lithium-induced Nephrogenic Diabetes Insipidus. Acta Physiol (Oxf). 2015; 214(2):176-88.

Radó JP, Simatupang T, Boer P, Dorhout Mees EJ. Pharmacologic studies in Bartter's syndrome: effect of DDAVP and indomethacin on renal concentrating operation. Part II. Int J Clin Pharmacol Biopharm. 1978; 16(1):22-6.

Radó JP, Zdravkova S. Lithium-induced chronic water-metabolism disorder (nephrogenic diabetes insipidus)]. Orv Hetil. 1991; 132:1987-90.

Radó JP, Zdravkova S. Effect of Indomethacine and Calcitonin During Administration of 1-Deamino-8-D-Arginin-Vasopressin (desmopressin) on Free Water Clearance in Nephrogenic Diabetes Insipidus (NDI). XIIth International Congress of Nephrology. June 13–18, 1993 Jerusalem, Israel.

Radó J. Final comment (Use of modern antidiuretic agents in the treatment of permanent lithium-induced nephrogenic diabetes insipidus [Barry Blackwell: The lithium controversy. A historical autopsy]). inhn.org.collated. January 25, 2018a.

Radó J. Addition to final comment: Calcitonin in lithium-induced nephrogenic diabetes insipidus (Barry Blackwell: The lithium controversy. A historical autopsy) inhn.org.collated. September 13, 2018b.

Radó J. Desmopressin may counteract polyuria in lithium-induced nephrogenic diabetes insipidus (Review of the literature) inhn.org.controversies. June 27, 2019a.

Radó J. Renal Toxicity of Lithium in Historical Perspective with Special Reference To Nephrogenic Diabetes Insipidus and its Treatment. inhn.org.controversies. May 2, 2019b.

Rybakowski J. Final comment: Half a Century of Inspiring Lithium Controversy (Barry Blackwell: The Lithium controversy: A historical autopsy. Collated by Olaf Fjetland). inhn.org.collated. September 30, 2017.

Severus E, Taylor MJ, Sauer C, Pfennig A, Ritter P, Bauer M, Geddes JR. Lithium for prevention of mood episodes in bipolar disorders: systematic review and meta-analysis. Int J Bipolar Disord. 2014; 2:15.

Warnes H. Comment on Janos Radó's additional final comment:

Calcitonin in lithium-induced nephrogenic diabetes insipidus (Barry Blackwell: The lithium controversy. A historical autopsy) inhn.org.collated. January 17, 2019.

Zhang Y, Pop I, Carlson NG, Kishore BK. Genetic deletion of the P2Y12 receptor offers significant resistance to development of lithium-induced polyuria accompanied by alterations in PGE2 signaling. Am J Physiol Renal Physiol 2012; 302:F70–F77.

Zhang Y, Li L, Kohan DE, Ecelbarger CM, Kishore BK. Attenuation of lithium-induced natriuresis and kaliuresis in P2Y12 receptor knockout mice. Am J Physiol Renal Physiol. 2013; 305(3):F407-16.

Zhang Y, Peti-Peterdi J, Müller CE, Carlson NG, Baqi Y, Strasburg DL, Heiney KM, Villanueva K, Kohan DE, Kishore BK. P2Y12 Receptor Localizes in the Renal Collecting Duct and Its Blockade Augments Arginine Vasopressin Action and Alleviates Nephrogenic Diabetes Insipidus. J Am Soc Nephrol. 2015; 26(12):2978-87.

Zhang Y, Peti-Peterdi J, Heiney KM, Riquier-Brison A, Carlson NG, Müller CE, Ecelbarger CM, Kishore BK. Clopidrogel attenuates lithium-induced alterations in renal water and sodium channels/transporters in mice. Purinergic Signal. 2015;11(4):507-18.

Zhang Y, Peti-Peterdi J, Brandes A, Riquier-Brison A, Carlson NG, Müller CE, Ecelbarger CM, Kishore BK. Prasugral suppresses development of lithium-induced nephrogenic diabetes insipidus in mice. Purinergic Signal. 2017;13(2):239-48.

Zhang Y, Riquier-Brison A, Liu T, Huang Y, Carlson, NG, Peti-Peterdi J, Kishore BK. Genetic Deletion of P2Y12 Receptor Offers Long-Term (5 Months) Protection Against Lithium-Induced Polyuria, Natriuresis, Kaliuresis, and Collecting Duct Remodeling and Cell Proliferation. Front Physiol. 2018; 9:1765.

Zhang Y, Hansson K M, Liu T, Kishore B. Genetic Deletion of ADP-activated P2Y12 Receptor Ameliorates Lithium-induced Nephrogenic

Thomas A. Ban

Diabetes Insipidus in Mice. Acta Physiol (Oxf). 2019; 225(2):e13191.

July 4, 2019

JANOS RADÓ: CALCITONIN IN LITHIUM-INDUCED NEPHROGENIC DIABETES INSIPIDUS

In our previous studies the favorable antidiuretic action of Desmopressin was counteracted by the concomitant administration of Calcitonin in Lithium-induced permanent nephrogenic diabetes insipidus (Radó 2018). However, the exact mechanism of the abolishment of Desmopressin-induced antidiuresis by Calcitonin was not clear. As the opinions in the literature are rather divided concerning the basic water metabolic action of Calcitonin, further considerations may have significance.

Calcitonin is a "tricky" hormone, having both diuretic and antidiuretic properties. Diuretic effect of Calcitonin was an observation mainly in the older literature (Carney and Thompson 1981; Keeler, Walker and Copp 1970) and is in harmony with our published data on a water mobilizing action (Radó 1991, 1993, 2018). On the other hand, a water retaining action was found by the de Rouffignac group (Elalouf, Roinel and de Rouffignac 1986) in response to human Calcitonin in rats during micropunture studies simulating the changes induced by Desmopressin. The results of these investigations were later confirmed by elegant sophisticated methods (Bouley 2011) indicating that Calcitonin has a vasopressin-like action, indeed. Calcitonin was even recommended - though purely on theoretical basis - for the treatment of nephrogenic diabetes insipidus, i.e., in a vasopressin resistant condition (Bouley et al. 2011).

An alternative explanation to the complicated water effects of Calcitonin may be provided by supposing that both Desmopressin and have an effect on the same renal tubular site on the vasopressin (V2) receptor, but the effect of Calcitonin is weaker than that of Desmopressin. So, Calcitonin, by occupying the receptors, can have a competitive antagonism with the Desmopressin molecule. Further studies are necessary to confirm or exclude the possible competitive antagonism between Desmopressin and Calcitonin.

References:

Bouley R, Lu HA, Nunes P, Da Silva N, McLaughlin M, Chen Y, Brown D. Calcitonin Has a Vasopressin-like Effect on Aquaporin-2 Trafficking and Urinary Concentration. J Am Soc Nephrol. 2011; 22(1):59-72

Carney S, Thompson L. Acute effect of calcitonin on rat renal electrolyte transport. Am J Physiol 1981; 240:F12–F16.

Elalouf JM, Roinel N, de Rouffignac C. Effects of human calcitonin on water and electrolytemovements in rat juxtamedullary nephrons: inhibition of medullary K recycling. Pflugers Arch. 1986; 406(5):502-8.

Radó JP, Zdravkova S. Lithium-induced chronic water-metabolism disorder (nephrogenic diabetes insipidus). Orv Hetil. 1991;132, 1987-90.

Radó JP, Zdravkova S. Effect of Indomethacine and Calcitonine During Administration of 1-Deamino-8-D-Arginin-Vasopressin (dDAVP) on Free Water Clearance in Nephrogenic Diabetes Insipidus (NDI). XIIth International Congress of Nephrology. June 13–18, 1993, Jerusalem, Israel.

Radó J. Use of modern antidiuretic agents in the treatment of permanent lithium induced nephrogenic diabetes insipidus. (Administration of excessive doses of desmopressin resulted in clinically relevant antidiuresis, enhanced by indomethacine and abolished by calcitonine). inhn.org.controversies. January 25, 2018. (Janos Radó's final comment on Barry Blackwell The lithium controversy. A historical autopsy. Collated by Olaf Fjetland).

September 13, 2018

JANOS RADÓ: RENAL TOXICITY OF LITHIUM IN HISTORICAL PERSPECTIVE WITH SPECIAL REFERENCE TO NEPHROGENIC DIABETES INSIPIDUS AND ITS TREATMENT

ABSTRACT

Renal toxicity of lithium is a highly important subject which may jeopardize the use of an agent needed by millions suffering from recurrent episodes of bipolar disorder. Lithium may cause profound changes in the previously normal kidney functions and structure leading to end stage kidney disease. The recent use of lower serum lithium levels, however, almost eliminated the risk of lithium-induced renal failure.

In the present report we deal with disturbances of the normal concentrating operation of the kidney; lithium-induced concentrating defect and nephrogenic diabetes insipidus (NDI); and treatment of the lithium-induced disorders.

Treatment of the lithium-induced NDI consists of the thiazides, indomethacine and other non-steroid anti-inflammatory compounds as well as the administration of large doses of desmopressin, amiloride and combinations thereof. Administration of very high doses of desmopressin has resulted in clinically relevant antidiuresis, enhanced by indomethacine. Amiloride is a very special antikaluretic diuretic drug which can abolish several lithium-induced abnormalities. In such an important form of psychiatric treatment as lithium, a serious disturbance of water metabolism can be alleviated by the clever use of modern antidiuretic interventions.

Introduction

"Lithium is a simple ion that remains the best, safest and least expensive treatment for the prevention of recurrent episodes of bipolar disorder" (Blackwell 2018). However, long term administration of lithium has been associated with nephrotoxic effects, altering the structure or/and function of the kidney. Although chronic lithium therapy can cause advanced renal disease, most cases of nephrotoxicity are limited only to narrowed renal concentrating operation. Even in cases with the lithium-induced most severe disturbance of water metabolism, i.e., NDI, there are some therapeutic measures which can alleviate, to some extent, the patient's suffering. Decreasing the polyuria may secure some rest for the patients during the night. Treatment options for the lithium-induced NDI were not fully considered in a recent review of lithium nephrotoxicity (Davis, Desmond and Berk 2018). More extensive analysis of these options is the purpose of the present article, with special reference to historical points of views.

Lithium Induced Nephropathy

General toxicity was a concern even for John Cade, the discoverer of the lithium therapy in 1947 (Cade 1949). The strongest propagator of this treatment, Morgens Schou, was also frightened of the side effects, considering that his loved brother's health was at stake (Schou 1958). Gordon Johnson investigated the influence of lithium treatment on the endogenous creatinine clearance and found that "overall, glomerular filtration rate fell within the established normal range" (Johnson 1984). However, Hestbech, Hansen and Amdisen (1977); Bendz (1983); Bendz, Aurell, Balldin et al. 1994; Bendz, Schön, Attman and Aurell (2010); and Boton, Gauiria and Battle (1987) found chronic renal lesions following long-term treatment with lithium. Chronic lithium therapy produces progressive interstitial fibrosis, hyperplastic changes in the medullary collecting ducts, distal tubule dilatation and microcyst formation (Croft, Bedford, Leader and Walker 2018). Renal failure occurs in chronic lithium treatment but is uncommon (Bendz Schön, Attman and Aurell 2010; Johnson 1998). Davis, Desmond and Berk (2018) developed a search strategy using the most valuable electronic databases to identify the most pertinent questions of lithium- induced nephropathy. They confirmed that there was no correlation between the duration of therapy and decreases in eGFR. At least 20 years or more is necessary for the development of lithium-induced end stage kidney disease. Nevertheless, the incidence of the latter is not more than 0,2-0,7 % (according to Shine, McKnight, Leaver and Geddes [2015], 0,5-1%). Not only duration of therapy but other factors may also be relevant to the development lithium-induced nephropathy, such as age, female gender, other diseases favoring nephropathy (diabetes mellitus and hypertension), use of nephrotoxic drugs, prior episodes of acute lithium toxicity, etc. (Davis, Desmond and Berk 2018; Johnson 2018). However, Aiff, Attman P, Aurell et al. (2014) stress that the recent use of lower serum lithium levels almost eliminated the risk of lithium-induced renal failure.

Disturbances in the Renal Concentrating Operation

In healthy people urine concentration can exceed that of plasma which is ca 290 mOsm/Kg. The osmolal concentration of the urine can be as high as 1200 mOsm/Kg during prolonged thirst. During water conservation the renal medullary interstitial tissue is hypertonic, due to the accumulated sodium and urea in consequence of the active sodium reabsorption in the ascending limb of the loop of Henle transporting the sodium into the medullary interstitium. Its osmolality is as high as that of the concentrated urine. The presence of vasopressin-induced increase of collecting tubular permeability allows diffusion of water back into the medullary interstitium down the established medullary osmotic gradient resulting in maximally concentrated urine. Lithium diminishes the osmotic gradient in the renal medulla reflected in a marked reduction in both osmolyte and urea content. Decrease in the renal medullary interstitial hypertonicity results in lower urinary concentration, polyuria and polydipsia. Amiloride, by increase in medullary osmolytes, restores the renal medullary interstitial hypertonicity, resulting in normalization of the renal concentrating mechanism and less and more concentrated urine. (Bedford, Leader, Jing et al. 2008b)

During ad libitum fluid as intake in healthy people the average urine osmolality is ca 600 mOsm/Kg. During water diuresis however, the urinary osmolality is ca 100 mOsm/Kg or less. The lowest value I observed in my human pharmacology studies was 40 mOm/Kg after water loading. In prolonged polyuria the osmotic concentration in the renal medulla decreases due to the "washout" effect with the consequence of reduced concentrating power.

In some patients with neurohypophyseal (central) diabetes insipidus the value of urine osmolality can be as high as 300 mOsm/Kg or more, though in most cases it is as in water diuresis. The osmolal concentration of the urine increases at least 9 % in response to vasopressin (Miller Moses test), so differentiation from the NDI - at least in the full cases - is simple. In congenital NDI the urine osmolality figures are the same as in central DI but are not responding to the antidiuretic hormone (ADH, vasopressin).

The diagnosis may be difficult in patients with the partial form of the diseases. Fortunately, sophisticated molecular genetic studies provide exact methods for successful differentiation. The identification, characterization and mutational analysis of the two different genes, the arginine vasopressin receptor 2 gene (AVPR2) and the vasopressin-sensitive water channel gene (aquaporin 2 [AQP2]), provide the basis for understanding the two hereditary forms of renal diabetes insipidus: the X-linked NDI (relatively frequent) and the non x-linked NDI (very rare) (Fujiwara and Bichet 2005). The two types of NDI result from mutation in the structure either of the V2 receptor or AQP2 which causes impaired arginine-vasopressin induced signal transduction (Canfield, Tamarappoo, Moses et al. 1997). "All families with hereditary diabetes insipidus (the X-linked NDI and the non x-linked NDI) should have their molecular defect identified" (Fujiwara and Bichet 2005).

The concentrating process normally starts with the binding of arginine-vasopressin to the V2 receptors on the basolateral surface of the principal cells in the collecting duct. It stimulates adenyl cyclase and influences the content of the intracellular vesicles, the AQP2 protein which is the "water channel" to be inserted in the apical membrane in the luminal site of the principal cell in the collecting duct. Vasopressin stimulation results in the 20-fold increase in water permeability of responsive principle cells.

Although the mechanisms of the development of inherited and acquired forms of diabetes insipidus are entirely different, therapy of the two types is surprisingly similar. In the patients with the full (complete) form of the inherited disease the vasopressin resistance may be absolute. However, many patients with congenital NDI suffer only in a partial form of the disease (Boccalandro, De Mattia, Guo et al. 2004). In such patients administration of large doses of DDAVP can alleviate somewhat the suffering. It is interesting that within one family huge interindividual variations can be observed in the degree of vasopressin resistance. On this basis the effectiveness of large doses of DDAVP can be significantly different within one family. Figure 1 shows our personal observations in such a family.

In a five- member congenital NDI family who were investigated during thirst and administration of lysin-vasopressin urine, osmolality values were 207 mOsm/Kg, 236 mOsm/Kg, 296 mOsm/Kg, 322 mOsm/Kg, and 405 mOsm/Kg. (Radó, Szende 1995). In Figure 1 only data of four members are depicted.

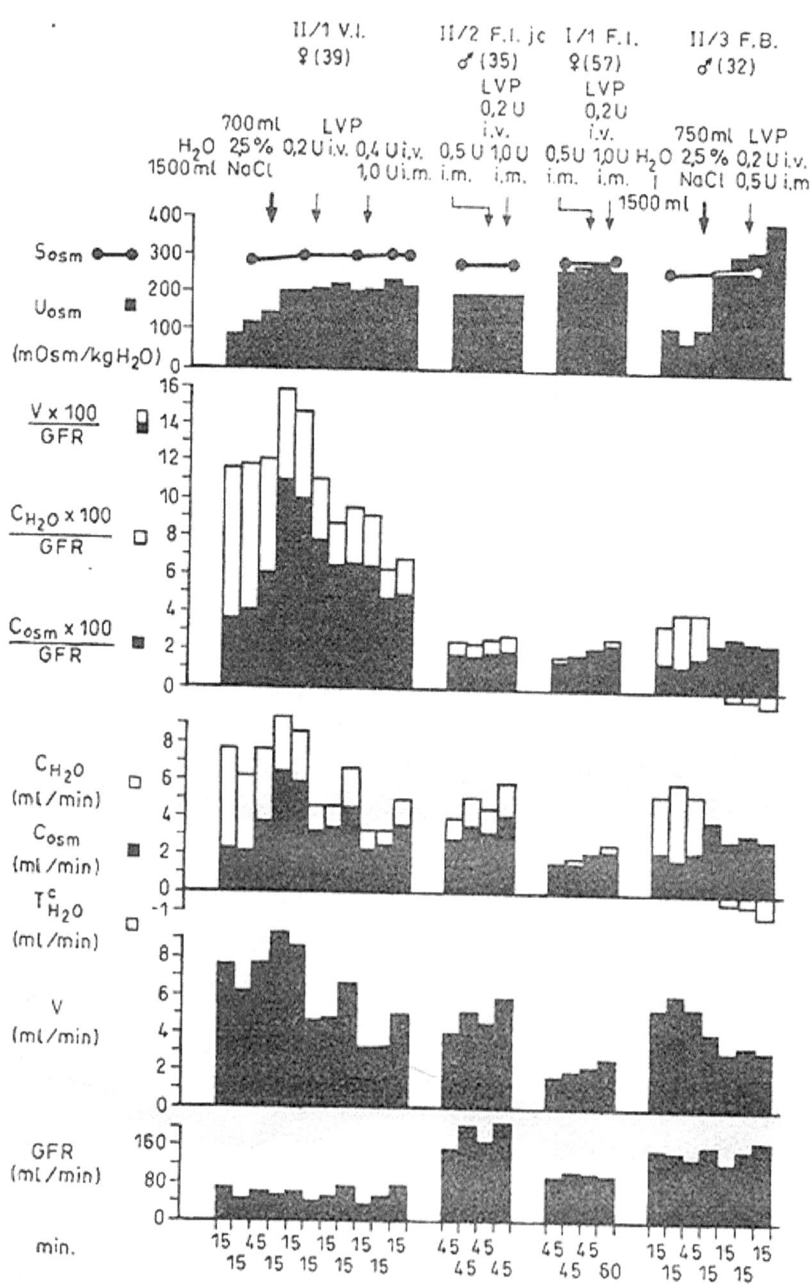
II/1 V.I.
♀ (39)
II/2 F.I. jc
♂ (35)
I/1 F.I.
♀ (57)
II/3 F.B.
♂ (32)
LVP
0,2 U
i.v.
LVP
0,2 U
i.v.
700 ml
LVP
H₂O 2,5 % 0,2 U i.v. 0,4 U i.v.
1500 ml NaCl
1,0 U i.m.
0,5 U 1,0 U
i.m. i.m.
0,5 U 1,0 U
i.m. i.m.
750 ml LVP
H₂O 2,5 % 0,2 U i.v.
NaCl 0,5 U i.m.
1500 ml
400
Sosm
300
Uosm
200
100
(mOsm/kg H₂O)
0
16
V x 100
GFR
14
12
10
C_H₂O x 100
GFR
8
6
4
Cosm x 100
GFR
2
0
C_H₂O
(ml/min)
8
6
Cosm
(ml/min)
4
2
T^c_H₂O
0
(ml/min)
-1
8
V
(ml/min)
6
4
2
0
GFR
(ml/min)
160
80
0
min.
15 45 15 15 15 15
15 15 15 15 15
45 45
45 45
45 45
45 60
15 45 15 15
15 15 15

Investigational data of the congenital NDI family (Mother /I/1 F.I./ and three siblings). The effect of thirst and administration of lysine-vasopressin (doses are indicated above the figure) without or with infusion of hypertonic saline. It can be seen that in the first two members urine osmolality remains definitely lower than that of plasma. In the third member urine osmolality reaches that of plasma, while in the fourth member surpasses it.

Free water clearance (CH2O) increases during hypertonic sodium chloride infusions while in response to administration of lysine-vasopressin it decreases. Only in the fourth family member is free water clearance turned into free water reabsorption (TcH2O). Changes are similar in the free water clearance expressed in the percentage of glomerular filtration rate (CH2Ox100/ GFR). Osmolal clearance (Cosm) as well as Cosmx100/GFR markedly increased during hypertonic sodium chloride infusion in the first member of the family. Parallel changes were seen in urine flow (V)) and free water clearance.

The values of the glomerular filtration rate (GFR) were normal in three members of the family.

The lowest numbers indicate the duration of the individual clearance periods.

Lithium – Induced Concentrating Defect

The lithium-induced disturbance in renal concentrating operation begins shortly after the introduction of the drug. Lithium entering the principal cells of the collecting duct through the sodium epithelial channel abolishes the formation of cyclic AMP and by that the vasopressin mediated insertion of the water channel protein aquaporin 2 into the apical membrane of the cells. Down regulation of AQP2 reduces water reabsorption because of decreasing water permeability of the tubules. Lithium therapy reduces also the organic osmolyte content of the renal medulla (Bedford, Leader, Jing et al. 2008b). Dissipation of the high solute content of the renal medulla, the decrease in renal medullary hypertonicity, is the other cause of the lithium polyuria. Amiloride restores renal medullary osmolytes and hypertonicity improving by that the renal concentrating operation (Bedford, Weggery, Ellis et al. 2008a; Bedford, Leader, Jing et al. 2008b).

The concentrating defect progressively increases during further administration of lithium. In Gordon Johnson's patient material (after 12 hr thirst and administration of pitressin) the average maximal urine concentration was of about 400 mOsm/kg in 11 patients treated two years with lithium, while it was only 200 mOsm/kg in three patients treated 10-20 years (Johnson 1984).

The concentrating defect can be demonstrated at least in 50% of all patients. It is questionable whether in any patient the renal concentrating operation can remain intact during administration of lithium for several decades. Also a difficult question where is the limit between "narrowed" concentration and NDI. NDI can be only "functional" or in all cases lithium induced morphological structural alterations are present. On the basis of modern studies we may account perhaps in all patients lithium-induced "remodeling" of cells in the cortical and medullary renal tubules. "The cellular effects of lithium treatment are broad and complex" (Nielsen, Hoffert, Knepper et al. 2008).

Lithium-induced NDI

Nephrogenic diabetes insipidus is a clinical condition characterized with vasopressin-resistant polyuria and polydipsia. One of the most frequent causes of acquired NDI is chronic administration of lithium; it develops after 10 years of treatment with lithium in more than 10% of the patients. Disturbance of water metabolism is the most characteristic alteration in lithium- induced NDI; increased sodium excretion and hyperchloremic metabolic acidosis is also present. Decreased abundances of vasopressin governed aquaporin 2 and 3 water channels in the collecting duct is responsible for the insufficient tubular water reabsorption. Increased sodium excretion is caused by the reduced expression of the epithelial sodium channel in the cortical and outer medullary collecting duct. Lithium-induced increased expression of H+ATPase in the collecting duct is associated with the impaired excretion of acid. (There are other mechanisms too, also leading to renal tubular acidosis.) Nielsen, Hoffert, Knepper et al. (2008) performed "proteomic analysis" of lithium-induced NDI and found previously unknown mechanisms for aquaporin down regulation as well as cellular proliferation. Their model system was the inner medullary collecting duct isolated from lithium treated rats. Their most important finding was that lithium treatment affected proteins involved in cell death, apoptosis and cell proliferation. Several signaling pathways were activated by lithium treatment, as well as the increased intracellular accumulation of beta-catenin and phosphorylated glycogen synthase kinase type 3beta. The authors remark that similar targets may have lithium in the brain. It should be stressed again that the author's conclusion is "that the cellular effects of lithium treatment are broad and complex, and as such a single pathway leading to reduced AQP2 expression and subsequent polyuria is unlikely."

Treatment of Lithium-induced NDI

Before the era of Modern Pharmacology congenital NDI could be treated only by providing water. "Adjuvant" therapy was the restriction of sodium and protein in the patient's diet, thus decreasing the excreted osmols and water

Chlorothiazide, the first thiazide diuretic, was introduced into clinical medicine in 1958. Crawford, Kennedy and Hill discovered in 1960 that in patients with central diabetes insipidus the high urine volume can be halved by the administration of the new drug. In our several studies we could corroborate the original results of these authors and extended those with other classes of diuretics (Radó, Bános, Marosi et al. 1968). The thiazide diuretic acts by inhibiting sodium reabsorption in the distal convoluted tubule which interferes with urine dilution, on the one hand, and (indirectly) enhances sodium reabsorption in the proximal tubules on the other. This latter mechanism decreases the delivery of the filtrate to the distal nephron and enhances there the reabsorption of sodium and water reducing by that the excreted volume of urine (Earley and Orloff 1962; Osio, Robertson, Norgard and Juul 2013). Modern studies proved that the antidiuretic effect of hydrochlorothiazide in lithium-induced NDI is associated with upregulation of the aquaporin 2, the Na-Cl cotransporter and the epithelial sodium channel (Kim, Lee, Oh et al. 2004). *In the paradoxical thiazide antidiuresis finally sodium reabsorption (and water reabsorption) is increasing both in the proximal and distal nephron.*

Thiazides can be combined with amiloride, indomethacine, DDAVP etc. Congenital NDI was treated successfully with a thiazide combined with large doses of DDAVP (Mizuno, Fujimoto, Sugiyama et al. 2003)

Indomethacine, a prostaglandin synthetase inhibitor was also found to have antidiuretic properties in NDI. The efficiency is dependent upon inhibition of prostaglandin synthesis. Prostaglandins antagonize the effect of vasopressin. Indomethacine therefore increases concentrating capacity. According to Osio, Robertson, Norgard and Juul (2013) indomethacine probably acts by inhibiting the retrieval of acquaporin 2 water channels from the apical membrane of the principal cells. Simon, Garber and Arieff used indomethacine in lithium-induced NDI in 1977; Libber, Harrison and Spector administered it in 1986; Allen, Jackson, Winchester et al. in 1989; Vierhapper in 1990; Radó and Zdravkova in 1991 and 1993; and Thompson, France and Baylis in 1997. We administered indomethacine together with desmopressin in a patient with Bartter syndrome, and found a dramatic antidiuretic effect (Radó, Simatupang, Boer et al.1978). In our recent study (Radó 2018) we found that indomethacine had a more pronounced antidiuretic effect than piroxicam, another non-steroid anti-inflammatory compound.

For *Desmopressin (1-Deamino-8-D-Arginine Vasopressin: DDAVP),* structural alterations of the vasopressin molecule resulted in increased antidiuretic potency, longer duration of action and lacking pressor effect due to decreased vasoconstrictor activity. In our studies carried out over 40 years we have demonstrated a relationship between the dose and both the magnitude and the duration of the antidiuretic effect (Radó et al. 1975c, 1976c). Robertson and his coworkers (Osio, Robertson, Norgard and Juul 2013) wrote about our early investigations that "in patients with neurohypophyseal diabetes insipidus rapid infusion of 1 /ug DDAVP increased urine osmolality to a maximum of 700-800 mOm/Kg; further increases in dosage only prolonged the duration of action from an average of 26 hours after 1 /ug to 46 hours after 8 /ug." Our further studies revealed large interindividual variability in the magnitude and duration of the antidiuretic response of DDAVP, which was contributed -at least in part- to the interindividual differences in renal concentrating power (Radó et al. 1976a). The long duration of action of DDAVP is attributed mainly to its slow metabolic (enzymatic) degradation, and both shortened duration of action (Radó et al. 1976b) and lengthened duration of action (Radó et al 1975b) were reported under varying pharmacological circumstances. . Comparison of the antidiuretic effects of single intravenous and intranasal doses of DDAVP in diabetes insipidus was also an important part of our investigations (Radó, Marosi and Fischer 1977). Intranasal administration of DDAVP was at that time a comfortable way of administration and proved to be reliable. Today DDAVP therapy can be carried out by oral melting tablets. We have elaborated a diagnostic procedure for the differentiation of the various concentrating defects by intranasal administration of DDAVP, the "DDAVP concentrating test" (Radó 1978).

"Vasopressin-like" antidiuretic action has been reported after administration of carbamazepine, even leading to water intoxication (Radó 1973). Clofibrate has also a similar effect. The development of a drug-induced inappropriate secretion of antidiuretic hormone syndrome has been described after combined administration of carbamazepine and clofibrate (Radó, Juhos and Sawinsky 1975a). Combination of carbamazepine and chlorpropamide was effective in the treatment of "hyporesponder" diabetes insipidus (Radó et al 1974a). Antidiuretic effect of small doses of DDAVP could be enhanced by the coadministration of carbamazepine or/and clofibrate and can be inhibited by glyburide (Radó 1974b,c).

Indomethacine and DDAVP was used for the first time in lithium induced NDI in 1990 by and Weinstock and Moses and in 1991 by Stasior, Kikeri, Duel and Seifter. We used successfully excessive doses of DDAVP combined with indomethacine or piroxicam for the alleviation of polyuria in lithium induced NDI (Radó and Zdravkova 1993; Radó 2018)

Amiloride is a potassium retaining (antikaluretic) diuretic. Polyuria and polydipsia due to lithium-induced NDI decreases during administration of amiloride. Amiloride improved responsiveness to arginine-vasopressin stimulated translocation of AQP 2 to the apical membrane of the principal cell and increased AQP2 excretion as well as maximal urinary osmolality (Bedford Leader, Jing et al. 2008b). Inhibiting the lithium- induced epithelial sodium channel in the collecting duct with amiloride reduces the lithium induced down-regulation of the acquaporin 2 expression. Amiloride reduces transcellular lithium transport, intracellular lithium concentration and lithium-induced inactivation of GSK-3-beta (Kalra, Zargar, Sunil et al. 2016). Amiloride therapy alleviated also the chronic lithium therapy produced progressive interstitial fibrosis and hyperplastic changes in the medullary collecting ducts (Croft, Bedford, Leader and Walker 2018).

A Vasopressin–analogue (DDAVP) in NDI a "Vasopressin-Resistant" Condition?
Yes, In Large Doses in NDI.

Per definition, NDI is a vasopressin-resistant condition. In two congenital cases of Moses, Scheinman and Oppenheim (1984), however, NDI responded to large doses of DDAVP. Though 25-50 times as resistant to DDAVP nasal spray as Radó's patients with central diabetes insipidus (Radó 1975c) these patients could be treated effectively with large doses of the nasal spray. Our dosage protocol is in total agreement with the calculation of Moses, Scheinman and Oppenheim. We gave 250-300 /ug DDAVP nasal spray to our lithium induced NDI patient, which is ca 25 times more than a normal 10 /ug dose (Radó 2018). In our patient with lithium- induced NDI (Radó 2018) 24 hr urine osmolality before treatment was 175 mOsm/Kg, while under treatment with excessive doses of DDAVP plus indomethacine it was 280 mOsm/Kg. Others have similar experiences (Osio, Robertson, Norgard and Juul 2013; Mizuno, Fujimoto, Sugiyama et al. 2003; Stasior, Kikeri, Duel and Seifter 1991; Weinstock and Moses 1990).

Conclusions

Lithium is important for the world's millions of patients with recurrent episodes of bipolar disorder -- based on the works of Ban 2017, Blackwell 2014 and 2018, Rybakowski 2017, Severus 2014 and others. Lithium remains a key treatment, although its use needs monitoring and a safety-conscious approach is needed (Shine, McKnight, Leaver and Geddes 2015). The burden of the not too uncommon side effect, the lithium-induced NDI can be alleviated somewhat by the clever use of modern antidiuretic agents (indomethacine combined with excessive doses of desmopressin), including also the use of amiloride, and thiazides.

References:

Aiff H, Attman P, Aurell M, Bendz H, Schön S, Svedlund J. The impact of modern treatment principles may have eliminated lithium-induced renal failure. Journal of Psychopharmacology. 2014; 28:151-4.

Ban TA. Neuropsychopharmacology in Historical Perspective. Education in the Field in the Post-Neuropsychopharmacology Era. Prologue. inhn.org.education. September 18, 2017.

Bedford JJ, Weggery S, Ellis G, McDonald FJ, Joyce PR, Leader JP, Walker RJ. Lithium-induced nephrogenic diabetes insipidus: renal effects of Amiloride. Clin J Am Soc Nephrol 2008a; 3:1324-31.

Bedford JJ, Leader JP, Jing R, Walker RJ, Klein JD, Sands JM, Walker RJ. Amiloride restores renal medullary osmollytes in lithium-induced nephrogenic diabetes insipidus. Am. J. Physiol. Renal. Physiol. 2008b; F812-F820.

Bendz H. Kidney function in lithium treated patients. Acta Psychiat

Scand 1983; 68:303.

Bendz H, Aurell M, Balldin J, Mathe A, Sjodin I. Kidney damage in long term lithium patients: A cross sectional study of patients with 15 years or more on lithium. Nephrol Dial Transplant 1994; 9:1250-4.

Bendz H, Schön S, Attman P, Aurell M. Renal failure occurs in chronic lithium treatment but is uncommon. Kidney International 2010; 77:219-24.

Blackwell B. Lithium Controversy. A historical autopsy. inhn.org.controversies. June 19, 2014.

Blackwell B. Final reply to Janos Radó's final comment. inhn.org.controversies. May 10, 2018.

Boccalandro C, De Mattia F, Guo DC, Xue L, Orlander P, King TM, Gupta P, Deen PM, Lavis VR, Milewicz DM. Characterization of an aquaporin-2 water channel gene mutation causing partial nephrogenic diabetes insipidus in a Mexican family: Evidence of increased frequency of the mutation in the town of origin. J Am Soc Nephrol 2004; 15:1223-31.

Boton R, Gauiria M, Battle D. Prevalence, pathogenesis, and treatment of renal dysfunction associated with chronic lithium therapy. Amer. J Kidney Dis 1987; 10:329- 45.

Cade JP. Lithium salts in the treatment of psychotic excitement. Med J Australia 1949; 2:349-52.

Canfield MC, Tamarappoo BK, Moses AM, Verkman AS, Holtzman EJ. Identification and characterization of aquaporin-2 water channel mutations causing nephrogenic diabetes insipidus with partial vasopressin response. Human Molecular Genetics 1997; 6:1865-71.

Crawford JD, Kennedy GC, Hill LE. Clinical results of treatment of diabetes insipidus with drugs of the chlorothiazide series. N Engl J Med 1960; 262:739-42.

Croft PK, Bedford JJ, Leader JP, Walker RJ. Amiloride modifies the progression of lithium-induced renal interstitial fibrosis. Nephrology (Carlton). 2018; 3(1):20-30.

Davis J, Desmond M, Berk M. Lithium and nephrotoxicity: a literature review of approaches to clinical management and risk stratification. BMC Nephrology 2018; 19:305.

Fujiwara TM, Bichet DG. Molecular Biology of hereditary diabetes insipidus. J Am Soc Nephrol 2005; 16:2836-46.

Earley LE, Orloff J. The mechanism of antidiuresis associated with the administration of hydrochlorothiazide to patients with vasopressin resistant diabetes insipidus. J Clin Invest 1962; 41:1988-97.

Hestbech J, Hansen HE, Amdisen A. Chronic renal lesions following long-term treatment with lithium. Kidney Int 1977; 12:205-13.

Johnson G. Lithium early development, toxicity and renal function Neuropsychopharmacology 1998; 19:200-5

Johnson G, Glenn E, Hunt G, Duggin G, Horvath JS, Tiller DJ. Renal function and lithium treatment: initial and follow up tests in Manic - Depressive patients. J. Affective Disorders 1984; 6:249-63.

Johnson G. Comment on Janos Radó's (January 25, 2018) final comment (Barry Blackwell: The Lithium Controversy. A historical autopsy). inhn.org.collated. July 5, 2018.

Kalra S, Zargar AH, Sunil MJ, Bipin S, Chowdhury S, Singh AK, Thomas N, Unnikrishnan AG, Thakkar PB, Malve H. Diabetes insipidus: The other diabetes. Indian J Endocr Metab 2016; 20:9-21.

Kim GH, Lee JW, Oh YK, Chang HR, Joo KW, Na KY, Earm JH, Knepper MA, Han JS. Antidiuretic effect of hydrochlorothiazide in lithium-induced nephrogenic diabetes insipidus is associated with upregulation of aquaporin 2, Na-Cl cotransporter and epithelial sodium channel. J Am Soc Nephrol 2004; 15:2836-43.

Libber S, Harrison M, Spector D. Treatment of Nephrogenic diabetes insipidus with prostaglandin synthesis inhibitors. J Pediatr 1986; 108:305-11.

Mizuno H, Fujimoto S, Sugiyama Y, Kobayashi M, Ohro Y, Uchida S, Sasaki S, Togari H. Successful treatment of partial nephrogenic diabetes insipidus with thiazide and desmopressin. Horm Res. 2003; 59:297-300.

Moses AM, Scheinman SJ, Oppenheim A. Marked hypotonic polyuria resulting from nephrogenic diabetes insipidus with partial sensitivity to vasopressin. J Clin Endocrinol Meta.1984; 59:1044–9.

Nielsen J, Hoffert JD, Knepper MA, Agre P, Nielsen S, Fenton RA. Proteomic analysis of lithium-induced nephrogenic diabetes insipidus: Mechanisms for aquaporin 2 down-regulation and cellular proliferation. PNAS 2008; 105:3634-9.

Osio Y, Robertson GL, Norgard JP, Juul KV. Clinical review: Treatment of neurohypophyseal diabetes insipidus. J Clin Endocrinol Metab 2013; 98:3958-67.

Radó J. Final comment (Use of modern antidiuretic agents in the treatment of permanent lithium-induced nephrogenic diabetes insipidus [Barry Blackwell: The lithium controversy. A historical autopsy]). inhn.org.collated. January 25, 2018.

Radó JP. Water intoxication during carbamazepine treatment. Brit Med J. 1973; 3:479.

Radó JP. Combination of carbamazepine and chlorpropamide in the treatment of "hyporesponder" diabetes insipidus. J Clin Endocrinol Metab 1974; 1:38.

Radó JP. 1-desamino-8-D-arginine vasopressin (DDAVP) concentration test. Am J Med Sci 1978; 275:43-52.

Radó JP, Bános Cs, Marosi J, Borbély L, Takó. Investigation on diuretic and antidiuretic properties of furosemide in diabetes insipidus. Endokrinologie 1968; 53:253-60.

Radó JP, Juhos É, Sawinsky I. Dose-response relations in drug-induced inappropriate secretion of ADH: Effects of clofibrate and carbamazepine. Int J Clin Pharmacol 1975a; 12:315-19.

Radó JP, Marosi J. Prolongation of duration of action of 1-deamino-8-D-arginine vasopressin (DDAVP) by ineffective doses of clofibrate in diabetes insipidus. Horm Metab Res 1975b; 7:527-8.

Radó JP, Marosi J, Borbely L, Tako J. Individual differences in the antidiuretic response induced by single doses of 1-deamino-8-D-arginine-vasopressin (DDAVP) in patients with pituitary diabetes insipidus. Int J Clin Pharmacol Biopharm 1976a; 14:259-65.

Radó JP, Marosi J, Fischer J. Shortened duration of action of 1-deamino-8-D-arginine vasopressin (DDAVP) in patients with diabetes insipidus requiring high doses of peroral antidiuretic drugs. J Clin Pharmacol 1976b; 16:518-24.

Radó JP, Marosi J, Fischer J. Comparison of the antidiuretic effects of single intravenous and intranasal doses of DDAVP in diabetes insipidus. Pharmacology 1977; 15:40-5.

Radó JP, Marosi J, Fischer J, Tako J, Kiss N. Relationship between the dose of 1-deamino-8-d-arginine vasopressin (DDAVP) and the antidiuretic response in man. Endokrinologie 1975c; 66:184-95.

Radó JP, Marosi J, Szende L, Borbely L, Tako J, Fischer J. The antidiuretic action of 1-deamino-8-D-arginine vasopressin (DDAVP) in man. Int J Clin Pharmacol Biopharm 1976c; 13:199-209.

Radó JP, Szende L, Marosi J. Influence of glyburide on the antidiuretic response induced by 1-deamino-8-d-arginine vasopressin in patients with pituitary diabetes insipidus. Metabolism 1974b; 23:1057-1063.

Radó JP, Simatupang T, Boer P, Dorhout Mees EJ. Pharmacologic studies in Bartter's syndrome: effect of DDAVP and indomethacin on renal concentrating operation. Part II. Int J Clin Pharmacol Biopharm 1978; 16:22-6.

Radó JP, Szende L. Simultaneous familial occurrence of distal renal tubular acidosis, polycystic kidney and nephrogenic diabetes insipidus. Orvosi Hetilap 1995; 136:995-1001.

Radó JP, Szende L, Marosi J, Juhos É, Sawinsky I, Takó J. Inhibition of the diuretic action of glibenclamide by clofibrate, carbamazepine and 1-deamino-8-D-arginin vasopressin (DDAVP) in patients with pituitary diabetes insipidus. Acta Diabetologia Latina 1974c; 11:179-97.

Radó JP, Zdravkova S. Lithium-induced chronic water-metabolism disorder (nephrogenic diabetes insipidus)]. Orv Hetil. 1991; 132:1987-90.

Radó JP, Zdravkova S. Effect of Indomethacine and Calcitonin During Administration of 1-Deamino-8-D-Arginin-Vasopressin (dDAVP) on Free Water Clearance in Nephrogenic Diabetes Insipidus (NDI). XIIth International Congress of Nephrology. June 13–18, 1993 Jerusalem, Israel.

Rybakowski J. Final comment: Half a Century of Inspiring Lithium Controversy. Barry Blackwell: The Lithium controversy: A historical autopsy. Collated by Olaf Fjetland. inhn.org.collated. September 30, 2017.

Schou M. Lithium studies. 1. Toxicity Acta Pharmacol Toxicol 1958; 15:70-84.

Shine B, McKnight RF, Leaver L, Geddes JR. Long term effects of lithium on renal, thyroid, and parathyroid function: retrospective analysis of laboratory data. The Lancet 2015; 386:461-8.

Severus E, Taylor MJ, Sauer C, Pfennig A, Ritter P, Bauer M, Geddes

JR. Lithium for prevention of mood episodes in bipolar disorders: systematic review and meta-analysis. International Journal of Bipolar Disorders 2014; 2:15.

Simon NM, Garber E, Arieff AJ. Persistent nephrogenic diabetes insipidus after lithium carbonate. Ann Int Med 1977; 86:446-7.

Stasior DS, Kikeri D, Duel B, Seifter JL. Nephrogenic diabetes insipidus responsive to indomethacine plus dDAVP. New Eng J Med 1991; 324:850-1.

Thompson CJ, France AJ, Baylis PH. Persistent nephrogenic diabetes insipidus following lithium therapy. Scottish Medical Journal 1997; 42:16-7.

Vierhapper H. Indomethacine in the treatment of lithium-induced nephrogenic diabetes insipidus. Arch Int Med 1990; 150:2419.

Weinstock RS Moses AM. Desmopressin and indomethacine therapy for nephrogenic diabetes insipidus in patients receiving lithium carbonate. South Med J 1990; 83:1475-7.

May 2, 2019

JANOS RADÓ: DESMOPRESSIN MAY COUNTERACT POLYURIA IN LITHIUM-INDUCED NEPHROGENIC DIABETES INSIPIDUS

REVIEW OF THE LITERATURE

ABSTRACT

Lithium is a simple ion that remains the best, safest and least expensive treatment for the prevention of recurrent episodes of bipolar disorder. However, in many patients administration of lithium is associated with renal side effects. The most frequent side effect is a defect in urinary concentration which may lead to permanent lithium-induced nephrogenic diabetes insipidus. In the older literature this problem was treated with great attention; in the most recent publications, however, lithium-induced nephrogenic insipidus is hardly mentioned. Patients suffer from a disturbed night therefore it is an eminent goal to secure them some rest.

In our previous work administration of excessive doses of desmopressin resulted in clinically relevant antidiuresis in lithium-induced nephrogenic insipidus enhanced by indomethacine (Radó and Zdravkova 1991; Radó 2018a,b; Radó 2019). The purpose of the present paper is to review the literature concerning the use of desmopressin in lithium-induced nephrogenic diabetes insipidus.

Introduction

Lithium is a simple ion that remains the best, safest and least expensive treatment for the prevention of recurrent episodes of bipolar disorder (Blackwell 2018). This concept is supported by many reports, among them those of Ban (2017); Gupta, Kripafani, Khastgir and Reilly (2013); Rybakowski (2017); and Severus, Taylor, Sauer et al. (2014). However, its use has gradually declined and many less-established drugs are preferred. It is underused because of its low therapeutic index, the need for regular blood tests and perceptions about its adverse effects, including renal problems (Gupta, Kripafani, Khastgir, Reilly 2013)

The most frequent renal problem encountered is the disturbance in water metabolism due to lithium-induced insufficiency in renal concentrating operation resulting in polyuria and polydipsia. Daily urine volume increases, in many cases more than 3-5 liters a day (Johnson 2018; Warnes 2019), but we have seen a patient, in whom in a stage of her long history it was more than 10 liters. Patients suffer from a disturbed night. Therefore, it is an eminent goal to secure some rest for them. In the older literature this problem seemed to be very important (Johnson, Glenn, Hunt et al. 1984; Johnson 1998; Radó and Zdravkova 1991) and was treated with great attention. In the most recent publications, however, lithium-induced nephrogenic insipidus is hardly mentioned (Gupta and Khastgear 2017; Davis, Desmond and Berk 2018). The recommended drugs are mostly a thiazide diuretic (Mizuno, Fujimoto, Sugiyama et al. 2003), indomethacine (Weinstock and Moses 1990) and amiloride (Croft, Bedford, Leader and Walker 2018).

A Short Pharmacology of Desmopressin

Structural alterations of the vasopressin molecule resulted in 1-deamino-8-D-arginine vasopressin (DDAVP) or desmopressin, with increased antidiuretic potency, longer duration of action and lacking a pressor effect due to decreased vasoconstrictor activity. In our studies carried out over 40 years we have demonstrated a relationship between the dose and both the magnitude and the duration of the antidiuretic effect (Radó, Marosi, Fischer et al. 1975a; Radó, Marosi, Szende et al.1976c). Robertson and his coworkers (Oiso, Robertson, Norgard and Juul 2013) wrote about our early investigations that "in patients with neurohypophyseal diabetes insipidus rapid infusion of 1 micgr desmopressin increased urine osmolality to a maximum of 700-800 mOm/Kg; further increases in dosage only prolonged the duration of action from an average of 26 hours after 1 micgr to 46 hours after 8 micgr."

Our further studies revealed large interindividual variability in the magnitude and duration of the antidiuretic response of desmopressin, which was contributed - at least in part - to the interindividual differences in renal concentrating power (Radó, Marosi, Borbely and

Tako 1976a). The long duration of action of desmopressin is attributed mainly to its slow metabolic (enzymatic) degradation and both shortened duration of action (Radó, Marosi and Fischer 1976b) and lengthened duration of action (Radó and Marosi 1975b) were reported under varying pharmacological circumstances.

The effect of desmopressin was inhibited by glyburide, an antidiabetic compound, probably by competitive antagonism (Radó, Szende and Marosi 1974a; Radó, Szende, Marosi et al. 1974b) A similar antagonism by calcitonine was discovered later (Radó 2018ab). Comparison of the antidiuretic effects of single intravenous and intranasal doses of desmopressin in diabetes insipidus was also an important part of our investigations (Radó, Marosi and Fischer 1977). Intranasal administration of desmopressin was at that time a comfortable way of administration and proved to be reliable and today desmopressin therapy can be carried out by ingesting dissolving tablets (Walle, Stockner, Raes and Nørgaard 2007).

We have elaborated a diagnostic procedure for the differentiation of the various concentrating defects by intranasal administration of desmopressin, the "desmopressin concentrating test" (Radó 1978). When we started our studies with desmopressin a "supramaximal" dose was 300 microgr given intranasally. In these early human pharmacology investigations 320 mcg was given as a quasi "single dose" during one hour to patients with neurohypophyseal (central) diabetes insipidus (Radó and Marosi 1975b). When we used desmopressin for nephrogenic diabetes insipidus 300 microgr was given during 24 hrs. (Radó and Zdravkova 1991). In the meantime, however, it became known desmopressin may also be effective in hematologic disorders; for these disorders, in certain cases, desmopressin was given in very extreme doses. The industry produced desmopressin preparations containing very high concentrations of desmopressin intended to act on the blood clotting mechanism for bleeding disorders. By using such a preparation (Octim Nasal Spray Ferring Pharmaceuticals Ltd) administration of 300 micrgr (150 micrgr into both nostrils) as a single dose is easily feasible. To the best of my knowledge this preparation has not been tried, up to now, in the therapy of the lithium-induced permanent nephrogenic diabetes insipidus.

Desmopressin Administered Alone in Nephrogenic Diabetes Insipidus

Although nephrogenic diabetes insipidus is said to be "vasopressin resistant," on the basis of ours and others' previous investigations we did not exclude the use of certain vasopressin derivatives in this condition because vasopressin resistance in many cases is not absolute (Canfield, Tamarappoo, Moses et al. 1997; Fujiwara and Bichet 2005; Khanna 2006; Oiso, Robertson, Norgard and Juul 2013; Moses, Scheinman and Oppenheim 1984). Large doses of desmopressin were successfully given to patients with congenital nephrogenic diabetes insipidus for antidiuretic purposes (Boccalandro, De Mattia, Guo et al. 2004; Canfield, Tamarappoo, Moses et al. 1997; Khanna 2006; Oiso, Robertson, Norgard and Juul 2013; Moses, Scheinman and Oppenheim 1984). The effectiveness of relatively large doses of vasopressin (and also excessive doses of desmopressin) can be significantly different even within one family with congenital nephrogenic diabetes insipidus (Radó and Szende 1995; Radó 2019). Probably the degree of resistance to vasopressin (desmopressin) may differ among the family members: one family member was treated successfully with desmopressin for decades and the case was published because the (congenital nephrogenic) diabetes insipidus was later associated with diabetes mellitus (Radó 2011). In our previous work we found that in a patient with lithium-induced permanent nephrogenic diabetes insipidus in response to excessive desmopressin doses free water excretion (expressed in the percentage of glomerular filtration rate (CH2Ox100/GFR)) significantly decreased and urine osmolality significantly increased (Radó 2018a).

A very special observation

Müller, Marr, Ankermann et al. (2002) investigated two unrelated families in which two children had inherited primary nocturnal enuresis and nephrogenic diabetes insipidus; they had mutations in the aquaporin-2 gene. The mutant proteins were inactive, suggesting that administration of desmopressin could not concentrate the urine in these patients. However, treatment with desmopressin resolved primary nocturnal enuresis completely.

Combination of Desmopressin with Other Antidiuretic Agents in Nephrogenic Diabetes Insipidus

Mizuno, Fujimoto, Sugiyama et al. (2003) treated a seven-year-old boy suffering from congenital nephrogenic diabetes insipidus who had demonstrated a partial response to desmopressin. Neither a low salt diet and a thiazide nor a large dose of desmopressin was effective in reduction of daily urine volume. However combination of thiazide and a large dose of desmopressin resulted in a decrease in urine volume and disappearance of nocturia.

Indomethacine and desmopressin was used for the first time in lithium induced nephrogenic diabetes insipidus in 1990 by Weinstock and Moses. They found in their two patients that indomethacine alone was practically ineffective, but in combination with large doses of desmopressin urine volume decreased by 47% and 63% respectively, while urine osmolalities increased by200% and 227% respectively.

Stasior, Kikeri, Duel and Seifter (1991) reported a patient with lithium-induced nephrogenic diabetes insipidus who was responsive to desmopressin in the presence of indomethacine, but not to desmopressin or indomethacine alone. A single dose of 6 micgr desmopressin subcutaneously (not a too large dose!) without indomethacine caused an increase in urine osmolality from 187 mOsm/Kg to 270 mOsm/Kg (44%). However, in response to the same dose of desmopressin in the presence of indomethacine urine osmolality increased from106 mOsm/Kg to 384 mOsm/Kg (262%).
In our patient urine volume and free water clearance significantly decreased while urine osmolality significantly increased after administration of the combination of indomethacine and

desmopressin as compared to desmopressin administered alone (Radó 2018a).

In our further studies piroxicam plus desmopressin, as compared to desmopressin (administered alone), was also antidiuretic: urine volume and free water excretion decreased while urine osmolality increased without any consistent change in osmolal clearance, glomerular filtration rate and serum osmolality. These results support the contention that indomethacine is not the only nonsteroidal anti-inflammatory compound which can be used in the antidiuretic therapy. However, piroxicam seemed to be less antidiuretic than indomethacine by 20-30%.

Antidiuretic properties have been demonstrated for chlorpropamide, carbamazepine and clofibrate which potentiate the effect of desmopressin (Radó 2019). From these compounds probably only carbamazepine may be useful in a limited extent in the treatment of the lithium-induced nephrogenic insipidus. Statins (Bonfrate, Procino, Wang et al. 2015; Milano, Carmoniso, Gerbino and Procino 2017); metformin (Efe, Klein, LaRocque et al. 2016); sildenafil and calcitonine (Milano, Carmoniso, Gerbino and Procino 2017); prasugrel (Zhang, Peti-Peterdi, Brandes et al. 2017); and clopidrogel (Zhang, Peti-Peterdi, Heiney et al. 2015) were also shown to have some antidiuretic capabilities. Only calcitonine was combined with desmopressin (Radó 2018 a,b). In our hands, however, it was not an antidiuretic factor.

Administration of excessive doses of desmopressin resulted in clinically relevant antidiuresis, enhanced by indomethacine and abolished by calcitonine (Radó 2018a). Calcitonine is a "tricky" hormone, having both diuretic and antidiuretic properties. Diuretic effect of calcitonine was an observation found mainly in the older literature and is in harmony with our published data on a water mobilizing action (Radó 1991, 1993, 2018a). On the other hand, water retaining action was found (Elalouf, Roinel and de Rouffignac 1986) in response to human calcitonine in rats during micropuncture studies simulating the changes induced by desmopressin. Calcitonin was recommended as a possible treatment for hereditary nephrogenic diabetes insipidus by Milano, Carmoniso, Gerbino and Procino (2017).

Combinations of hydrochlorothiazide with indomethacine, amiloride with thiazide diuretics have additive antidiuretic effects (Milano, Carmoniso, Gerbino and Procino 2017). All could have been combined - at least theoretically - with desmopressin to have a really potentiated antidiuretic intervention for the treatment of lithium-induced nephrogenic diabetes insipidus.

Conclusion

It is important to save lithium treatment for millions of people suffering from bipolar disorder and other psychiatric abnormalities in an age when its use has gradually declined and many less-established drugs are preferred (Gupta, Kripafani, Khastgir, Reilly 2013.) This can be done (at least partly) by demonstrating that treatment of lithium-induced permanent nephrogenic diabetes insipidus is not so hopeless as it appears from some recent articles dealing with lithium induced nephrotoxicity. Our therapeutic armamentarium include several drugs, thiazide diuretics, nonsteroid anti-inflammatory drugs, amiloride and desmopressin. In this article we dealt with desmopressin administered alone and in combination with other drugs in the treatment of congenital, as well as lithium-induced nephrogenic diabetes insipidus. On the basis of the available literature desmopressin alone and in combination with other antidiuretic drugs seemed to be an effective means in counteracting lithium-induced polyuria.

References:

Ban TA: Neuropsychopharmacology in Historical Perspective. Education in the Field in the Post-Neuropsychopharmacology Era. Prologue. inhn.org.education. September 18, 2017.

Blackwell B. Lithium Controversy. A historical autopsy. inhn.org.controversies. June 19, 2014.

Blackwell B. Final reply to Janos Radó's final comment.

inhn.org.controversies. May 10, 2018.

Boccalandro C, De Mattia F, Guo DC, Xue L, Orlander P, King TM, Gupta P, Deen PM, Lavis VR, Milewicz DM. Characterization of an aquaporin-2 water channel gene mutation causing partial nephrogenic diabetes insipidus in a Mexican family: Evidence of increased frequency of the mutation in the town of origin. J Am Soc Nephrol 2004; 15:1223-31.

Bonfrate L, Procino G, Wang DQ-H, Svelto M, Portincasa P. A novel therapeutic effect of statins in nephrogenic diabetes insipidus. J Cell Mol Med 2015;19:265-82.

Canfield MC, Tamarappoo BK, Moses AM, Verkman AS, Holtzman EJ. Identification and characterization of aquaporin-2 water channel mutations causing nephrogenic diabetes insipidus with partial vasopressin response. Human Molecular Genetics 1997; 6: 1865-171.

Croft PK, Bedford JJ, Leader JP, Walker RJ. Amiloride modifies the progression of lithium-induced renal interstitial fibrosis. Nephrology (Carlton). 2018 Jan;23(1):20-30.

Davis J, Desmond M, Berk M. Lithium and nephrotoxicity: a literature review of approaches to clinical management and risk stratification. BMC Nephrology 2018; 19:305.

Efe O, Klein JD, LaRocque LM, Ren H, Sands JM. Metformin improves urine concentration in rodents with nephrogenic diabetes insipidus. JCI Insight. 2016 Jul 21;1(11).

Elalouf JM, Roinel N, de Rouffignac C. Effects of human calcitonin on water and electrolyte movements in rat juxtamedullary nephrons: inhibition of medullary K recycling. Pflugers Arch. 1986; 406:502-8.

Fujiwara TM, Bichet DG. Molecular Biology of hereditary diabetes insipidus. J Am Soc Nephrol 2005; 16:2836-46.

Gupta S, Kripafani M, Khastgir U, Reilly J. Management of the renal adverse effects of lithium. Advances in psychiatric treatment. 2013; 19, 457–66.

Gupta S, Khastgear U. Drug information update. Lithium and chronic kidney disease: debate and dilemmas. BJPsych Bulletin 2017;41:216-20.

Johnson G. Lithium early development, toxicity and renal function Neuropsychopharmacology 1998; 19:200-5

Johnson G, Glenn E, Hunt G, Duggin G, Horvath JS, Tiller DJ. Renal function and lithium treatment: initial and follow up tests in Manic-Depressive patients. J. Affective Disorders 1984; 6: 249-63.

Johnson G. Comment on Janos Radó's final comment. In: Blackwell B. The Lithium Controversy. A historical autopsy. inhn.org.collated. July 5, 2018.

Khanna A. Acquired nephrogenic diabetes insipidus. Semin Nephrol 2006;26: 244-8.

Milano S, Carmoniso M, Gerbino A, Procino G. Hereditary nephrogenic diabetes insipidus: Pathophysiology and possible treatment. An Update. Int J Mol Sci. 2017 Nov 10;18(11).

Mizuno H, Fujimoto S, Sugiyama Y, Kobayashi M, Ohro Y, Uchida S, Sasaki S, Togari H. Successful treatment of partial nephrogenic diabetes insipidus with thiazide and desmopressin. Horm Res. 2003;59(6):297-300.

Moses AM, Scheinman SJ, Oppenheim A. Marked hypotonic polyuria resulting from nephrogenic diabetes insipidus with partial sensitivity to vasopressin. J Clin Endocrinol Meta.1984; 59:1044–9.

Müller D, Marr N, Ankermann T, Eggert P, Deen PMT. Desmopressin for nocturnal enuresis in nephrogenic diabetes insipidus. Lancet 2002;359 (9305) 495-7.

Oiso Y1, Robertson GL, Nørgaard JP, Juul KV. Clinical review: Treatment of neurohypophyseal diabetes insipidus. J Clin Endocrinol Metab. 2013 Oct;98(10):3958-67.

Radó JP. 1-desamino-8-D-arginine vasopressin (desmopressin) concentration test. Am J Med Sci 1978; 275: 43-52.

Radó J. Diabetes mellitus és (nephrogen) diabetes insipidus együttes előfordulása. Hypertonia és Nephrologia 2011;15:183-7.

Radó J. Final comment (Use of modern antidiuretic agents in the treatment of permanent lithium-induced nephrogenic diabetes insipidus. In Blackwell B: The lithium controversy. A historical autopsy inhn.org.controversies. inhn.org.collated. January 25, 2018a.

Radó J. Addition to final comment. Calcitonin in lithium-induced nephrogenic diabetes insipidus. In Blackwell B. The lithium controversy. A historical autopsy. inhn.org.collated Sept.13, 2018b.

Radó J. Renal Toxicity of Lithium in Historical Perspective with Special Reference To Nephrogenic Diabetes Insipidus and its Treatment. inhn.org.collated May 2, 2019.

Radó JP, Marosi J. Prolongation of duration of action of 1-deamino-8-D-arginine vaso(desmopressin) by ineffective doses of clofibrate in diabetes insipidus. Horm Metab Res 1975b; 7: 527-8.

Radó JP, Marosi J, Borbely L, Tako J. Individual differences in the antidiuretic response induced by single doses of 1-deamino-8-D-arginine-vasopressin (desmopressin) in patients with pituitary diabetes insipidus. Int J Clin Pharmacol Biopharm 1976a; 14: 259-65.

Radó JP, Marosi J, Fischer J. Shortened duration of action of 1-deamino-8-D-arginine vasopressin (desmopressin) in patients with diabetes insipidus requiring high doses of peroral antidiuretic drugs. J Clin Pharmacol 1976b; 16: 518-24.

Radó JP, Marosi J, Fischer J. Comparison of the antidiuretic effects of single intravenous and intranasal doses of desmopressin in diabetes insipidus. Pharmacology 1977; 15: 40-5.

Radó JP, Marosi J, Fischer J, Tako J, Kiss N. Relationship between the dose of 1-deamino-8-d-arginine vasopressin (desmopressin) and the antidiuretic response in man. Endokrinologie 1975a; 66: 184-95.

Radó JP, Marosi J, Szende L, Borbely L, Tako J, Fischer J. The antidiuretic action of 1-deamino-8-D-arginine vasopressin (desmopressin) in man. Int J Clin Pharmacol Biopharm 1976c; 13: 199-209.

Radó JP, Szende L, Marosi J. Influence of glyburide on the antidiuretic response induced by 1-deamino-8-d-arginine vasopressin in patients with pituitary diabetes insipidus. Metabolism 1974a; 23:1057-63.

Radó JP, Simatupang T, Boer P, Dorhout Mees EJ. Pharmacologic studies in Bartter's syndrome: effect of desmopressin and indomethacin on renal concentrating operation. Part II. Int J Clin Pharmacol Biopharm 1978; 16:22-6.

Radó JP, Szende L. Simultaneous familial occurrence of distal renal tubular acidosis, polycystic kidney and nephrogenic diabetes insipidus. Orvosi Hetilap 1995; 136:995-1001.

Radó JP, Szende L, Marosi J, Juhos É, Sawinsky I, Takó J. Inhibition of the diuretic action of glibenclamide by clofibrate, carbamazepine and 1-deamino-8-D-arginin vasopressin (desmopressin) in patients with pituitary diabetes insipidus. Acta Diabetologia Latina 1974b;11:179-97.

Radó JP, Zdravkova S. Lithium-induced chronic water-metabolism disorder (nephrogenic diabetes insipidus). Orv Hetil. 1991;132, 1987-90.

Rybakowski J. Final comment: Half a Century of Inspiring Lithium Controversy. Barry Blackwell: The Lithium controversy: A historical autopsy. Collated by Olaf Fjetland. inhn.org. collated. September 30, 2017.

Severus E, Taylor MJ, Sauer C, Pfennig A, Ritter P, Bauer M, Geddes JR. Lithium for prevention of mood episodes in bipolar disorders: systematic review and meta-analysis. International Journal of Bipolar Disorders 2014; 2:15.

Stasior DS, Kikeri D, Duel B, Seifter JL. Nephrogenic diabetes insipidus responsive to indomethacine plus desmopressin. New Eng J Med 1991; 324: 850-1.

Vierhapper H. Indomethacine in the treatment of lithium-induced nephrogenic diabetes insipidus. Arch Int Med 1990; 150: 2419.

Walle JV, Stockner M, Raes A, Nørgaard JP. Desmopressin 30 years in clinical use: A safety review. Curr Drug Saf. 2007 2:232-8.

Warnes H. Comment on Janos Radó's additional final comment: Calcitonin in lithium-induced nephrogenic diabetes insipidus. In: Blackwell B: The lithium controversy. A historical autopsy. inhn.org.collated. January 16, 2019.

Weinstock RS, Moses AM. Desmopressin and indomethacine for nephrogenic diabetes insipidus in patients receiving lithium carbonate. South Med J 1990; 83: 1475-7.

ZhangY, Peti-Peterdi J, Brandes A, Riquier-Brison A, Carlson NG, Müller CE, Ecelbarger CM, Kishore BK. Prasugral suppresses development of lithium-induced nephrogenic diabetes insipidus in mice. Purinergic Signalling 2017; 13:239-48.

ZhangY, Peti-Peterdi J, Heiney KM, Riquier-Brison A, Carlson NG, Müller CE, Ecelbarger CM, Kishore BK. Clopidrogel attenuates lithium-induced alterations in renal water and sodium channels/transporters in mice. Purinergic Signalling 2015; 11:507-8.

June 27, 2019

JANOS RADÓ: USE OF MODERN ANTIDIURETIC AGENTS IN THE TREATMENT OF PERMANENT LITHIUM-INDUCED NEPHROGENIC DIABETES INSIPIDUS (ADMINISTRATION OF EXCESSIVE DOSES OF DESMOPRESSIN RESULTED IN CLINICALLY RELEVANT ANTIDIURESIS, ENHANCED BY INDOMETHACINE AND ABOLISHED BY CALCITONIN)

ABSTRACT

Recent views about lithium therapy ("Lithium has been firmly established as the first-choice drug for preventing mood episodes in bipolar disorders, meeting all requirements of the Evidence-Based Medicine" [Rybakowsky 2017]) made it worthwhile to seek further solutions for the alleviation of the side effects resulting from this therapy, first of all in the disturbance of water metabolism, occurring almost in every case of the patient population during long-term therapy. These views prompted us to publish our data concerning the use of modern antidiuretic agents in the treatment of "vasopressin resistant" lithium induced polyuria (permanent nephrogenic diabetes insipidus). We found that the administration of very high doses of Desmopressin resulted in clinically relevant antidiuresis, enhanced by Indomethacine and abolished by Calcitonine. Piroxicam, another nonsteroidal anti-inflammatory compound, also seemed to be antidiuretic, though in a less extent than indomethacine. The message of our writing is: in such an important form of psychiatric treatment as Lithium is, a serious disturbance of water metabolism can be alleviated by the clever use of modern antidiuretic interventions.

Introduction

Lithium was introduced into clinical medicine (again) by Cade in 1949, for the treatment of certain psychiatric disorders. This type of therapy spread worldwide, became the "gold standard" and then gave its place to other psychotropic, and later neuropsychopharmacologic compounds (Ban 2017). Differing from the fate of many other drugs, however, lithium did not disappear totally from the palette. From time to time it appears from the dark as a "gold standard in its time," and as a possibility to treat "refractory conditions." In addition, lithium was declared many times not only a remedy of acute conditions, but as a prophylactic measure for the prevention of acute episodes of the bipolar disorder. The writer of these opinions met several patients whose Lithium treatment was going to be stopped by his or her psychiatrist, but they all were very unsatisfied with this decision. I think that the fact that the lithium carbonate molecule was too "simple" as compared to the modern drugs with more complicated chemical structures, and that therapy with Lithium was burdened with the need to determine blood levels several times in each case, as well as the number of serious side effects, not mentioning the known "corporate corruptions" in the industry producing and promoting more modern medicines (Blackwell 2017), all may have played a role in the decreasing use of Lithium.

Excellent experts of lithium therapy stress the significance of this treatment. "Although a number of drugs with mood-stabilizing properties already exist, none has so far surpassed lithium as far as prophylactic efficacy in bipolar illness is concerned, not even to mention a duration of such prophylaxis" (Rybakowsky 2017). "The evidence base for lithium in the long-term treatment of bipolar disorders has strengthened. With no other drug available having such ample and consistent evidence for its efficacy lithium remains the most valuable treatment option in this indication" (Severus 2014). Further opinions about Lithium therapy can be found in collated documents in the INHN webpages under the heading Lithium controversy (Blackwell 2014.) In any case, use of lithium proved to be a valuable way to treat certain psychiatric diseases, with the probable capability to prevent acute episodes. Therefore, further studies concerning both the effects and side effects of lithium are not useless efforts even in the "molecular genetic era" of neuropsychopharmacology (Ban 2017).

Our Studies Concerning the Effects of Modern Antidiuretic Agents

One of the side effects of lithium is a disorder in renal concentrating operation (Forrest 1974; Glick 1984). The disturbance in water metabolism is appearing almost in every patient treated with lithium on a long-term basis (Allen 1989). The abnormality is frequently mild, manifesting in increased urine volume and polydipsia of various degree because of the decreased water reabsorption in the distal nephron. (Boccalandro 2004; Cohen 2002; Haris and Radó 2008; Kazama 2007). Sometimes, however, marked polyuria, resembling "diabetes insipidus" can develop. As this polyuria is "vasopressin resistant" by definition it is named "nephrogenic diabetes insipidus" (Bedford 2008; Kalra 2016; Radó 1978, 1998; Thompson 1997). We have dealt with these abnormalities for several years and during our studies we found a 61-year-old women patient suffering from affective bipolar disorder in whom nephrogenic diabetes insipidus developed during lithium therapy lasting more than 10 years. Her serum calcium, potassium and glucose levels were normal, 10 ug dDAVP into both nostrils was ineffective and the water deprivation test was negative. Therefore, diabetes mellitus, central diabetes insipidus and psychic polyuria have been excluded from the polyuric disorders, as well as the calcium or potassium abnormality induced nephrogenic diabetes (Radó 1991, 1993). As the polyuria did not cease after discontinuation of lithium it was named "permanent lithium induced nephrogenic diabetes insipidus" (Guirguis 2000; Neithercut 1990; Simon 1977). Although nephrogenic diabetes insipidus is said to be "vasopressin resistant," on the basis of our and others' previous investigations (Boccalandro 2004; Moses 1984; Radó 1978/b, 1995, 2004, 2007, 2011; Stasior 1991; Weinstock and Moses 1990), we did not exclude the use of certain vasopressin derivatives in this condition.

In our above-mentioned patient, polyuria developed during Lithium treatment; the average 24hr urine volume was 5483 ml, while the 24hr glomerular filtration rate (endogenous creatinine clearance) was only 31,5 ml/min. Alleviating polyuria is a very important immediate task in such patients: having a less disturbed night's rest. As mentioned above, despite the theoretical vasopressin resistant condition we gave excessive supramaximal doses of a very powerful antidiuretic compound, desmopressin (1-deamino-8-d-arginine – vasopressine, dDAVP). This vasopressin derivative molecule has an extremely strong antiuretic capability combined with a uniquely long duration of action (Radó 1975a,b, 1976a,b,c,d, 1977, 1978a). dDAVP was also given in certain cases of congenital and acquired nephrogenic diabetes insipidus for antidiuretic purposes (Boccalandro 2004; Moses 1984; Radó 1995). The administered doses were generally less then given by us. Nonsteroidal anti-inflammatory compounds have also been successfully administered in some cases of similar conditions. These drugs were administered also in Lithium induced polyuria (Allen 1989; Radó 1991, 1993, 1995; Weinstock and Moses 1990; Vierhapper 1990). However, in several cases of these disorders with excessive polyuria, administration of nonsteroidal drugs failed or the effect was not satisfactory as shown in our patient presented here. The combination of dDAVP and nonsteroidal drugs also have been tried (Weinstock and Moses 1990). In such cases we used a combination of nonsteroidal drugs with excessive - supramaximal doses of dDAVP. A way to administer these two drugs is reported here.

As our patient suffered too from very severe arthritic and osteogenic pains, Calcitonin was also given. During these studies we discovered that co-administration of Calcitonin with dDAVP can abolish the antidiuretic effect of the latter (Radó 1991,1993). Surprisingly, the original condition of the nephrogenic diabetes insipidus is restored when adding Calcitonin to the continued administration of dDAVP. One of our main purposes is to describe this interaction between dDAVP and Calcitonine.

Investigations Performed During Maintained Lithium Therapy

We studied our patient both during maintained lithium carbonate treatment and again several months after the discontinuation of lithium. During maintained lithium therapy the investigated parameters can be seen in Figures 1, 2 and 3. Standard methods were used in the laboratory determinations as well as in the statistics. The patient was allowed to drink water "ad libitum." Daily sodium intake was 100 mmol, potassium intake was 40 mmol. dDAVP was given 30-30 ug into both nostrils 5 times a day, at 8 am, 12 am, 4 pm, 8 pm, and 12 pm.

Urine was collected in 24hr clearance periods. After a 7-day "no drug" period, indomethacine (75 mg per day) was given for six days. After a wash-out period, dDAVP was administered for five consecutive days. After that, indomethacine and dDAVP were given in combination for a 6-day period. (Duration of investigational periods are indicated with "N" in the figures.) The combination of calcitonin and dDAVP was studied in a 11-day period (daily 100 IU calcitonin was given).

Results are Summarized in Figures 1-3 and in the Table

We can see in Figure 1 that indomethacine (administered alone) as compared to "no drug" did not cause significant change in urine volume and osmolality.

However, dDAVP (administered alone) as compared to "no drug" significantly decreased ($p<0.05$) free water excretion expressed in the percentage of glomerular filtration rate (CH_2Ox100/GFR) and increased ($p<0.05$) urine osmolality.

In response to dDAVP (administered alone) as compared to

indomethacine (administered alone), urine volume (1 asterisk= p<0.05) and free water excretion decreased (3 asterisks= p<0.001) while urine osmolality increased (p<0.001).

After administration of the combination of indomethacine and dDAVP as compared to dDAVP (administered alone), urine volume (p<0.001) and free water excretion (p<001) decreased while urine osmolality increased (p<0.001).

Figure 1

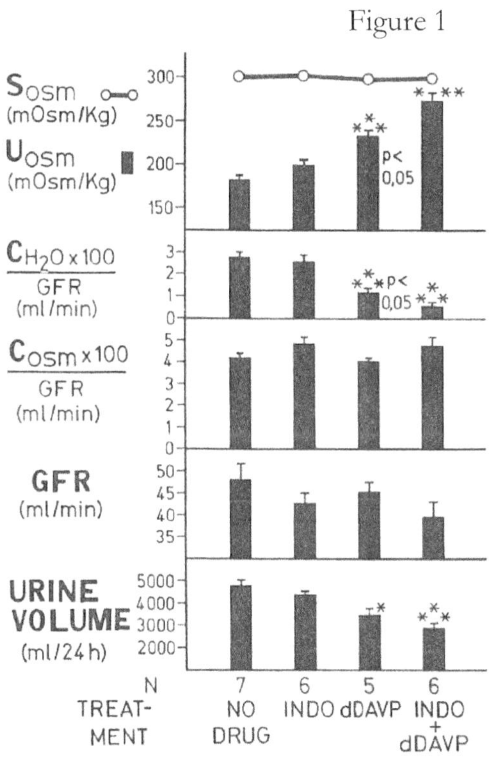

Legend to the Figure 1. The effects of various interventions (no drug, indomethacine, dDAVP (desmopressin), indomethacine and dDAVP) on specific renal functions were investigated in a patient with permanent lithium induced nephrogenic insipidus during maintained Lithium carbonate treatment. P>0.05= comparison with NO DRUG. ASTERISKS above dDAVP= comparison with INDO. ASTERISKS above INDO + dDAVP= comparison with dDAVP.

In Figure 2 we can see that dDAVP (administered alone) decreased urine volume (p<0.001) and free water excretion (p<0,01), while increased (p<0.05) urine osmolality as compared to "no drug" was seen. However, when calcitonin was combined with dDAVP urine volume (p<0.05) and free water excretion (p<0.001) increased and urine osmolality decreased (not significant) as compared to dDAVP (administered alone).

Figure 2

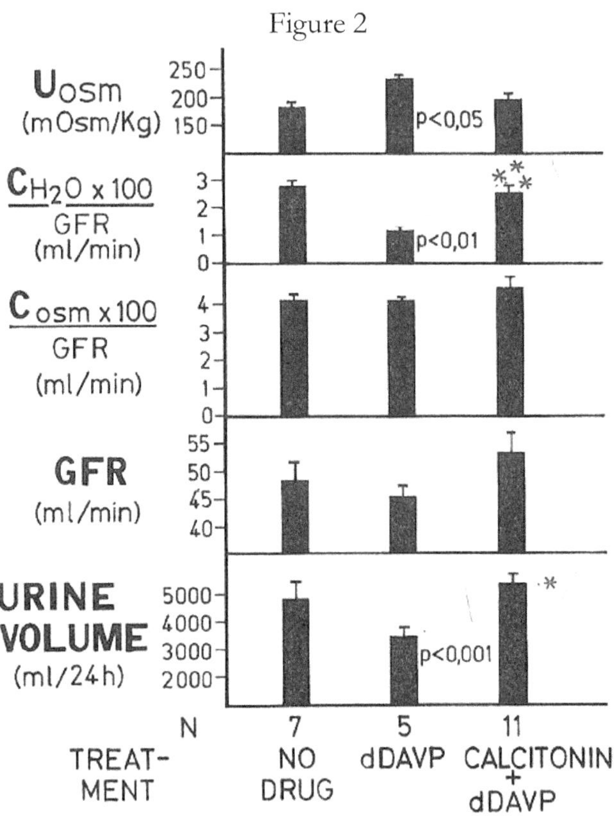

Legend to Figure 2. The effects of various interventions (no drug, dDAVP (desmopressin), Calcitonine and dDAVP) on specific renal functions were investigated in a patient with permanent Lithium induced nephrogenic insipidus during maintained lithium carbonate treatment. dDAVP induced a marked antidiuresis which has been abolished by Calcitonin despite further administration of dDAVP. ASTERISKS = comparison of CALCITONIN + dDAVP to dDAVP.

In Figure 3 changes of free water excretion (expressed in the percentage of glomerular filtration rate) can be seen. dDAVP (administered alone) caused a decrease, while co-administration of indomethacine and dDAVP potentiated this effect. Indomethacine (administered alone) was practically without any effect. Calcitonin abolished the effect of dDAVP.

Figure 3

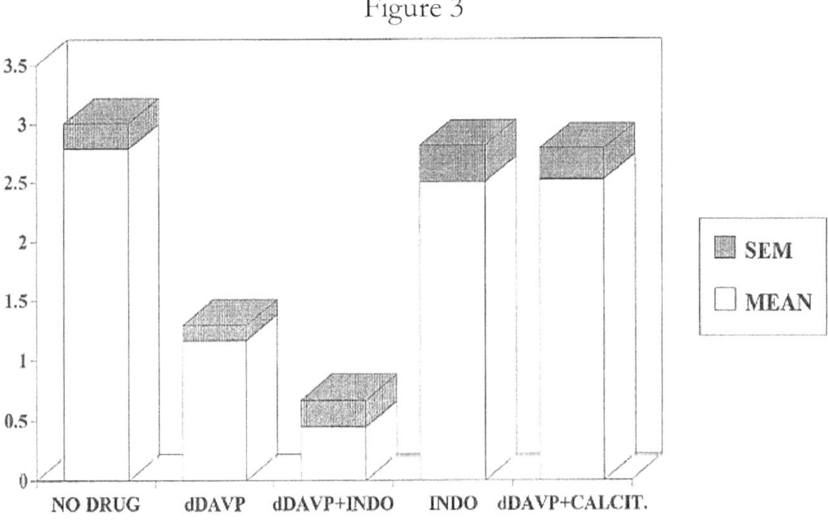

Legend to Figure 3. The effect of various interventions (no drug, dDAVP /desmopressin/, dDAVP and indomethacine, indomethacine, dDAVP and Calcitonin) on free water excretion expressed in the percentage of glomerular filtration was investigated in a patient with permanent lithium induced nephrogenic insipidus during maintained Lithium carbonate treatment. CH2Ox100/GFR ml/min mean values and standard error of the mean are given.

TABLE

DRUG	URINE VOLUME (ml/min)	Cosmxl00/ GFR (ml/min)	CH2OX1OO/ GFR (ml/min)
NO	4778+335	4.17+0.21	2.78+0.22
INDO	4350+180	4.76+0.31	2.50+0.32

dDAVP'	3480+299X	4.13+0.16	1.16+0.13XXX
INDO+dDAVP	2875 +161xxx	4.71+0.40	0.44+0.22xxx Y
CALCIT+dDAVP	5363+283	4.59+0.38	2.52+0.27yyy

values are expressed as mean±SEM.

 x=p<O.O5; xxx = p< 0.001   as compared to "no drug" - Y= p< 0.05; YYY=p<O.OOl as compared to the single drug,

Abbreviations. dDAVP=1-deamino-8D-arginine vasopressin= desmopressin. INDO=indomethacine. CALCIT= calcitonine.

Cosm =osmolal clearance; CH2 O=- free water clearance; GFR=glomerular filtration rate.

As shown in the table above, changes in urine volume, osmolal clearance and free water excretion (expressed in the percentage of glomerular filtration) can be seen numerically. Indomethacine (administered alone) was practically without any effect, while desmopressin (administered alone) caused significant decrease both in urine volume and free water excretion, enhanced markedly by the co-administration of indomethacine. (In osmolal clearance no significant change occurred.).

We can summarize the results of the first part of our present studies by reporting that administration of excessive doses of Desmopressin resulted in clinically relevant antidiuresis, enhanced by Indomethacine and abolished by Calcitonin.

After performing these investigations, administration of lithium carbonate was discontinued.

Investigations Performed after Stopping Lithium Therapy

Polyuria remained and practically did not change during the next three years. Therefore, the diagnosis is: "permanent" lithium induced nephrogenic diabetes insipidus. Another interesting observation was that the glomerular filtration rate increased from the 31-47 ml/min value, found during lithium therapy, to 130 ml/min two months after the discontinuation of lithium and permanently remained at this level. The increase of glomerular filtration apparently did not enhance the polyuria. Polyuria was, however, partially sensitive to Desmopressin.

After stopping lithium therapy, two months later the patient was studied again. This time the effect of dDAVP (administered alone) – "as baseline" – was compared with that of the combinations of dDAVP and indomethacine, as well as dDAVP and piroxicam. (To have an ideal baseline, discontinuation of dDAVP was not possible because it would have been unethical and the patient definitely opposed it.) Urine volume, free water excretion, osmolal clearance, urine and serum osmolality, as well as glomerular filtration rate were determined.

It can be seen in Figure 4 that indomethacine plus dDAVP as compared to dDAVP (administered alone) was antidiuretic (urine volume [p<0.001] and free water excretion [p<0.001] decreased and urine osmolality [p<0.001] increased) without any consistent change in osmolal clearance, glomerular filtration rate and serum osmolality. Piroxicam plus dDAVP as compared to dDAVP (administered alone) was also antidiuretic (urine volume [p<0.01] and free water excretion [p<0.01] decreased and urine osmolality [p<0.1] increased) without any consistent change in osmolal clearance, glomerular filtration rate and serum osmolality. These results support the contention that indomethacine is not the only nonsteroidal anti-inflammatory compound which can be used in the antidiuretic therapy. However, piroxicam seemed to be less antidiuretic than indomethacine, by ca 20-30 %. It should be mentioned, that another nonsteroidal drug (aspirin) had no antidiuretic capability (Vierhapper 1990).

Figure 4

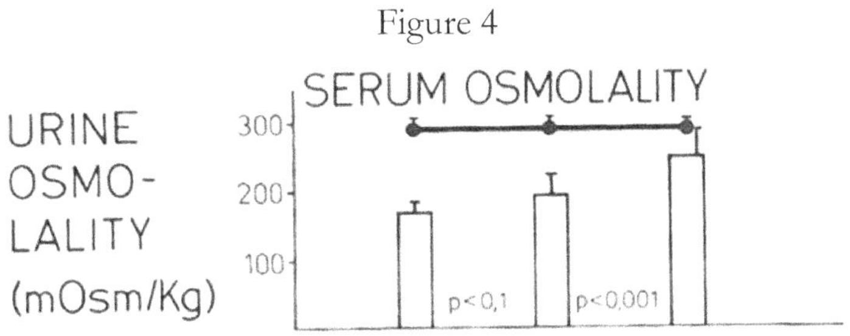

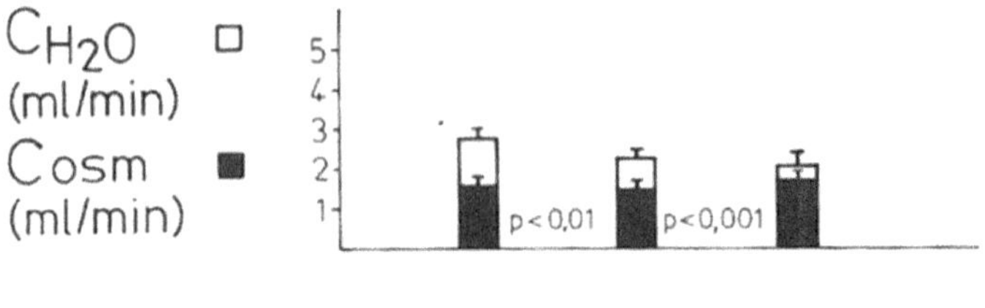

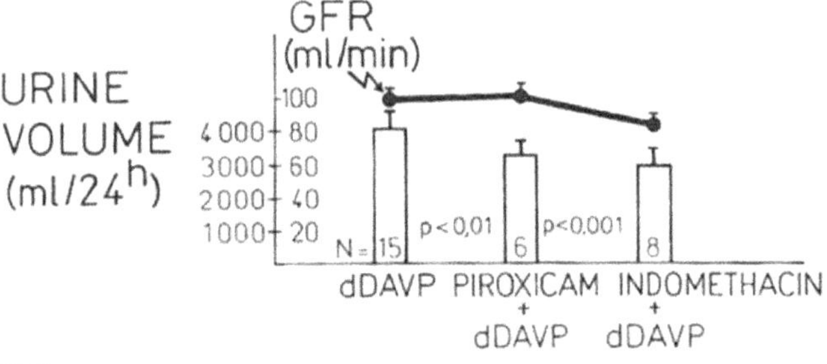

Legend to Figure 4. Two months after discontinuation of lithium carbonate treatment the effects of various interventions (dDAVP /desmopressin/, piroxicam and dDAVP, indomethacine and dDAVP) on specific renal functions were investigated in a patient with permanent lithium induced nephrogenic insipidus.

Conclusion

The message of our present writing is that in such an important form of psychiatric treatment as lithium is, a serious side effect, the disturbance of water metabolism, can be alleviated by clever use of modern antidiuretic interventions.

References:

Allen HM, Jackson RL, Winchester MD, Deck LV, Allon M. Indomethacin in the treatment of lithium-induced nephrogenic diabetes insipidus. Arch Intern Med. 1989; 149(5):1123-6.

Ban TA. Neuropsychopharmacology in Historical Perspective. Education in the Field in the Post-Neuropsychopharmacology Era. Prologue. inhn.org.education. September 18, 2017.

Bedford JJ, Weggery S, Ellis G, McDonald FJ, Joyce PR, Leader JP,

Walker RJ. Lithium-induced nephrogenic diabetes insipidus: renal effects of Amiloride. Clin J Am Soc Nephrol 2008; 3:1324-31.

Blackwell B. Lithium Controversy. A historical autopsy. inhn.org.controversies. June 19, 2014.

Blackwell B. Barry Blackwell: Corporate Corruption In: The Psychopharmaceutical Industry (Revised). inhn.org.controversies. March 16, 2017.

Boccalandro C, De Mattia F, Guo DC, Xue L, Orlander P, King TM, Gupta P, Deen PM, Lavis VR, Milewicz DM. Characterization of an aquaporin-2 water channel gene mutation causing partial nephrogenic diabetes insipidus in a Mexican family: Evidence of increased frequency of the mutation in the town of origin. J Am Soc Nephrol 2004; 15:1223-31.

Cade JP. Lithium salts in the treatment of psychotic excitement. Med J Australia 1949; 2:349-52.

Cohen M, Post GS. Water Transport in the Kidney and Nephrogenic Diabetes Insipidus J Vet Intern Med 2002; 16:510-7.

Felsenfeld AJ, Levine BS. Calcitonin, the forgotten hormone: does it deserve to be forgotten? Clin Kidney J 2015; 8:180-7.

Forrest JN Jr, Cohen AD, Torretti J, Himmelhoch JM, Epstein FH. On the mechanism of Lithium-induced diabetes insipidus in man and the rat. J Clin Invest. 1974; 53(4):1115-23.

Glick IS, Janowsky D, Salzman C, Shader R. APPENDIX B Lithium: A clinical update 1984. A Model Psychopharmacology Curriculum for Psychiatric Residents An Ad Hoc Committee of the American College of Neuropsychopharmacology. inhn.org.archives. February 9, 2017.

Guirguis AF, Taylor HC. Nephrogenic diabetes insipidus etc. Endocrine Practice 2000; 6:324-328.

Haris Á, Radó J.   A víz-és elektrolitháztartás zavarai. Budapest: Medicina; 2008

Kalra S, Zargar AH, Jain SM, Sethi B, Chowdhury S, Singh AK, Thomas N, Unnikrishnan AG, Thakkar PB, Malve H. Diabetes insipidus: The other diabetes. Indian J Endocr Metab 2016; 20:9-21.

Kazama I, Arata T, Michimata M, Hatano R, Suzuki M, Miyama N, Sanada S, Sato A, Satomi S, Ejima Y, Sasaki S, Matsubara M. Lithium effectively complements vasopressin V2 receptor antagonist in the treatment of hyponatraemia of SIADH rats Nephrology Dialysis Transplantation 2007; 22: 68-76.

Kittikulsuth W, Friedman PA, van Hoek A, Gao Y, Kohan DE. Identification of adenylyl cyclase isoforms mediating parathyroid hormone- and calcitonin-stimulated cyclic AMP accumulation in distal tubule cells. BMC Nephrology 2017; 18:292.

Moses AM, Scheinman SJ, Oppenheim A. Marked hypotonic polyuria resulting from nephrogenic diabetes insipidus with partial sensitivity to vasopressin. J Clin Endocrinol Meta.1984; 59:1044-9.

Neithercut WD, Spooner RJ, Hendry A, Dagg JH. Persistent nephrogenic diabetes insipidus, tubular proteinuria, aminoaciduria and parathyroid hormone resistance following long term lithium administration. Postgrad Med J 1990; 66:479-82.

Radó JP.   1-desamino-8-D-arginine vasopressin (DDAVP) concentration test. Am J Med Sci 1978; 275:43-52.

Radó JP. Nephrogenic diabetes insipidus. Orv Hetil 1998; 139:559-63.

Radó JP. Nephrogen diabetes insipidus. In: Kakuk G. szerk. Klinikai nephrologia. Budapest: Medicina; 2004, p. 375.

Radó JP. Humán farmakológiai kutatásaink desmopressinnel és más készítményekkel neurohypophyseális és nephrogen diabetes insipidusban: I. Neurohypophyseális diabetes insipidus és II.

nephrogen diabetes insipidus. Hypertonia és Nephrologia 2007; 11:181-98 and 244-56.

Radó JP. Diabetes mellitus és (nephrogen) diabetes insipidus együttes előfordulása Hypertonia és Nephrologia 2011; 15:183-7.

Radó JP, Marosi J. Prolongation of duration of action of 1-deamino-8-D-arginine vasopressin (DDAVP) by ineffective doses of clofibrate in diabetes insipidus. Horm Metab Res 1975; 7:527-8b.

Radó JP, Marosi J, Borbely L, Tako J. Individual differences in the antidiuretic response induced by single doses of 1-deamino-8-D-arginine-vasopressin (DDAVP) in patients with pituitary diabetes insipidus. Int J Clin Pharmacol Biopharm 1976; 14:259-65d.

Radó JP, Marosi J, Borbely L, Tako J. Individual differences in the antidiuretic response induced by DDAVP in diabetes insipidus. Horm Metab Res 1976; 8:155-6a.

Radó JP, Marosi J, Fischer J. Shortened duration of action of 1-deamino-8-D-arginine vasopressin (DDAVP) in patients with diabetes insipidus requiring high doses of peroral antidiuretic drugs. J Clin Pharmacol 1976; 16:518-24c.

Radó JP, Marosi J, Fischer J. Comparison of the antidiuretic effects of single intravenous and intranasal doses of DDAVP in diabetes insipidus. Pharmacology 1977; 15:40-5.

Radó JP, Marosi J, Fischer J, Tako J, Kiss N. Relationship between the dose of 1-deamino-8-darginine vasopressin (ddavp) and the antidiuretic response in man. Endokrinologie 1975; 66:184-95a.

Radó JP, Marosi J, Szende L, Borbely L, Tako J, Fischer J. The antidiuretic action of 1-deamino-8-D-arginine vasopressin (DDAVP) in man. Int J Clin Pharmacol Biopharm 1976; 13:199-209b.

Radó JP, Simatupang T, Boer P, Dorhout Mees EJ. Pharmacologic studies in Bartter's syndrome: effect of DDAVP and indomethacin on renal concentrating operation. Part II. Int J Clin Pharmacol Biopharm 1978; 16:22-6b.

Radó JP, Szende L. Simultaneous familial occurrence of distal renal tubular acidosis, polycystic kidney and nephrogenic diabetes insipidus] Orvosi Hetilap 1995; 136:995-1001.

Radó JP, Zdravkova S. [Lithium-induced chronic water-metabolism disorder (nephrogenic diabetes insipidus)]. Orv Hetil. 1991; 132:1987-90.

Radó JP, Zdravkova S. Effect of Indomethacine and Calcitonin During Administration of 1-Deamino-8-D-Arginin-Vasopressin (dDAVP) on Free Water Clearance in Nephrogenic Diabetes Insipidus (NDI). XIIth International Congress of Nephrology. June 13–18, 1993 Jerusalem, Israel.

Rybakowski J. Final comment: Half a Century of Inspiring Lithium Controversy. Barry Blackwell: The Lithium controversy: A historical autopsy. Collated by Olaf Fjetland. inhn.org.collated. September 30, 2017.

Severus E, Taylor MJ, Sauer C, Pfennig A, Ritter P, Bauer M, Geddes JR. Lithium for prevention of mood episodes in bipolar disorders: systematic review and meta-analysis. International Journal of Bipolar Disorders 2014; 2:15.

Simon NM, Garber E, Arieff AJ. Persistent nephrogenic diabetes insipidus after lithium carbonate. Ann Int Med 1977; 86:446-7.

Stasior DS, Kikeri D, Duel B, Seifter JL. Nephrogenic diabetes insipidus responsive to indomethacine plus dDAVP. New Eng J Med 1991; 324:850-1.

Thompson CJ, France AJ, Baylis PH. Persistent Nephrogenic diabetes insipidus following lithium therapy. Scottish Medical Journal 1997; 42:16-7.

Vierhapper H. Indomethacine in the treatment of lithium-induced nephrogenic diabetes insipidus. Arch Int Med 1990; 150: 2419.

Weinstock RS Moses AM: Desmopressin and indomethacine therapy for nephrogenic diabetes insipidus in patients receiving lithium carbonate. South Med J 1990; 83:1475-7.

Acknowledgment. The author expresses his sincere thanks to Dr. Zdravkova Sznyeska, nephrologist, for her contribution in collecting data and handling the statistical analysis.

January 25, 2018

CHAPTER 7.

ACTION

Thomas A. Ban

MAGDA MALEWSKA-KASPRZAK, AGNIESZKA PERMODA-OSIP, JANUSZ RYBAKOWSKI: DISTURBANCES OF THE PURINERGIC SYSTEM IN AFFECTIVE DISORDERS AND SCHIZOPHRENIA*

ABSTRACT

The purinergic system plays a role in the regulation of many psychological processes, including mood and activity. It consists of P1 receptors, with adenosine as the agonist, and P2 receptors, activated by nucleotides (e.g., adenosine 5'-triphosphate – ATP).

Propounded disturbances of uric acid in affective disorders were related to the introduction of lithium for the treatment of these disorders in the 19th and 20th century. At the beginning of the 21st century, new evidence was accumulated concerning a role of uric acid in the pathogenesis and treatment of bipolar disorder (BD). In patients with BD, higher prevalence of gout and increased concentration of uric acid have been found, as well as the therapeutic activity of allopurinol, used as an adjunct to mood stabilizers, has been demonstrated in mania.

In recent years, the research on the role of the purinergic system in the pathogenesis and treatment of affective disorders and schizophrenia focuses on the role of adenosine (P1) receptors and nucleotide (P2) receptors. Activation of adenosine receptors is related to an antidepressant activity. Alterations of P2 receptors are also significant for the pathogenesis of affective disorders. The role of the purinergic system in schizophrenia is related to the effect of adenosine and nucleotide receptors on dopaminergic and glutamatergic neurotransmission. A lot of data indicate that schizophrenia is related to a deficit of the adenosine system. Changes in the purinergic system are also significant for psychopathological symptoms of schizophrenia and for the action of antipsychotic drugs.

Purinergic system and its role in the central nervous system functioning

Uric acid is the final metabolite of purine bases, derived from food, synthesis de novo and metabolism of endogenous nucleic acids. It has been found that both uric acid and some purines (e.g., adenosine) may play a role in the regulation of psychological processes, including mood and activity.

In the central nervous system, adenosine 5'-triphosphate (ATP), other nucleotides and adenosine are stored and released into extracellular space from various types of cells: neurons (Fields 2011), astrocytes (Koizumi 2010), and microglia cells (Imura, Morizawa, Komatsu et al. 2013). Mechanisms of ATP release have been described as an exocytotic vesicular release from nerve terminals (Bodin and Burnstock 2001), involving, among others, calcium ions (Lalo, Palygin, Rasooli-Nejad et al. 2014). In vitro studies showed that the activity of astrocytes depends on the release of transmitters, such as glutamate, ATP, and adenosine (Zhang, Chen, Zhou et al. 2007).

The extracellular concentration of ATP increases during neuronal activity under the influence of psychostimulant drugs and in oxygen-glucose deprivation models (OGD) during seizures, as well as inflammations or injuries of the brain (Burnstock, Krügel, Abbracchio and Illes 2011; Pintora, Alberto Porrasb, Francisco Morab and Miras-Portugal 1993). Mitochondrial dysfunctions of ATP synthesis may be significant for the pathogenesis of neurological and psychiatric illnesses.

Nucleotide receptors, discovered in the 1970s by a British scientist Geoffrey Burnstock, were initially called "purinergic receptors." When it was found that their activation involves both purine and pyrimidine nucleotides, their name was changed into "nucleotide receptors" and they were divided into two groups, P1 and P2; P1 receptors' agonist is a purine nucleoside – adenosine. Adenosine receptors were divided into A1, A2 and A3 subtypes. P2 receptors, further divided into P2X and P2Y subgroups, are activated by nucleotides. P2X receptors are ionotropic receptors, forming a channel in the cell membrane and activated by ATP. P2Y receptors are metabotropic receptors, G-protein coupled (similarly to P1), activated by ATP, adenosine diphosphate (ADP), uridine triphosphate (UTP), uridine diphosphate (UDP) and sugar derivatives of UDP (Barańska 2014). The release of adenosine, ATP and ADP into the extracellular space exerts an effect on P1 and P2 receptors, localized on neurons and on non-neuronal cells, such as astrocytes, oligodendrocytes, microglia cells and endothelial cells (Fields and Burnstock 2006).

Purinergic transmission plays a significant role in various physiological processes, as well as in numerous pathological states. Purinergic receptors are widely spread in the central nervous system, in neurons and glia cells of the cerebral cortex, in the hypothalamus, basal ganglia, hippocampus and other parts of the limbic system (Burnstock 2008). Purinergic system dysfunctions have been found in many neuropsychiatric conditions, including affective disorders and schizophrenia (Gomes, Kaster, Tomé et al. 2011). The current review presents the recent knowledge on the role of the purinergic system in affective disorders and schizophrenia, based on the research performed in the last two decades.

Purinergic system dysfunctions in affective disorders
The relations between BD and purinergic system dysfunction concerned initially the disturbances of uric acid. This was related to the introduction of lithium as a treatment for affective disorders. A Danish scientist, Carl Lange, suggested in 1886 that an excess of uric acid played a role in the pathogenesis of depression and proposed a therapeutic use of lithium, as lithium urate is one of best soluble urates. In 1949, an Australian psychiatrist, John Cade, introduced lithium as a treatment for manic states, suggesting beforehand that these states are characterized by increased excretion of urates (Malewska, Jasińska and Rybakowski 2016).

The premises for a significance of uric acid in the pathogenesis of bipolar disorder are epidemiological, clinical and therapeutic. An epidemiological study performed by Chung, Huang and Lin (2010) in

Action

Taiwan, covering 24,262 patients with BD and 121,310 patients in the control group, and followed up during the period of 2000-2006, found that gout occurred among 16.4% of the patients with BD and in 13.6% of the patients of the control group. The risk of developing gout during the 6-year follow-up period was 1.19% higher for patients with BD than for the control group (95% confidence interval (CI) = 1.10-1.24, p<0.001).

Salvadore, Viale, Lucke et al. (2010) observed that patients with the first episode of mania had increased levels of uric acid which might indicate that the purinergic system dysfunctions may occur even in the early phases of BD. Recent analyses, performed by Bartoli, Crocamo, Mazza et al. (2016), Bartoli, Crocamo, Clerici and Carrà (2017) and Bartoli, Crocamo, Dakanalis et al. (2017) found that patients with BD have a significantly increased concentration of uric acid in comparison with healthy control subjects and with patients suffering from depression. Albert, De Cori, Aguglia et al. (2015) reported a significantly higher concentration of uric acid in BD in comparison with obsessive-compulsive disorder or schizophrenia. In patients with BD, no difference between acute phase and remission was observed. A recent study has shown that the concentration of uric acid is significantly higher in people with the first episode of mania compared to the control group and negatively correlates with the improvement of the clinical state after one month of treatment (Chatterjee, Ghosal, Mitra et al. 2018). In our study, comparing uric acid concentration in patients with BD during mania, depression and remission, no significant differences were found. However, hyperuricemia was observed in more than one-third of patients during depressive episode (Malewska, Permoda-Osip, Kasprzak et al. 2017).

Allopurinol, used for the treatment of gout, acts by inhibiting the enzyme, xanthine oxidase, which results in reducing the level of uric acid. In a double-blind, randomized, placebo-controlled trial, including patients with mania (moderate to acute), it was found that addition of allopurinol to lithium or haloperidol, during eight weeks, resulted in a greater reduction of agitation and symptoms of mania, assessed by the

Young Mania Rating Scale (YMRS), compared to the control group, where placebo was added (Akhondzadeh, Milajerdi, Amini and Tehrani-Doost 2006). The study performed by Machado-Vieira, Soares, Lara et al. (2008) estimated the efficacy and tolerance to allopurinol (600 mg/day) and dipyridamole (200 mg/day) combined with lithium in the treatment of acute manic episode. The study lasted four weeks, was randomized and double-blind, placebo controlled. The results indicated that obtained reduction in the YMRS scale was significantly greater in case of added allopurinol than dipyridamole or placebo. Antimanic effects of allopurinol correlated with a decrease of uric acid concentration. The results of these two studies suggest that allopurinol may by synergistic with lithium in the treatment of manic episodes in patients with BD.

The study of Jahangard, Soroush, Haghighi et al. (2014) including 57 patients with manic episode investigated potential benefits of allopurinol (600 mg/day) compared with placebo for augmenting the antimanic effect of sodium valproate (15-20 mg/kg/day). Compared to the control group receiving placebo, both symptoms of mania and uric acid concentration decreased significantly in the group of patients where allopurinol was added. The probability of remission after four weeks of treatment was 23 times higher in the group receiving allopurinol and lower uric acid concentration after four weeks was associated with symptom improvement. Thus, in the treatment of acute mania, allopurinol could act in synergy with sodium valproate.

Experimental studies also showed an antidepressant effects of allopurinol. Özgür, Aksu, Birincioğlu and Dost (2015) compared the effects of allopurinol with these of fluoxetine in a forced swimming test in rats after 14 days of drug administration. Both allopurinol and fluoxetine caused a decrease in the duration of immobility, with similar efficacy. However, no significant differences in the antidepressant effect between the combined therapy versus single drug therapy were found. A meta-analysis of Bartoli, Crocamo, Clerici and Carrà (2017) and Bartoli, Crocamo, Dakanalis et al. (2017) proved the beneficial effect of using allopurinol for an augmentation of the treatment of mania.

Current research on the role of the purinergic system in the pathogenesis of affective disorders has been mainly focused on the abnormalities of adenosine receptors (P1) and nucleotide receptors (P2) (Ortiz, Ulrich, Zarate and Machado-Vieira 2015). The activation of adenosine receptor causes a reduction of neuronal excitability, a decrease of uric acid concentration and inhibition of calcium-dependent release of excitatory neurotransmitters. Experimental studies found that lithium increases the level of adenosine by inhibiting the activity of ectonucleotidase (Oliveira, Seibt, Rico et al. 2011). It was also found that the agonists of adenosine system, cyclohexyladenosine (CHA) and (N6-[2-(3.5-di-methoxyphenyl)-2-(2-methylphenyl)-ethyl] adenosine (DMPA), exert an antidepressant effect in the forced swimming test (Kaster, Rosa, Rosso et al. 2004). Sleep deprivation causes an increase of adenosine signaling in the brain. S-adenosyl-l-methionine, a precursor of adenosine, has a similar effect (De Berardis, Marini, Serroni et al. 2013).

Both sleep deprivation and electroconvulsive therapy cause an increase in adenosine A1 receptors (Elmenhorst, Meyer, Winz et al. 2007). The activation of A1 receptors has an inhibiting effect on N-methyl-D-aspartate (NMDA) receptors. Experimental studies demonstrated that such an effect is associated with antidepressant activity and activation of neuronal plasticity. Adenosine A2 receptors modulate dopaminergic signaling in subcortical structures of the brain and their activation is associated with the weakening of motivational and motor skills. In turn, inhibition of these receptors, e.g., by bupropion, is associated with an antidepressant effect. Thus, the antidepressant effect can be obtained both by adenosine A1 receptors activation and A2 receptors inhibition. In turn, Gubert, Jacintho Moritz, Vasconcelos-Moreno et al. (2016) showed that the concentration of adenosine is lower in bipolar patients compared to the control group and pointed to its negative correlation with the severity of depression. It was also found that a greater functional impairment was associated with lower levels of adenosine.

Some research also found that P2 receptors, activated by extracellular ATP, are of significance for the pathogenesis of BD. Gubert, Fries, Wollenhaupt de Aguiar et al. (2013) presented the role of the P2X7 receptor which mediates in the processes of apoptosis, proliferation and release of proinflammatory cytokines, as well as in mechanisms of neurotransmission and neuromodulation. The release of proinflammatory cytokines may be important for the pathogenesis of BD, most significantly with the microglia P2X7 receptor activation. The gene of the P2X7 receptor is located on the chromosome 12q23-24, which is described as a potential susceptibility locus for affective disorders (Abkevich, Camp, Hensel et al. 2003). Moreover, it was found that specific genotypes of the P2X7 receptor, e.g., two haplotypes containing A348T, might increase the risk for affective disorders. Recent animal studies have shown that P2X7 receptor is associated with learned helplessness model of depression in mice (Otrokocsi, Kittel and Sperlágh 2017).

There is also data concerning the pathogenetic role of the P2Y1 receptor in affective disorders. This receptor, located on astrocytes, modulates presynaptic, calcium-dependent release of glutamine. The experimental research found that P2Y1 receptors on neurons play a role in motivational processes (Krügel, Spies, Regenthal et al. 2004) and are important for antidepressant and anxiolytic effects (Kittner, Franke, Fischer et al. 2003).

Purinergic system dysfunctions in schizophrenia

The role of the purinergic system in schizophrenia is related to the effects of adenosine and nucleotide receptors on dopaminergic and glutamatergic signaling. Many data have indicated that schizophrenia may be related to a deficit in the adenosine system (Deckert, Brenner, Durany et al. 2003). As early as 20 years ago, the association between polymorphism of adenosine A2A receptor gene, located on chromosome 22q, and susceptibility to schizophrenia was reported (Deckert, Nöthen, Bryant et al. 1997).

Stimulation of adenosine system exerts an anti-dopaminergic and pro-glutamatergic effect. Adenosine and A2A receptor agonists have similar activity as dopamine antagonists (Ferré, Fredholm, Morelli et al. 1997; Ferré, Ciruela, Quiroz et al. 2007; Rimondini, Ferré, Ogren and Fuxe 1997; Shen, Coelho, Ohtsuka et al. 2008; Villar-Menéndez, Díaz-Sánchez, Blanch et al. 2014). On the other hand, adenosine antagonists, such as caffeine, exert similar effects to those of psychostimulants by increasing dopamine concentration in the striatum. By forming the A2A / D2 heteromers, a decrease of adenosine may cause an increase in dopamine. A reduction of the A2A receptors at the level of transcription and DNA methylation, coding the A2A receptor gene, was found in schizophrenic patients. In some papers, it was shown that dipyridamole and allopurinol, which enhance adenosine system by inhibiting cellular uptake and metabolic elimination of adenosine, can potentiate the effects of antipsychotic drugs in schizophrenia (Akhondzadeh, Shasavand, Jamilian et al. 2000; Weiser, Gershon, Rubinstein et al. 2012; Wonodi, Gopinath, Liu et al. 2011).

In animal models, A1 and A2A receptor agonists decrease behavioral activity caused by NMDA receptor antagonists (Popoli and Pepponi 2012; Sills, Azampanah and Fletcher 1999) and agonists of A2A receptors enhance glutamate release in glutamatergic neuronal endings of the striatum (De Mendonça, Sebastião and Ribeiro 1995). A post-mortem study of schizophrenia patients found that an increase of mRNA glutamine transporter in astrocytes is associated with the functioning of the A2A receptors (Matute, Melone, Vallejo-Illarramendi and Conti 2005; Smith, Haroutunian, Davis and Meador-Woodruff 2001). Recent in vivo studies concerning A2A receptors indicate that glutamatergic system dysfunctions may depend on impaired signaling from astrocytes to neurons. In the study of mice with A2A receptors removed from astrocytes, inhibition of psychomotor functions and memory after administration of the NMDA receptor antagonist, MK-801, as well as suppression of glutamine transporter activity were observed (Matos, Shen, Augusto et al. 2015).

Zhang, Abdallah, Wang et al. (2012) assessed a relationship between the adenosine gene A2A receptor expression and the results of sensory gating in schizophrenia patients, before and after 6-week antipsychotic treatment, compared with healthy subjects. Before treatment, schizophrenia patients exhibited sensory gating impairment in comparison with healthy patients. However, there was no difference in A2A receptors expression. After treatment, schizophrenia patients had increased expression of the receptors (up-regulation) which correlated with the initial amplitude of P50, the measure of sensory gating. Recently, Turčin, Dolžan, Porcelli et al. (2016) studied an association between genes of adenosine A1, A2A, and A3 receptors and psychopathological symptoms and antipsychotic drugs side effects in 127 chronic schizophrenia patients. Association with psychopathological effects was found in relation to A1 and A2A receptors, whereas the association with akathisia was related to all three receptors. Association with tardive dyskinesia was found about the A3 receptor.

Besides adenosine receptors, much data also points to a significance of nucleotide receptors in the pathogenesis and treatment of schizophrenia. In contrast to adenosine receptors, stimulation of nucleotide receptors exerts a pro-dopaminergic and anti-glutamatergic effect. Experimental studies found that stimulation of the P2 receptors causes behavioral activation and their inhibition prevents such an activation. Stimulation of P2Y1 receptors in the prefrontal cortex is related to an increase in dopamine release from the ventral tegmental area (Guzman, Schmidt, Franke et al. 2010). Activation of these receptors also causes the hypofunction of NMDA receptors in the prefrontal cortex (Gonzalez-Burgos and Lewis 2008). It was demonstrated that antipsychotic drugs, such as haloperidol and chlorpromazine, inhibit ATP-evoked stimulation via P2X receptors without blocking the D2 dopamine receptors. In contrast, application of ATP or non-selective P2X/Y receptor agonist, 2-methylthio ATP, into the rat striatum increases dopamine levels and exerts a euphorigenic effect, similar to that of dopamine (Krügel, Kittner and

Action

Illes 1999; Zhang, Yamashita, Ohshita et al. 1995). Stimulation of P2 receptors via endogenous ATP probably plays a role in an activating effect of amphetamine. On the other hand, blocking P2 receptors may contribute to preventing the development of dopaminergic hyperactivity. Koványi, Csölle, Calovi et al. (2016) examined for the first time the role of P2X7 in an animal model of schizophrenia. Using the phencyclidine induced schizophrenia model, they showed that P2X7 can make a potential therapeutic target in schizophrenia.

The research on uric acid concentration in schizophrenia patients can also be mentioned. In some studies, an increased concentration of uric acid during acute phase of the illness was found (Nagamine 2010). Recent research has pointed out to a relationship between increased uric acid concentration and the risk of metabolic syndrome in schizophrenia patients (Godin, Leboyer, Gaman et al. 2015; Rajan, Zalpuri, Harrington et al. 2016). In our own study, we did not find any differences in uric acid concentration in schizophrenia patients between an acute and remission phases of the illness. Uric acid concentration in schizophrenia patients did not also differ from the concentration in patients with bipolar disorder (Malewska, Permoda-Osip, Kasprzak et al. 2017).

Summary

Disturbances of purinergic system in affective disorders and schizophrenia are related to uric acid and adenosine and nucleotide receptors. Propounded disturbances of uric acid in affective disorders were related to the introduction of lithium for the treatment of these disorders in the 19th and 20th century. At the beginning of the 21st century, new evidence was found, for the role of uric acid in pathogenesis and treatment of BD. The more frequent occurrence of gout and increased concentration of uric acid was found in patients with BD. The efficacy of allopurinol, used as an augmentation of mood stabilizers in mania, was also observed.

In recent years, the research on the role of the purinergic system in the pathogenesis and treatment of affective disorders and schizophrenia has mainly focused on the role of adenosine (P1) receptors and nucleotide (P2) receptors. Adenosine receptors activation is related to an antidepressant activity. Alterations in P2 receptors are also significant for the pathogenesis of affective disorders. The role of the purinergic system in schizophrenia is related to the effects of adenosine and nucleotide receptors on dopaminergic and glutamatergic signaling. Much data have indicated that schizophrenia is related to a deficit of the adenosine system. Alterations in the purinergic system are also significant for psychopathological symptoms of schizophrenia and the effects of antipsychotic drugs.

References:

Abkevich V, Camp NJ, Hensel CH, Neff CD, Russell DL, Hughes DC, Plenk AM, Lowry MR, Richards RL, Carter C, Frech GC, Stone S, Rowe K, Chau CA, Cortado K, Hunt A, Luce K, O'Neil G, Poarch J, Potter J, Poulsen GH, Saxton H, Bernat-Sestak M, Thompson V, Gutin A, Skolnick MH, Shattuck D, Cannon-Albright L. Predisposition locus for major depression at chromosome 12q22-12q23.2. Am J Hum Genet 2003; 73: 1271–81.

Akhondzadeh S, Milajerdi MR, Amini H, Tehrani-Doost M. Allopurinol as an adjunct to lithium and haloperidol for treatment of patients with acute mania: a double-blind, randomized, placebo-controlled trial. Bipolar Disord 2006; 8:485–9.

Akhondzadeh S, Shasavand E, Jamilian H, Shabestari O, Kamalipour A. Dipyridamole in the treatment of schizophrenia: adenosine-dopamine receptor interactions. J Clin Pharm Ther. 2000; 25:131-7.

Albert U, De Cori D, Aguglia A, Barbaro F, Bogetto F, Maina G. Increased uric acid levels in bipolar disorder subjects during different phases of illness. J Affect Disord 2015;173: 170-5.

Barańska J. Nucleotide receptors - structure and functions, history and perspectives (in Polish). Post Biochem 2014; 60: 424–37.

Action

Bartoli F, Crocamo C, Clerici M, Carrà G. Allopurinol as add-on treatment for mania symptoms in bipolar disorder: systematic review and meta-analysis of randomised controlled trials. Br J Psychiatry 2017; 210:10-5.

Bartoli F, Crocamo C, Dakanalis A, Brosio E, Miotto A, Capuzzi E, Clerici M, Carrà G. Purinergic system dysfunctions in subjects with bipolar disorder: A comparative cross-sectional study. Compr Psychiatry 2017;73:1-6.

Bartoli F, Crocamo C, Mazza MG, Clerici M, Carrà G. Uric acid levels in subjects with bipolar disorder: A comparative meta-analysis. J Psychiatr Res 2016;81:133-9.

Bodin P, Burnstock G. Purinergic signalling: ATP release. Neurochem Res 2001; 26:959-69.

Burnstock G. Purinergic signalling and disorders of the central nervous system. Nat Rev Drug Discov 2008; 7: 575–90.

Burnstock G, Krügel U, Abbracchio MP, Illes P. Purinergic signalling: from normal behavior to pathological brain function. Prog Neurobiol. 2011; 95:229-74.

Chatterjee SS, Ghosal S, Mitra S, Mallik N, Ghosal MK. Serum uric acid levels in first episode mania, effect on clinical presentation and treatment response: Data from a case control study. Asian J Psychiatr 2018;35:15-7.

Chung KH, Huang CC, Lin HC. Increased risk of gout among patients with bipolar disorder: a nationwide population-based study. Psychiatry Res 2010; 180: 147-50.

De Berardis D, Marini S, Serroni N, Rapini G, Iasevoli F, Valchera A, Signorelli M, Aguglia E, Perna G, Salone A, Di Iorio G, Martinotti G, Di Giannantonio M. S-Adenosyl-L-Methionine augmentation in patients with stage II treatment-resistant major depressive disorder: an open label, fixed dose, single-blind study. Scientific World Journal 2013; 2046-9.

De Mendonça A, Sebastião AM, Ribeiro JA. Inhibition of NMDA receptor-mediated currents in isolated rat hippocampal neurones by adenosine A1 receptor activation. Neuroreport 1995;6:1097-100.

Deckert J, Brenner M, Durany N, Zöchling R, Paulus W, Ransmayr G, Tatschner T, Danielczyk W, Jellinger K, Riederer P. Up-regulation of striatal adenosine A(2A) receptors in schizophrenia. Neuroreport 2003;14:313-6.

Deckert J, Nöthen MM, Bryant SP, Schuffenhauer S, Schofield PR, Spurr NK, Propping P. Mapping of the human adenosine A2a receptor gene: relationship to potential schizophrenia loci on chromosome 22q and exclusion from the CATCH 22 region. Hum Genet 1997;99:326-8.

Elmenhorst D, Meyer PT, Winz OH, Matusch A, Ermert J, Coenen HH, Basheer R, Haas HL, Zilles K, Bauer A. Sleep deprivation increases A1 adenosine receptor binding in the human brain: a positron emission tomography study. J Neurosci 2007;27:2410-5.

Ferré S, Fredholm BB, Morelli M, Popoli P, Fuxe K. Adenosine-dopamine receptor-receptor interactions as an integrative mechanism in the basal ganglia. Trends Neurosci 1997;20:482-7.

Ferré S, Ciruela F, Quiroz C, Luján R, Popoli P, Cunha RA, Agnati LF, Fuxe K, Woods AS, Lluis C, Franco R. Adenosine receptor heteromers and their integrative role in striatal function. Scientific World Journal. 2007; 7:74-85.

Fields RD, Burnstock G. Purinergic signalling in neuron-glia interactions. Nat Rev Neurosci 2006; 7:423-6.

Fields RD. Nonsynaptic and nonvesicular ATP release from neurons and relevance to neuron-glia signaling. Semin Cell Dev Biol 2011;

22:214-9.

Godin O, Leboyer M, Gaman A, Aouizerate B, Berna F, Brunel L, Capdevielle D, Chereau I, Dorey JM, Dubertret C, Dubreucq J, Faget C, Gabayet F, Le Strat Y, Llorca PM, Misdrahi D, Rey R, Richieri R, Passerieux C, Schandrin A, Schürhoff F, Urbach M, Vidalhet P, Girerd N, Fond G; FACE-SZ group. Metabolic syndrome, abdominal obesity and hyperuricemia in schizophrenia: Results from the FACE-SZ cohort. Schizophr Res. 2015;168:388-94.

Gomes CV, Kaster MP, Tomé AR, Agostinho PM, Cunha RA. Adenosine receptors and brain diseases: neuroprotection and neurodegeneration. Biochem Biophys Acta. 2011;1808:1380-99.

Gonzalez-Burgos G, Lewis DA. GABA neurons and the mechanisms of network oscillations: implications for understanding cortical dysfunction in schizophrenia. Schizophr Bull 2008;34:944-61.

Gubert C, Fries GR, Wollenhaupt de Aguiar B, Ribeiro Rosa A, Busnello JV, Ribeiro L, Bueno Morrone F, Oliveira Battastini AM, Kapczinski F. The P2X7 purinergic receptor as a molecular target in bipolar disorder. Neuropsychiatr Neuropsychol 2013; 8: 1-7.

Gubert C, Jacintho Moritz CE, Vasconcelos-Moreno MP, Quadros Dos Santos BTM, Sartori J, Fijtman A, Kauer-Sant'Anna M, Kapczinski F, Battastini AMO, Magalhães PVDS. Peripheral adenosine levels in euthymic patients with bipolar disorder. Psychiatry Res. 2016;246:421-6.

Gürbüz Özgür B, Aksu H, Birincioğlu M, Dost T. Antidepressant-like effects of the xanthine oxidase enzyme inhibitor allopurinol in rats. A comparison with fluoxetine. Pharmacol Biochem Behav.2015;138:91-5.

Guzman SJ, Schmidt H, Franke H, Krügel U, Eilers J, Illes P, Gerevich Z. P2Y1 receptors inhibit long-term depression in the prefrontal cortex. Neuropharmacology 2010;59:406-15.

Imura Y, Morizawa Y, Komatsu R, Shibata K, Shinozaki Y, Kasai H, Moriishi K, Moriyama Y, Koizumi S. Microglia release ATP by exocytosis. Glia. 2013; 61:1320-30.

Jahangard L, Soroush S, Haghighi M, Ghaleiha A, Bajoghli H, Holsboer-Trachsler E, Brand S. In a double-blind, randomized and placebo-controlled trial, adjuvant allopurinol improved symptoms of mania in in-patients suffering from bipolar disorder. Eur Neuropsychopharmacol.2014;24:1210-21.

Kaster MP, Rosa AO, Rosso MM, Goulart EC, Santos AR, Rodrigues AL. Adenosine administration produces an antidepressant-like effect in mice: evidence for the involvement of A1 and A2A receptors. Neurosci Lett 2004; 355: 21–4.

Kittner H, Franke H, Fischer W, Schultheis N, Krugel U, Illes P. Stimulation of P2Y1 receptors causes anxiolytic-like effects in the rat elevated plus-maze: implications for the involvement of P2Y1 receptor-mediated nitric oxide production. Neuropsychopharmacology 2003, 28: 435–44.

Koizumi S. Synchronization of Ca2+ oscillations: involvement of ATP release in astrocytes. FEBS J. 2010; 277:286-92.

Koványi B, Csölle C, Calovi S, Hanuska A, Kató E, Köles L, Bhattacharya A, Haller J, Sperlágh B. The role of P2X7 receptors in a rodent PCP-induced schizophrenia model. Sci Rep 2016;6:366-80.

Krügel U, Kittner H, Illes P. Adenosine 5'-triphosphate-induced dopamine release in the rat nucleus accumbens in vivo. Neurosci Lett. 1999;265:49-52.

Krügel U, Spies O, Regenthal R, Illes P, Kittner H. P2 receptors are involved in the mediation of motivation-related behavior. Purinergic Signal 2004; 1: 21–29.

Lalo U, Palygin O, Rasooli-Nejad S, Andrew J, Haydon PG, Pankratov

Y. Exocytosis of ATP from astrocytes modulates phasic and tonic inhibition in the neocortex. PLoS Biol. 2014; 12:e1001747.

Machado-Vieira R, Soares JC, Lara DR, Luckenbaugh DA, Busnello JV, Marca G, Cunha A, Souza DO, Zarate CA Jr, Kapczinski F. A double-blind, randomized, placebo-controlled 4-week study on the efficacy and safety of the purinergic agents allopurinol and dipyridamole adjunctive to lithium in acute bipolar mania. J Clin Psychiatry 2008; 69: 1237–45.

Malewska M, Permoda-Osip A, Kasprzak P, Niemiec A, Rybakowski J. A study of uric acid concentration in bipolar disorder and schizophrenia. Pharmacother Psychiatry Neurol 2017; 33: 181-7.

Malewska MK, Jasińska A, Rybakowski J. The therapeutic effects of lithium, a concept of purinergic theory in affective disorders. Pharmacother Psychiatry Neurol 2016; 32: 97–109.

Matos M, Shen HY, Augusto E, Wang Y, Wei CJ, Wang YT, Agostinho P, Boison D, Cunha RA, Chen JF. Deletion of adenosine A2A receptors from astrocytes disrupts glutamate homeostasis leading to psychomotor and cognitive impairment: relevance to schizophrenia. Biol Psychiatry 2015;78:763-74.

Matute C, Melone M, Vallejo-Illarramendi A, Conti F. Increased expression of the astrocytic glutamate transporter GLT-1 in the prefrontal cortex of schizophrenics. Glia. 2005;49:451-5.

Nagamine T. Abnormal laboratory values during the acute and recovery phases in schizophrenic patients: a retrospective study. Neuropsychiatr Dis Treat. 2010;6:281-8.

Oliveira Rda L, Seibt KJ, Rico EP, Bogo MR, Bonan CD. Inhibitory effect of lithium on nucleotide hydrolysis and acetylcholinesterase activity in zebrafish (Danio rerio) brain. Neurotoxicol Teratol 2011; 33: 651–7.

Ortiz R, Ulrich H, Zarate CA, Machado-Vieira R. Purinergic system dysfunction in mood disorders: a key target for developing improved therapeutics. Prog Neuropsychopharmacol Biological Psychiatry 2015; 57: 117–31.

Otrokocsi L, Kittel Á, Sperlágh B. P2X7 Receptors drive spine synapse plasticity in the learned helplessness model of depression. Int J Neuropsychopharmacol 2017;20:813-22.

Pintora J, Alberto Porrasb A, Francisco Morab F, Miras-Portugal MT. Amphetamine-induced release of diadenosine polyphosphates - Ap4A and Ap5A - from caudate putamen of conscious rat. Neurosci Lett.1993;150:13-6.

Popoli P, Pepponi R. Potential therapeutic relevance of adenosine A2B and A2A receptors in the central nervous system. CNS Neurol Disord Drug Targets 2012;11:664-74.

Rajan S, Zalpuri I, Harrington A, Cimpeanu C, Song X, Fan X. Relationship between serum uric acid level and cardiometabolic risks in nondiabetic patients with schizophrenia. Int Clin Psychopharmacol 2016;31:51-6.

Rimondini R, Ferré S, Ogren SO, Fuxe K. Adenosine A2A agonists: a potential new type of atypical antipsychotic. Neuropsychopharmacology 1997;17:82-91.

Salvadore G, Viale CI, Luckenbaugh DA, Zanatto VC, Portela LV, Souza DO, Zarate CA Jr, Machado-Vieira R. Increased uric acid levels in drug-naive subjects with bipolar disorder during a first manic episode. Prog Neuropsychopharmacol Biol Psychiatry 2010; 34: 819–21.

Shen HY, Coelho JE, Ohtsuka N, Canas PM, Day YJ, Huang QY, Rebola N, Yu L, Boison D, Cunha RA, Linden J, Tsien JZ, Chen JF. A critical role of the adenosine A2A receptor in extrastriatal neurons in modulating psychomotor activity as revealed by opposite phenotypes of striatum and forebrain A2A receptor knock-outs. J Neurosci 2008;28:2970-5.

Sills TL, Azampanah A, Fletcher PJ. The adenosine A1 receptor agonist N6-cyclopentyladenosine blocks the disruptive effect of phencyclidine on prepulse inhibition of the acoustic startle response in the rat. Eur J Pharmacol 1999;369:325-9.

Smith RE1, Haroutunian V, Davis KL, Meador-Woodruff JH. Expression of excitatory amino acid transporter transcripts in the thalamus of subjects with schizophrenia. Am J Psychiatry. 2001;158:1393-9.

Turčin A, Dolžan V, Porcelli S, Serretti A, Plesničar BK. adenosine hypothesis of antipsychotic drugs revisited: Pharmacogenomics variation in nonacute schizophrenia. OMICS.2016;20:283-9.

Villar-Menéndez I, Díaz-Sánchez S, Blanch M, Albasanz JL, Pereira-Veiga T, Monje A, Planchat LM, Ferrer I, Martín M, Barrachina M. Reduced striatal adenosine A2A receptor levels define a molecular subgroup in schizophrenia. J Psychiatr Res 2014;51:49-59.

Weiser M, Gershon AA, Rubinstein K, Petcu C, Ladea M, Sima D, Podea D, Keefe RS, Davis JM. A randomized controlled trial of allopurinol vs. placebo added on to antipsychotics in patients with schizophrenia or schizoaffective disorder. Schizophr Res 2012;138:35-8.

Wonodi I, Gopinath HV, Liu J, Adami H, Hong LE, Allen-Emerson R, McMahon RP, Thaker GK. Dipyridamole monotherapy in schizophrenia: pilot of a novel treatment approach by modulation of purinergic signalling. Psychopharmacology (Berl). 2011; 218:341-5.

Zhang J, Abdallah CG, Wang J, Wan X, Liang C, Jiang L, Liu Y, Huang H, Hong X, Huang Q, Wu R, Xu C. Upregulation of adenosine A2A receptors induced by atypical antipsychotics and its correlation with sensory gating in schizophrenia patients. Psychiatry Res. 2012; 30: 126-

32.

Zhang YX, Yamashita H, Ohshita T, Sawamoto N, Nakamura S. ATP increases extracellular dopamine level through stimulation of P2Y purinoceptors in the rat striatum. Brain Res 1995;691:205-12.

Zhang Z, Chen G, Zhou W, Song A, Xu T, Luo Q, Wang W, Gu XS, Duan S. Regulated ATP release from astrocytes through lysosome exocytosis. Nat Cell Biol. 2007;9:945-53.

*From the Department of Adult Psychiatry and Department of Child and Adolescent Psychiatry, Poznan University of Medical Sciences, Poznan, Poland.

December 13, 2018

JANUSZ K. RYBAKOWSKI'S ADDITIONAL INFORMATION
A COMMENTARY ON WALTER FELBER'S PAPER ON LITHIUM PREVENTION OF DEPRESSION 100 YEARS AGO -- AN INGENIOUS MISCONCEPTION, PUBLISHED IN 1987

Werner Felber's paper, Die Lithiumprophylaxe der Depression vor 100 Jahren - ein genialem Irrtum, was published a year after the 100th anniversary of Carl Lange's treatise on the periodic depressive states: Om Periodiske Depressionstilstande og deres Patogenese (Lange 1886). Lange's monograph was reproduced nine years later in German, translated by Hans Kurella, as Periodische Depressionzustände und ihre Pathogenesis auf dem Boden der harnsauren Diathese (On periodical depressions and their pathogenesis in the context of uric acid abnormality) (Lange 1895). Johan Schioldann's English translation appeared more than a 100 years later, in the beginning of the 21st century (Schioldann 2001).

Felber's paper consists of six parts: 1) Preface; 2) Short biography of Carl Lange and the German translator of his book, Hans Kurella; 3) Remarks on Lange's description of periodic depression; 4) Practical aspects of lithium therapy as performed by Carl Lange; 5) The reasons for the oblivion of epochal achievement; and 6) The pathway to lithium re-discovery.

In the preface, Felber underlined the significance of the Carl Lange's treatise of 1886 which became known to the wider public several years later thanks to German translation by Hans Kurella. The "uric acid diathesis" concept put forward in Lange's treatise provided the basis for long-term lithium administration in periodic depression. Felber estimates that during the 20 years of his psychiatric ambulatory practice Lange treated about 2,000 of such patients with lithium.

In the second part, the short biographies of Carl Lange (1834-1900) and Hans Kurella (1858-1916) were provided. The latter, a German psychiatrist promoted by Karl Kahlbaum, was a keen translator of neurological, psychiatric, anthropological and sociopolitical works of foreign authors, among them Scandinavian and Italian.

The remarks on Lange's description of periodic depression pay great tribute to the clinical astuteness of the Danish physician. Mental and somatic symptoms of depression were delineated, most of which comply with contemporary diagnostic criteria of depression. Among the first are, among others, mental stiffness or paralysis, inability to initiate motor or mental activity, lack of spirits and concomitant anxiety. Within the second group, variable painful symptoms, vegetative disturbances, loss of weight and abnormalities of sleep are listed. In his treatise, Lange also points at circadian mood changes, with the worse mood in the morning in a majority of patients. Felber also mentions Lange's observations on the periodicity and natural course of the illness which are to a great extent similar to contemporary views on the major depressive disorder of mild to moderate intensity.

In the fourth part, Felber describes lithium administration outlined by Carl Lange, regarding dose and method of administration. The drug was given as lithium carbonate powder, 8-40 mmol lithium per day, in 3-4 doses. The daily amount of lithium is therefore comparable to what is used today. Lithium carbonate was dissolved in water or lemonade. In the end, Felber quotes Lange's statement that long-term treatment with lithium caused a disappearance or decrease of depressive episodes with significant prolongation of remission, although in most cases, the illness was not fully cured.

In the fifth part of the paper, Felber argues that the forgotten reason for introducing lithium into treatment of mood disorders by Lange was that the idea of uric acid diathesis behind it was false and was refuted by both psychiatrists and practitioners of general medicine where this kind of diathesis was a basis for using lithium in the treatment of rheumatic diseases.

In his final part (6), Felber mentions John Cade who related to Garrod's work on using lithium in gout on account of the suspected excess of uric acid in this condition (Garrod 1859). However, he did not mention the full story of Cade's experiments which gave rise to the introduction of lithium into contemporary psychiatry. One of Cade's premises was based on the excess of uric acid in manic patients. In the last paragraph of the paper, in relation to Carl Lange's work, Felber speculates about the discrepancy between theory and practice, showing how a false theory could sometimes result in a spectacular clinical achievement.

However, as far as pathogenesis of psychiatric disorders is concerned, the situation nowadays is entirely different from that of 30 years ago when Falber was writing his paper. In the recent two decades it has been found that both uric acid, as the final metabolite of purine bases, and some purines (e.g., adenosine), may play a role in the regulation of psychological processes, including mood and activity. Concomitantly, new evidence has been accumulated concerning a role of uric acid in the pathogenesis and treatment of bipolar disorder (BD). In patients with BD, a higher prevalence of gout and increased concentration of uric acid have been found, and the therapeutic efficacy of allopurinol, used as an adjunct to mood stabilizers, has been demonstrated in mania. In recent years, research on the role of the purinergic system in the pathogenesis and treatment of mood disorders (and also schizophrenia) has focused on the role of adenosine (P1) receptors and nucleotide (P2) receptors. Activation of adenosine receptors is related to antidepressant activity. Alterations of P2 receptors (mostly P2X7 receptors) has been found significant for the pathogenesis of mood disorders, especially bipolar disorder (Malewska-Kasprzak, Permoda-Osip, Rybakowski 2018). Therefore, a direct connection between uric acid and bipolar disorder, and indirectly with lithium, as the main therapeutic modality in this disorder can no longer be denied.

References:

Cade JFK. Lithium salts in the treatment of psychotic excitement. Med J Aust 1949; 2; 612-23.

Felber W. Die Lithiumprophylaxe der Depression vor 100 Jahren - ein genialem Irrtum. Fortschr Neurol Psychiatr 1987; 55: 141-4.

Garrod AB. The Nature and Treatment of Gout and Rheumatic Gout. London: Walton and Maberly; 1859.

Lange C. Om Periodiske Depressionstilstande og deres Patogenese. Copenhagen: Lund; 1886.

Lange C. Periodische Depressionzustände und ihre Pathogenesis auf dem Boden der harnsäuren Diathese. Hamburg/Leipzig: Verlag von Leopold Voss; 1895.

Malewska-Kasprzak M, Permoda-Osip A, Rybakowski J. Disturbances of the purinergic system in affective disorders and schizophrenia. Psychiatr Pol 2018; 52.

Schioldann J. In commemoration of the century of the death of Carl Lange. The Lange theory of 'periodical depressions.' A landmark in the history of lithium therapy. Adelaide: Academic Press; 2001.

February 21, 2019

CHAPTER 8.

INDICATIONS

THOMAS A. BAN: DEVELOPMENT OF THE DIAGNOSIS OF MANIC-DEPRESSIVE PSYCHOSIS IN EMIL KRAEPELIN'S CLASSIFICATIONS

In 44 years, from 1883 to 1927, Emil Kraepelin's Compendium of Psychiatry grew from about 400 pages into a 1,425-page Textbook of Psychiatry in which his syndromic classifications in the first three editions (1883, 1886 and 1889) were replaced by his disease-oriented classification. The shift from syndromic to disease-oriented classification was completed by 1899 with the introduction of the diagnostic concept of manic-depressive psychosis (insanity) in the 6th edition (Pichot 1983).

Tracking the development that led to the diagnostic concept of manic-depressive psychosis, an episodic disease with full remission between episodes, one finds the following chain of events (Menninger, Mayman and Pruyser 1968):

- 1st edition, 1883: Depression (simple melancholia and melancholia with delirium); excitement (melancholia active and mania); and periodic psychoses (periodic mania, periodic melancholia and circular states).
- 2nd edition, 1886: Melancholia (activa, simplex, attonita); mania; periodical insanity (mania, melancholia) and circular insanity.
- 3rd edition, 1889: Mania; melancholia; periodical mental disease (delirious form, manic form, circular form and depressive form).
- 4th edition, 1893: Mania; melancholia; periodical mental disease (delirious form, manic form, circular form and depressive form).
- 5th edition, 1896: Involutional melancholia; periodic psychosis (mania, circular psychosis and depression).
- 6th edition, 1899: Involutional melancholia; manic-depressive psychosis (manic states, depressive sates and mixed states).
- 7th edition, 1903-4: Involutional melancholia; manic-depressive psychosis.

Indications

- 8th edition, 1909 -15: Manic-depressive psychosis.
- 9th edition, 1927: Manic-depressive psychosis.

Kraepelin's all-embracing diagnostic concept of "manic-depressive psychosis" was first fully presented in 1913 in the third volume of the 8th edition of his textbook in which, on the basis of his own comprehensive observations with consideration of earlier German and French research, he united in this diagnosis "the entire realm of periodic and circular insanity, uncomplicated mania, the majority of illness entities taken for 'melancholia,' and a non-negligible quantity of 'amentia' cases," as well as "certain mild, partly periodic, partly chronic morbid mood modifications, which, on the one hand are to be considered as preliminary stages of more severe disorders, on the other as blending into the realm of individual nature" (Berner, Gabriel, Katschnig et al. 1983).

References:

Berner P, Gabriel E, Katschnig H, Kieffer W, Koehler K, Lenz G, Simhandl CH. Diagnostic Criteria for Schizophrenia and Affective Psychoses. World Psychiatric Association; 1983.

Kraepelin E. Compendium der Psychiatrie. Leipzig: Barth; 1883.

Kraepelin E. Compendium der Psychiatrie. Leipzig: Barth; 1889.

Kraepelin E. Psychiatrie. Ein Lehrbuch für Studierende und Ärzte. 4 Aufl. Leipzig: Barth; 1893.

Kraepelin E. Psychiatrie. Ein Lehrbuch für Studierende und Ärzte. 5 Aufl. Leipzig: Barth; 1896.

Kraepelin E. Psychiatrie. Ein Lehrbuch für Studierende und Ärzte. 6 Aufl. Leipzig: Barth; 1899.

Kraepelin E. Psychiatrie. Ein Lehrbuch für Studierende und Ärzte. 7 Aufl. Leipzig: Barth; 1903-1904.

Kraepelin E. Psychiatrie. Ein Lehrbuch für Studierende und Ärzte. 8 Aufl. Leipzig: Barth; 1908-1915.

Kraepelin E. Psychiatrie. Ein Lehrbuch für Studierende und Ärzte. 9 Aufl. Leipzig: Barth; 1927.

Menninger K, Mayman M, Pruyser P. The Vitla Balance. New York: Viking Press; 1969.

Pichot P. A Century of Psychiatry. Paris: Roger Dacosta; 1983.

November 5, 2015

THOMAS A. BAN: FROM EMIL KRAEPELIN'S MANIC-DEPRESSIVE PSYCHOSIS TO KARL LEONHARD'S PHASIC AND CYCLOID PSYCHOSES

The "insanity" that was to become Kraepelin's (1899) "manic-depressive psychosis" (MDP) was first described by Aretaeus, "The Incomparable," of Cappadocia toward the end of the 1st century (Menninger, Mayman and Pruyser 1968). It was separated from other "insanity in the mid-19th century in France independently by Julius

Indications

Baillarger (1854) and Jean-Pierre Falret (1854). To characterize the "insanity," Baillarger (1845) coined the term la fôlie a duble forme ("insanity in double form") while Falret (1854) used la fôlie circulaire ("circular insanity"). A somewhat similar diagnostic concept to Falret's (1954) cyklisches irresein ("cyclothymia") was introduced in 1882 in Germany by Karl Kahlbaum. The signal difference between Falret's (1854) diagnostic concept and Kahlbaum's (1882) was that "circular insanity" affected the whole mental apparatus, whereas "cyclothymia" was restricted to emotional life and left drive and intellect unaffected (Healy 2008; Shorter 2005).

Until Kraepelin's introduction of his diagnostic concept of MDP in 1899, "mania" and "melancholia" were perceived as distinct forms of illness from "cyclothymia" and "circular insanity" (Kahlbaum 1863; Meynert 1884; Ziehen 1894).

The Zeitgeist in psychiatry during the second part of the 19th century was dominated by two major discoveries: the linking of "motor aphasia" to a lesion of the posterior part of the frontal lobe by Paul Broca in 1861 in France and the linking of "sensory aphasia" to the posterior part of the temporal lobe by Carl Wernicke in 1874 in Germany. These breakthrough discoveries about the structures involved in speech, a unique human function, stimulated interest in research to study the relationship between mental and brain pathology; cross-sectional syndromes such as the "manic syndrome" and the "melancholic syndrome" seemed to provide more suitable clinical end-points for studying such relationships than "circular psychosis" and "cyclothymia."

Carl Wernicke

One of the leading proponents of studying the relationship between mental and cerebral pathology in the last quarter of the19th century was Wernicke (1900), himself. To facilitate the use and amplify the utility of syndromes for this research, he developed, in the 1890s, his "elementary symptom" approach for identifying (diagnosing) and classifying psychoses (Ban 2015; Krahl 2000; Wernicke 1893). It was with the use of "elementary symptoms," i.e., symptoms from which assumedly all other symptoms of a syndrome were derived, that Wernicke (1895) separated "anxiety psychosis," "psychic motility psychosis" and some other "psychoses" which by the end of the 19th century were engulfed by Kraepelin's (1899, 1913) diagnostic concept of MDP. By identifying these psychoses and recognizing their independence from each other, and from "circular psychosis" and "cyclothymia," Wernicke (1893) set the stage for a development that lead to the deconstruction of the diagnostic concept of MDP before the diagnostic concept was born (Leonhard 1957).

Wernicke (1900), in keeping with Wilhelm Wundt's (1874, 1896) teachings, perceived the brain as an associative organ and saw mental pathology as the result of "sejunction," i.e., "loosening of or detachment from the rigid structure of associations" (Franzek1990). Yet, as his conceptual framework was based on Griesinger's (1843) "psychic reflex," he used the components of the reflex path as reference points for classifying "psychoses." Accordingly, Wernicke (1900) recognized three classes of "psychoses": one displayed by "anesthesia," "hyperesthesia" or "paresthesia" that he perceived as the result of malfunctioning of the "psychosensory path" and corresponding brain areas; another, displayed by "afunction," "hyperfunction" or "parafunction," the result of malfunctioning of the "intrapsychic path" and corresponding "trans-cortical" brain areas; and a third, displayed by "akinesia," "hyperkinesia" or "parakinesia," the result of malfunctioning of the "psychomotor path" and corresponding brain areas (Ban 2013; Franzek 1990; Wernicke 1896, 1899, 1900).

To clinically refine further the site of malfunctioning, Wernicke (1900) divided consciousness (awareness) into consciousness (awareness) of the outside world (allopsyche), consciousness (awareness) of one's body (somatopsyche) and consciousness (awareness) of one's self-individuality (autopsyche) and distinguished among "allopsychoses," characterized by disorientation in the representation of the outside world, "somatopsychoses," characterized by disorientation in the representation of one's own body, and "autopsychoses," characterized by disorientation in the representation of one's own self and individuality. In his clinically-oriented alternative classification, he classified "delirium tremens," "Korsakoff psychosis" and "presbyophrenia" as "allopsychoses"; "anxiety psychosis" and "hypochondriacal psychoses" as "somatopsychoses"; and "mania" and "melancholia" as "autopsychoses." In describing "mania," Wernicke (1900) emphasized the presence of "ideas of grandeur," and in describing "melancholia," the presence of "ideas of indignity." He saw "manic" and "melancholic" psychoses as independent from each other but recognized that they frequently occur in the same patient (Angst and Grobler 2015; Menninger, Mayman and Pruyser 1968; Wernicke1896).

It was against this background that Kraepelin (1899) developed his diagnostic concept of MDP.

Emil Kraepelin

Instrumental to the development of Kraepelin's (1896, 1899) diagnostic concept of MDP was Thomas Sydenham's conceptualization of disease, in the late 17th century, as a "process" with a "natural history of its own" that "runs a regular and predictable course" (Ban 2000). The disease concept was dormant in psychiatry until Jean-Pierre Falret (1854), in the mid-19th century, identified la fôlie circulaire, on the basis of its "temporal characteristics," and stipulated that "a natural form of psychiatric illness implies a well-defined predictable course," and, vice versa, "a well-defined predictable course presupposes the existence of a natural species of disease with a specified pattern of development" (Falret 1864; Pichot 1983). A similar notion to Falret's was expressed in 1874 by Kahlbaum. Nevertheless, it was Kraepelin (1896, 1913) first who fully adopted Sydenham's concept of disease in psychiatry and by shifting emphasis from "cross-sectional" clinical manifestations to their "origin," "course of evolution" and "outcome" ("termination"), replaced syndromic classification by clinically- (disease) oriented classification.

His shift of emphasis resulted in a radical change, as in his clinically-oriented classification all the different syndromes of "endogenous psychoses" were engulfed by two broad diagnostic concepts: "dementia praecox" and MDP (Kraepelin 1896, 1899, 1913).

Tracing the development of the diagnostic concept of MDP in subsequent editions of Kraepelin's textbooks one finds that in the first five editions, published in 1883, 1887, 1889, 1891 and 1896, he perceived "mania," "melancholia" and "circular psychosis" as independent diagnoses. It was in the 6th edition, published in 1899, that he first introduced his diagnostic concept of MDP. The diagnostic concept was finalized only 15 years later, in 1913, in the third volume of the 8th edition of Kraepelin's textbook with the engulfment of "involutional melancholia" on the basis of G.E. Dreyfus' (1905) findings (Kraepelin 1909-1915). In the same edition, he defined MDP in terms of "etiology," an "endogenous psychosis whose appearance is generally unrelated to external circumstances"; he characterized it, in terms of "symptomatology," as an illness that becomes manifest in one of three states/forms: (1) "manic states" manifested by heightened mood, flight of ideas and increased drive; (2) "depressive states" manifested by sad or anxious mood, thought retardation and decreased drive; and (3) "mixed states," in which "signs of mania and depression appear simultaneously, so that pictures ensue whose traits correspond to those of both illnesses and yet they cannot be classified to either one"; and described it, in terms of "course," as an episodic, remitting and relapsing disease which "as a rule consists of separate attacks more or less sharply delimited from each other and from the normal state of health" (Berner, Gabriel, Katschnig et al. 1983).

Kraepelin's (1913) final diagnostic concept of MDP united the "entire realm of periodic and circular insanity, uncomplicated mania, the majority of illness entities taken from 'melancholia', and also a non-negligible quantity of amentia cases, including certain mild and moderate mood modifications, which on the one hand were considered as preliminary stages of more severe disorders, on the other were blending into the realm of individual nature." He argued for bringing all these varied conditions together under the diagnosis of MDP by pointing out that despite the differences in the clinical pictures, "some basic traits in all these illnesses recur, that the various illness forms merge into each other without recognizable boundaries, supersede each other in the same patient, have a uniform prognosis and can replace one another in genetic ascendency" (Berner, Gabriel, Katschnig et al. 1983).

The clinical features of the manic syndrome and the melancholic syndrome were based originally on information that Kraepelin (1899, 1913) collected on his "counting cards" (Zählenkarten), a symptom check list that included only 10 items: nervousness, restlessness, irritability, depression, psychomotor retardation, aggression, grandiosity, negativistic behavior, hallucinations and paranoid ideas (Bech 2012; Kraepelin 1909-15; Weber and Engstrom1997). But, as time passed the symptoms of the core syndromes of MDP, "mania" and "depression," were conceptualized in terms of Jasperian psychopathology and, by the 1960s, MDP was perceived as a group of "affective disorders" ("affective psychoses") with a primary disturbance of mood from which all other symptoms were derived (Jaspers 1923; Mayer-Goss, Slater and Roth 1960; Woodruff, Goodwin and Guze 1974). "Affective psychoses" are manifest by episodic recurrence of the "manic syndrome," characterized by "hyperthymia" (elated mood) with "acceleration of mental (including psychomotor) activity" and "sleep disturbance," or the "depressive (melancholic) syndrome," characterized by "dysthymia" (depressed mood) with "deceleration (slowing) of mental (including psychomotor) activity" and "sleep disturbance," or both, the "manic" and the "depressive" syndrome in the same patient. In all variations of "affective psychoses" there is full remission between episodes. In recognition of the variations in clinical (psychopathological) manifestations in the basic syndromes, several "manic syndromes" and several "depressive syndromes" were described. Included among them are: "anxious," "delirious," "dysphoric," "furious," "hypochondriacal," "querulous," "simple," "stuporous," "transitory" and "unproductive mania"; and "anxious," "agitated," "hypochondriacal," "simple" and "stuporous depression" (Nyiro 1962).

Kraepelin's (1913) broad "unitary concept" of MDP lingered on and as late as in 1977, in the 9th edition of the International Classification of Diseases, the five "affective psychoses" recognized were: "MDP manic type," "MDP depressed type," "MDP circular type, currently manic," "MDP circular type, currently depressed" and "MDP circular type, mixed" (World Health Organization 1977).

Karl Kleist

While Kraepelin's (1899) dichotomy of the "endogenous psychoses" into "dementia praecox" and MDP was becoming mainstream psychiatry, Wernicke's tradition was continued by Karl Kleist, one of his assistants during his short tenure (1904 to 1905) as professor of Neurology and Psychiatry in Halle, Germany.

By the time Kleist (1911) embarked on his research, the structural underpinning of the "reflex" was established and the emphasis in brain research shifted from pathological anatomy to neurohistology. Instrumental to this development were the contributions of Camillo Golgi (1874), an Italian histologist, who described multi-polar (Golgi) cells in the "olfactory bulb" with the employment of silver staining; Santiago Ramon y Cajal (1894), a Spanish histologist, who established the "neuron" as the morphological and functional unit of the nervous system; and Sir Charles Sherrington (1906), an English physiologist, who demonstrated that the "synapse" was the functional site of transmission from one neuron to another. Recognizing the potential that the neuronal network provides for studying the relationship between mental and neuronal processing in the brain, Kleist (1925, 1934), in Wernicke's (1900) tradition, attributed different clinical pictures in psychiatry to abnormalities at different sites in the functioning of this network (Teichmann 1990).

While Wernicke's contributions set the stage for the deconstruction of Kraepelin's (1899, 1913) diagnostic concept of MDP, Kleist (1911), on the basis of findings in his early research, challenged Kraepelin's

(1899) diagnostic concept of MDP and argued for the independence of "manic psychosis" from "melancholic psychosis." By using the terms "einpolig mania" that translates into English as "unipolar mania," and "einpolig melancholia" in reference to these distinct syndromes, Kleist (1911) set the stage for a development that led, in the 1940s, to the "unipolar-bipolar dichotomy" of "phasic psychoses" (Angst and Grobler 2015; Kleist 1943; Leonhard 1948). For Kleist (1928), "polarity" was a psychopathological concept. He perceived "bipolar psychosis" as a combination of two "unipolar psychoses," i.e., "manic psychosis" and "melancholic psychosis," that becomes manifest in a "polymorphous (multiform) psychosis." He continued all through his life to refer to "unipolar mania" and "unipolar melancholia" as "pure (monomorphous) mania" and "pure (monomorphous) melancholia," respectively, and to "bipolar (zweipolig) mania" and "bipolar (zweipolig) melancholia" as "polymorphous mania" and "polymorphous melancholia" (Kleist 1928, 1943; Leonhard 1943).

Similar to Wernicke (1900), Kleist (1911) also described several syndromes in which changes in "motility" were central (Shorter 2005). Included among them was the syndrome that was to become the diagnostic concept of "akinetic motility psychosis" and the syndrome that was to become the diagnostic concept of "hyperkinetic motility psychosis." Recognition of the affinity of this pair of "motility syndromes" to each other opened the path for the development of the diagnostic concept of "cycloid psychoses" in the mid-1920s (Kleist 1925). Kleist defined "cycloid psychoses" as a group of recurrent psychoses, with full remission between episodes, which circle between two "poles" as MDP but in which the dominant psychopathology is not "elated" or "melancholic" mood, as in MDP, but in another area of mental pathology. He also referred to the same group of psychoses as "marginal psychoses" (Randpsychosen) or "marginal degeneration (constitutional) psychoses" as he perceived them as psychoses which were bordering on "manic-depressive psychosis" (Kleist 1928; Teichmann 1990). By the mid-1930s Kleist recognized three "cycloid psychoses": "anxiety-ecstatic delusional psychosis," "excited-inhibited confusion psychosis" and "hyperkinetic-akinetic motility psychosis" (Fünfgeld 1935).

The distinctiveness of several "episodic psychoses" with full remission between episodes was supported by the findings of Edda Neele, a student of Kleist. She evaluated all "phasic sicknesses" diagnosed at Kleist's University Clinic in Frankfurt between 1938 and 1942 and presented the results of her "epidemiological genetic study" in 1949 in a monograph titled Die phasischen Psychosen nach ihrem Erscheinungs und Erbbild (The Phasic Psychoses According to Presentation and Family History). It was first in Neele's monograph that the "phasic psychoses" were separated into "pure phasic psychoses" which included "melancholia," "anxious melancholia," "anxious reference psychosis," "hypochondriacal depression," "depressive stupor," "mania," "ecstatic inspiration psychosis" and "hypochondriacal excitement"; and "polymorphous phasic psychoses" that included "manic-depressive illness of affect," "hyperkinetic-akinetic motility psychosis," "excited-stuporous confusion psychosis" and "anxious-ecstatic delusional psychosis" (Angst and Grober 2015; Shorter 2005; Teichmann 1990). Her classification of "phasic psychoses" was endorsed by Kleist (1953).

Karl Leonhard

The clinical tradition of Wernicke (1900) and Kleist (1953) continued with Karl Leonhard (1957), a member of Kleist's faculty from 1937 to 1954 at Goethe University in Frankfurt.

Leonhard (1931, 1934, 1936) began his research in the late 1920s and by 1936, the year he joined Kleist's Department of Psychiatry, he had already published some findings on "episodic psychoses," "atypical psychoses" and "defect schizophrenias" which were in line with Kleist's (1911, 1923, 1925, 1928).

During the Frankfurt years (1936-1954), Leonhard (1943) collaborated with Kleist (1943) and Neele (1949) in studying "phasic psychoses" and was instrumental in the conceptualization of findings

Indications

in this project (Kleist 1943; Leonhard 1943). It was in the course of this research that it was recognized that "polymorphous psychosis" was not restricted to "manic-depressive illness of affect" but included also the "psychoses" Kleist (1911, 1925, 1928, 1952) referred to as "cycloid psychoses" (Fünfgeld 1936; Leonhard 1939; Teichman1990). It was also in the course of this research that Leonhard (1948) introduced his concept of "polarity," a nosological organizing principle, and made his distinction between "unipolar depression" and "bipolar depression" based on this principle (Angst and Grobler 2015). Deconstruction of Kraepelin's (1913) diagnostic concept of MDP culminated in 1957 with the publication of Karl Leonhard's monograph, The Classification of Endogenous Psychoses. In his classification, Leonhard integrated the contributions of Wernicke, Kleist and his collaborators with his own findings and conceptualizations.

The concept of "polarity" became the central, but not the exclusive organizing principle in Leonhard's (1957) nosological re-evaluation of Kraepelin's (1913) MDP. While it was on the basis of "polarity" that he split MDP into "bipolar manic depressive disease" and "unipolar phasic psychoses," it was with consideration of Wernicke's (1899, 1900) "mental structure" that he separated the "cycloid psychoses" from "manic depressive disease" and divided the "cycloid psychoses" into "excited-inhibited confusion psychosis," "anxiety-happiness psychosis" and "hyperkinetic-akinetic motility psychosis." Furthermore, it was on the basis of "totality," the organizing principle introduced by William Cullen (1769, 1772, 1776), that he separated "pure mania" and "pure melancholia," both "universal" diseases, from the "pure euphorias" and "pure depressions," in which the "mental structure" was only "partially" affected. Finally, on the basis of Wernicke's (1893) "elementary symptoms," he distinguished five distinct forms of "pure mania": "unproductive," "hypochondriacal," "enthusiastic," "confabulatory" and "non-participatory"; and five distinct forms of "pure depression": "harried," "hypochondriacal," "self-torturing," "suspicious" and "non-participatory").

In 1957, at the time it was first published, Leonhard's classification had already some support from epidemiological genetic findings (Neele 1949). Yet, it was only in 1964, one year before the publication of the third edition of his text in 1965, that Leonhard succeeded in demonstrating that his diagnoses of "cycloid psychoses" were "catamnestically correct" (Leonhard and Trostorff 1964); and it was only in 1966, two years before the publication of the fourth edition in 1968, that Jules Angst (1966) and Carlo Perris (1966) independently demonstrated that "bipolar depression" and "unipolar depression" were distinct. The signal difference between the two populations was in "familiality": patients with "bipolar depression" had a significantly higher rate of "psychoses" among their relatives than patients with "unipolar depression." The distinctiveness of "unipolar depression" and "bipolar depression" in epidemiological genetic research was further substantiated, in 1969, by Winokur, Clayton and Reich.

It was well after the publication of the 6th edition of Leonhard's monograph in 1986, the last edition published during his lifetime, that findings relevant to the distinctiveness of "unipolar mania" and "bipolar mania" emerged. First, in three independent clinical epidemiological studies it was found that "unipolar mania" had an earlier onset and was characterized by fewer episodes and lower comorbidity with anxiety disorders than "bipolar mania" (Merikangas, Cui, Kattan et al. 2012; Pacheco Palha and Arrojo 2009; Young, Marek and Patterson 2009). Then, Yazici and Cakir (2012) noted that patients with "unipolar mania" were less responsive to lithium therapy than patients with "bipolar mania" and Grobler, Roos and Bekker (2014) reported that patients with "unipolar mania" were prescribed more "neuroleptics" than patient with "bipolar mania." Finally, in an epidemiological genetic study, Merikangas and associates (2014) found the familial aggregation of depression in relatives of "depressed probands" much lower than the familial aggregation of mania in the relatives of "manic probands," indicating the genetic independence of "mania" from "depression" (Angst and Grobler 2015; Hickie 2014).

With the exception of a "catalogue" of symptoms, presented

Indications

in1990, Leonhard (1957, 1986, 1990) offers little direct guidance for diagnosing the 16 forms (including 10 sub-forms) of illnesses that resulted from the deconstruction of Kraepelin's (1913) MDP. His monograph, "The Classification of Endogenous Psychoses," has remained through six editions a collection of case reports. Yet, Leonhard argues (1957) that within the "phasic psychoses" already in the first phase (episode) of the illness "bipolar manic-depressive disease" can be separated from "unipolar pure mania" and "unipolar pure melancholia," as well as from the "unipolar pure depressions" and "unipolar pure euphorias." He contends that the signal difference between "bipolar manic depressive disease" and the "unipolar forms of phasic psychoses" is that the "bipolar" form displays a more colorful appearance by varying not only between two poles, but by displaying in each phase, and even during a phase, different clinical pictures to the extent that no clear syndrome can be described. In contrast, the "unipolar" forms return in a periodic course with the same symptomatology, with every individual "unipolar" form characterized by a syndrome associated with no other form and not even related transitionally to any other forms. As the differentiation between "unipolar depression" and "bipolar depression" or "unipolar mania" and "bipolar mania" is not based on the presence or absence of a specific psychopathological symptom or syndrome in a point of time, but on the entire ("holistic") clinical picture in a permanently moving time (Pethö 1990), arguably it would provide a better guide for their recognition if they would be referred to as "polymorphous-" or "monomorphous depression" and "polymorphous-" or "monomorphous mania," as Kleist (1828, 1943) did, than "bipolar-" or "unipolar depression" and "bipolar-" or "unipolar mania." By doing so, one could restrict the use of "bipolar diagnosis" to those patients who already displayed both "poles" in their episodes and use the term "polymorphous" for those who display a "multiform" clinical picture in their episode but so far all their episodes were in the same direction.

Leonhard (1957) maintains that the "pure euphorias" and "pure depressions" can be differentiated from "pure mania" and "pure melancholia" on the basis of their psychopathology, as "pure euphorias" and "pure depressions" are exclusively affective diseases, whereas in "pure mania" and "pure melancholia" thought and desire are also disturbed. Thus, in "pure melancholia" and "pure mania" all three cardinal symptoms of the melancholic syndrome, i.e., depressed mood, psychomotor retardation and thought retardation, or of the manic syndrome, i.e. elated mood, accelerated thinking and increased psychomotor activity, are present; whereas in the "pure depressions" and "pure euphorias" thought and desire are not necessarily affected. In so far as "bipolar phasic" and "cycloid psychoses" are concerned, Leonhard's (1957) differentiation is based on the dominant "elementary symptom" pair, i.e., "depressed mood" or "elated mood," in case of "manic-depressive illness"; "anxious mood" or "ecstasy" in case of "anxiety-happiness psychosis"; "excited confusion" or "inhibited confusion" in case of "excited-inhibited confusion psychosis"; and "hyperkinesia" or "akinesia" in case of "hyperkinetic-akinetic motility psychosis."

Diagnostic instruments

The first diagnostic instrument that provided diagnoses relevant to Leonhard's (1957) classification was the KDK Budapest, developed by Pethö, Ban, Kelemen, Karczag, Ungvari, Bitter and Tolna. It was published in 1984, in the Hungarian periodical Ideggyogyaszati Szemle. The second diagnostic instrument was its English adaptation, the DCR Budapest-Nashville developed also in the mid-1980s by Pethö and Ban in collaboration with Kelemen, Ungvari, Karczag, Bitter, Tolna (Budapest), Jarema, Ferrero, Aguglia, Zuria and Fjetland (Nashville). The third, the Schedule for Operationalized Diagnosis for the Leonhard Classification (SODLC) was developed in the late 1980s by Fritze and Lanzig. Both, the DCR and the SODLC were published in Psychopathology, in 1987 and in 1990, respectively.

The DCR is based on diagnostic algorithms and its diagnostic process on a decision-tree model that leads to one diagnosis. The decision whether a diagnosis qualifies for a "unipolar" or a "bipolar"

Indications

illness, depends on the "presence or "absence" of five variables:

1. Unipolar episodic course: Course of illness is characterized by recurring shifts in mood and/or tempo of thoughts and/or psychomotor activity which is consistently in the same direction.
2. Bipolar episodic course: Course of disease is characterized by recurrent two-directional positive and negative shifts in mood and/or tempo of thought and/or psychomotor activity.
3. Monomorphous clinical picture: Well defined, pure, distinct disease picture which remains unchanged during the illness or at least within a single episode of the illness.
4. Polymorphous clinical picture: Variable disease picture in which different symptoms and/ or syndromes prevail at different times.
5. Polymorphous fluctuating disease picture: Multiform, variable disease picture in which different symptoms and/or syndromes prevail at different times. Behavior is characterized by its rapid and frequent variations alternating between extremes (opposite poles).

To qualify for a phasic or a cycloid "bipolar illness" subjects must qualify for one of the four diagnoses in addition to displaying a "polymorphous" or "polymorphous fluctuating clinical picture." The four diagnoses with qualifying criteria are:

1. Manic-depressive psychosis: At least three of the following five functional areas must be disordered: mood, drive, sex drive, sleep and psychomotility.
2. Anxiety-happiness psychosis: At least three of four from either one or the other sets of symptoms must be present: marked anxiety, marked tension, delusional perceptions and delusions of reference, or feelings of happiness, desire to make others happy, exaggerated self-esteem and misperceptions.
3. Excited–inhibited confusion psychosis: Incoherence must be present and at least three of four from either one or the other

sets of symptoms must be present: decreased talkativeness, decreased activity, reactive stupor and misperceptions, or increased talkativeness, increased activity, misperceptions and fragmentary hallucinations.

4. Hyperkinetic-akinetic motility psychosis: One of three from the following three symptoms must be present: akinesia, hypokinesia, hyperkinesia, as well as at least three of four from either one or the other sets of symptoms must be present: confused stupor, absence of purposeful activities, diminished reactive movements and diminished expressive movements, or increased reactive movements, increased expressive movements, agitation and speech characterized by short phrases and long pauses with occasional emotionally charged outbursts.

To qualify for a phasic "unipolar illness" subjects must qualify for one of 12 diagnoses in addition to displaying a "monomorphous" clinical picture. The 12 diagnoses with qualifying criteria are:

1. Pure mania: At least three of the following five symptoms must be present: hyperthymic mood, psychomotor agitation, flight of ideas, premature decisions and exaggerated self-esteem.

2. Pure melancholia: At least three of the following five symptoms must be present: dysthymic mood, psychomotor retardation, retarded thinking, indecisiveness and feelings of inadequacy.

3. Harried depression: At least three of the following five symptoms must be present: monomorphous clinical picture, motor restlessness, marked anxiety, driven complaintiveness and poor thematization.

4. Hypochondriacal depression: At least three of the following five symptoms must be present: monomorphous clinical picture, hypochondriasis, homonome bodily hallucinations, hopeless complaintiveness and corporization.

5. Self-torturing depression: At least three of the following five

symptoms must be present: monomorphous clinical picture, feelings of guilt, loss of self-esteem, lamentiveness and self-incrimination.

6. Suspicious depression: At least three of the following five symptoms must be present: monomorphous clinical picture, suspiciousness, ideas of reference, paranoid ideation and lack of hostility.

7. Non-participatory depression: At least three of the following five symptoms must be present: monomorphous clinical picture, lack of affective participation, abulia, anhedonia and feelings of alienation.

8. Unproductive euphoria: At least three of the following four symptoms must be present: monomorphous clinical picture, motiveless feeling of happiness, radiant facial expression and poor thematization.

9. Hypochondriacal euphoria: At last three of the following four symptoms must be present: monomorphous clinical picture, hypochondriasis, homonome bodily hallucinations and cheerful complaintiveness.

10. Enthusiastic euphoria: At least three of the following four symptoms must be present: monomorphous clinical picture, exaggerated self-esteem, happily enthused when talking about self-related topics and happily enthused when talking about topics related to others.

11. Confabulatory euphoria: At least three of the four following symptoms must be present: monomorphous clinical picture, confabulations with grandiose ideas, recounting happy experiences and lively talkativeness.

12. Nonparticipatory euphoria: At least three of the following four symptoms must be present: monomorphous clinical picture, lack of feeling of sympathy (with happiness), impoverishment of emotions (with happiness) and impoverishment of will (with happiness).

Neuropsychopharmacology

By the time of the publication of Leonhard's Classification of Endogenous Psychoses, in 1957, the "neuronal network" discovered around the turn of the 20th century was a functional entity and with the discovery of the presence of several neurotransmitters in the brain (serotonin, norepinephrine, dopamine), emphasis shifted in the understanding of the nature of synaptic transmission from a purely electrical to a chemically mediated event (Ban 2006; Montagu 1957; Twaog and Page 1953; Vogt 1954). Furthermore, introduction of the spectrophotofluorometer simultaneously with the first set of effective psychotropic drugs (lithium, chlorpromazine, imipramine) in the treatment of "endogenous psychoses in the1950s, provided a capability to measure the corresponding changes in the concentration of neurotransmitter monoamines and their metabolites with their therapeutic effects (Bowman, Caulfield and Udenfriend 1955; Cade 1949; Delay and Deniker 1952; Kuhn 1957.) With these developments, the only tangible obstacle in generating interpretable findings regarding the biochemical underpinning of manifest psychopathology was the pharmacological heterogeneity within the diagnoses derived by Kraepelin's (1909-15) nosology. In spite of this and the reasonable assumption that diagnoses derived by Leonhard's (1957) differentiated nosology would provide pharmacologically more homogenous populations than Kraepelin's (1913) MDP, Leonhard's (1957) "classification," with the exception of his distinction between unipolar and bipolar depression, remained isolated from main stream of psychiatry to date.

Pharmacotherapy

Developments, relevant to the pharmacotherapy of MDP, began in 1949 with John Cade's report that lithium was effective in controlling excitement in all 10 "manic" patients included in his study without any effect on his three depressed patients. Lithium, not even at the time, was a newcomer in psychiatry. In the late 19th century the substance was found effective in "periodic depression," but its use was

Indications

abandoned because of lithium toxicity (Lange 1886).

Cade's (1949) findings on the therapeutic effect of lithium in mania on 10 patients were further substantiated in 1951 by Noack and Trautner in a study that included several hundred patients. It was the historical study that rendered lithium treatment feasible by determining blood levels in which the substance could be safely administered with the employment of the flame-photometer. Still, another three years passed until, in 1954, Schou, Juel-Nielsen, Strömgren and Wolby demonstrated, in a placebo-controlled cross-over study, the therapeutic efficacy of lithium in "mania."

One would have thought that demonstration of lithium's therapeutic efficacy in mania would guarantee a smooth entry for lithium in the treatment of mania," but this was not the case. Attention to lithium and to Schou and his associates' (1954) findings was distracted by Lehmann and Hanrahan's (1954) report on the striking therapeutic effect of chlorpromazine in the treatment of "mania," published in the same year. It took about another 17 years until, in 1971, lithium found its place in the treatment of "mania," supported by findings in four placebo-controlled studies (Goodwin and Jamison 1990; Goodwin, Murphy and Bunney 1969; Maggs 1963; Stoke, Shamoian, Stoll and Patton 1971). Yet, without the identification of the treatment responsive subpopulation to lithium, the primary form of treatment in "mania" remained with neuroleptics.

Instrumental to lithium's further clinical development were the observations that continued treatment with lithium attenuated the severity and duration of subsequent episodes, regardless whether they were "manic" (Noack and Trautner's 1951) or both, "manic" and "depressive" (Schou et al 1954). Lithium's prophylactic effect on both "manic" and depressive" episodes, if they occurred in same patient, was supported by the findings of Gershon and Trautner in 1956; Vojtechowsky in 1957; Hartigan in 1963; Baastrup in 1964; and Baastrup and Schou in 1967.

Baastrup and Schou's (1967) report on the "propyhylactic effect" of lithium in MDP was challenged by Blackwell and Sheppard in 1968.

It was in response to this challenge that in 1970 Angst, Weis, Grof, Baastrup and Schou, and independently Baastrup, Poulsen, Schou and Thomsen, demonstrated the efficacy of "lithium prophylaxis" in patients diagnosed as "recurrent affective disorder" or MDP. Yet, without the identification of the treatment responsive subpopulation in which lithium could prevent relapse, by the dawn of the 21st century lithium has become one of many competing drugs with the primary indication of depression, psychosis and epilepsy, for prophylactic treatment in bipolar mood disorder.

It was in 1969, in the midst of the lithium controversy (1968 – 1970) about lithium's prophylactic effect, that Goodwin, Murphy and Bunney reported their findings of a placebo-controlled study on lithium's "unequivocal" therapeutic efficacy in "bipolar depression", i.e., in "typical "MDP patients, with a history of both, "manic |" and "depressive" episodes. Their findings were verified in a pooled analysis of seven placebo-controlled studies, including their own, in which response rate in "bipolar" patients was 79% and in "unipolar" depressed patients 36% (Baron et al 1975; Goodwin and Jamison 1990; Goodwin, Murphy and Bunney1969; Goodwin, Murphy, Dunner et al. 1972; Johnson 1974; Mendels 1975; Noyes, Dempsey, Blum and Cavanaugh 1974). Without a prior division of the population into "unipolar" and "bipolar depression," lithium's therapeutic potential for some depressed patients would have remained hidden.

The differential responsiveness to lithium between "unipolar" and "bipolar" patients is not restricted to "depression" but applies also to "mania." Already in the first placebo-controlled study it was noted that response rate in "mania" in "typical" patients, i.e., patients with both "manic" and "depressive" episodes, was considerably higher, 90%, than response rate in atypical patients (62%) (Schou, Juel-Nielsen, Strömgren and Voldby 1954). Similar differences in response rates in favor of "typical" over "atypical" patients were found in other studies by Goodwin and Ebert (1973) in their review of clinical trials and controlled studies with lithium in "mania." The difference is even more pronounced when response to lithium in "typical manic" patients and "schizoaffective manic" patients is compared. In Goodnick and Meltzer's (1984) study, "schizoaffective manic" patients required more than twice as long to achieve a full response to lithium than "typical manic" patients.

Re-evaluation

Reintroduction of lithium in psychiatry, in the mid-20th century, focused attention on the heterogeneity of responsiveness to the substance within Kraepelin's (1913) diagnostic concept of MDP. By the1960s clinical observations and findings indicated that dividing the population on the basis of "polarity" into "unipolar depression," "bipolar depression," "unipolar mania" and "bipolar mania" would provide, in "bipolar depression" and "bipolar mania," pharmacologically more homogenous populations in terms of responsiveness to acute, maintenance and prophylactic treatment with lithium than Kraepelin's (1899) MDP. Yet, it was also recognized that in the subpopulations derived by "polarity," the pharmacological heterogeneity was only reduced, not resolved. A full re-valuation was warranted with the separation within "bipolar psychoses" -- "cycloid psychosis" from "manic-depressive psychosis" -- and within "unipolar psychoses" -- "pure mania" from the "pure euphorias" -- and "pure melancholia" from the "pure depressions." This re-evaluation has not taken place to-date.

References:

Angst J. Zur Ätiologie und Nosologie endogener depressiver Psychosen. Eine genetische, soziologische und klinische Studie. Berlin/Heidelberg/ New York: Karger; 1966.

Angst J, Grobler Ch. Unipolar mania: a necessary diagnostic concept. Eur Arch Clin Neurosci 2015; 265:273-90.

Angst J, Weis P, Grof P, Baastrup PC, Schou M. Lithium prophylaxis in recurrent affective disorders. Br J Psychiatry. 1970; 116:604-14.

Baastrup PC. The use of lithium in manic-depressive psychosis. Compr Psychiatry. 1964; 5:396-408.

Baastrup PC, Poulsen JC, Schou M, Thomsen K. Prophylactic lithium: Double blind discontinuation in manic depressive and recurrent-depressive disorders. The Lancet. 1970; 2:326-30.

Baastrup PC, Schou M. Lithium as a prophylactic agent: Its effect against recurrent depressions and manic-depressive psychosis. Arch Gen Psychiat 1967; 16:162-7.

Baillarger J. De la folie a double forme. Annales medico-psychologique 1854; 6: 369-91.

Ban TA. Nosology in the teaching of psychiatry. J Bras Psiquiatr 2000; 49:39-49.

Ban TA. Academic psychiatry and the pharmaceutical industry. Progress in Neuro-Psychopharmacology and Biological Psychiatry 2006; 30:429-41.

Ban TA. Neuropsychopharmacology and the Forgotten Language of Psychiatry. Risskov: International Network for the History of Neuropsychopharmacology; inhn.org.ebooks. November 14, 2013.

Ban TA. Elementary symptoms. inhn.org.dictionary. October 8, 2015b.

Baron M, Gershon S, Rudy V, Jonas WZ, Buchsbaum M. Lithium carbonate response in depression. Prediction by unipolar/bipolar illness, averaged evoked response, catechol-O-methyl transferase and family history. Ach Gen Psychiatry 1975; 32:1107-11.

Bech P. Clinical Psychometrics. Copenhagen: Willey-Blackwell; 2012.

Blackwell B, Shepherd M. Prophylactic lithium: Another therapeutic myth? Lancet 1968; 1:968-71.

Bowman RL, Caulfield PA, Udenfriend S. Spectrophotometric assay in the visible and ultraviolet. Science 1955; 122:32-3.

Broca P. Remarques sur le siege de la faculte langage articule: suives d'une observation d'aphemie. Bull Soc Anal 1861; 6:330-57.

Cade JFJ. Lithium in the treatment of psychotic excitement. Med J Austr 1949; 2:349-52.

Cullen W. Synopsis Nosologiae Methodicae. Edinburgh: Kincaid & Creech; 1769.

Cullen W. Synopsis Nosologiae Methodicae. Edinburgh: Kincaid & Creech; 1772.

Cullen W. First Lines of the Practice of Physics. Edinburgh: Kincaid & Creech; 1777.

Delay J, Deniker P. 38 cas de psychoses traitèes par la cure prolongée et continué de 4560 RP. CR Congr Méd Alién Neurol (France) 1952; 50: 503–13.

Dreyfus GL. Die Melancholie ein Zustandsbild des Manisch-Depressiven Irreseins. Jena: Gustav Fischer; 1905.

Falret JP. De la Folie Circulaire. Thesis. 1854.

Falret JP. Mémoir sur la folie circulaire. Bulletin de l'Académie de Medicine 1854; 19; 382-415.

Falret JP. Des Maladies mentales et des asiles d'l alienes. Paris: J.B. Balliere et fils; 1864.

Franzek E. Influence of Carl Wernicke on Karl Leonhard's nosology. Psychopathology 1990; 23: 277-81.

Fritze J, Lanczik M. Schedule for operationalized diagnosis according to the Leonhard classification of endogenous psychoses. Psychopathology 1990; 23:303-15.

Fünfgeld E. Motilitätspsychosen und Verwirtheiten. Berlin: Karger; 1936.

Gershon S, Trautner EM. The treatment of shock-dependency by pharmacological agents. Med J Austr 1956; 43:783-7.

Goodnick PJ, Meltzer HY. Treatment of schizoaffective disorders. Schizophrenia Bulletin 1984; 10: 30-48.

Goodwin FK, Ebert M. Lithium in mania. Clinical trials and controlled studies. In: Gershon S, Shopsin B, editors. Lithium. Its role in psychiatric research and treatment. New York: Plenum Press 1973, pp. 237-52.

Goodwin FK, Jamison KR. Manic-Depressive Illness. Oxford: Oxford University Press; 1990.

Goodwin FK, Murphy DL, Bunney WE Jr. Lithium carbonate treatment in depression and mania: A longitudinal double-blind study. Arch Gen Psychiatry 1969; 21:486-96.

Goodwin FK, Murphy DL, Dunner DL, Bunney WE Jr. Lithium response in unipolar versus bipolar depression. Am J Psychiatry 1972; 129:44-7.

Griesinger W. Über psychische Reflexactionen. Archiv für Physiologische Heilkunde 1843; 2:76-112.

Grobbler C, Roos JL, Bekker P. Unipolar mania reconsidered evidence from a South African study. Afr J Psychiatry 2014: 17:473-91.

Hartigan GP. The use of lithium salts in affective disorders. Brit J Psychiat. 1963; 109:810-4.

Healy D. Mania. A Short History of Bipolar Disorder. Baltimore: The

Johns Hopkins University Press; 2008.

Hickie HB. Independence of mania and depression. Evidence for separate inheritance of mania and depression challenges current concepts of bipolar mood disorders. Mol Psychiatry 2014; 19: 153-5.

Jaspers K. Allgemeine Psychopathologie. Berlin: Springer; 1923.

Johnson G. Antidepressant effect of lithium. Compr Psychiatry 1974; 15:43-7.

Kahlbaum KL. Die Grouppierung der psychischen Krankheiten, Entwurf einer historisch-kritischen Darstellung der bisherigen Einteilungen und Versuch zur Anbahnung einer empirisch-wissentschaftlischen Grundlage der Psychiatrie als klinischer Disziplin. Danzig: A.W. Kaufman; 1863.

Kahlbaum KL. Die Katatonie oder das Spannungsirresein. Berlin: Hirschwald; 1874.

Kahlbaum KL. Über cyklisches Irresein. Der Irrenfreund-Psychiatrische Monatschrift für praktische Ärzte 1882; 24:145-57.

Kleist K. Die Streitfrage der akuten Paranoia. Ein Beitrag zur Kritik des manisch-depressiven Irreseins. Z. Ges Psychiatrie 1911; 5: 366-87.

Kleist K. Die Auffassung der Schizophrenien als psychische Systemkrankheiten (Heredodegenerationen). Vorl Mitteilung. Kl W Jg 1923; 21:962-3.

Kleist K. Die gegenwartigen Strömungen in der Psychiatrie. Allg Z Psychiat 1925; 82:1-41.

Kleist K. Über zykloide, paranoide und epileptoide Psychosen und über die Frage der Degenerationpsychosen. Schweiz Arch Neurol Neurochir Psychiat 1928; 23:3-37

Kleist K. Die Katatonien. Nervenarz. 1943; 16: 1-10.

Kleist K. Gliederung des neuropsychischen Erkrankungen. 1953; 125:526-54.

Kraepelin E: Compendium der Psychiatrie. Leipzig: Barth; 1883.

Kraepelin E: Compendium der Psychiatrie. 2 Aufl. Leipzig: Barth; 1886.

Kraepelin E: Compendium der Psychiatrie. Leipzig: Barth; 1889.

Kraepelin E. Psychiatrie. Ein Lehrbuch für Studierende und Ärzte. 4 Aufl. Leipzig: Barth; 1893.

Kraepelin E. Psychiatrie. Ein Lehrbuch für Studierende und Ärzte. 5 Aufl. Leipzig: Barth; 1896.

Kraepelin E. Psychiatrie. Ein Lehrbuch für Studierende und Ärzte. 6 Aufl. Leipzig: Barth; 1899.

Kraepelin E. Psychiatrie. Ein Lehrbuch für Studierende und Ärzte. 7 Aufl. Leipzig: Barth; 1903-1904.

Kraepelin E. Psychiatrie. Ein Lehrbuch für Studierende und Ärzte. 8 Aufl. Leipzig: Barth; 1909-1915.

Kraepelin E. Psychiatrie. Ein Lehrbuch für Studierende und Ärzte. III. Klinische Psychiatrie. 8. Auflage. Leipzig: Barth; 1913.

Kraepelin E. Psychiatrie. Ein Lehrbuch für Studierende und Ärzte. 9 Aufl. Leipzig: Barth; 1927.

Krahl A. Carl Wernicke's elementary symptom (Elementarsymptom). In: Franzek E, Ungvari GS, Ruther E, Beckmann H, editors. Progress in Differentiated Psychopathology. Wurzburg: International Wernicke-Kleist-Leonhard Society; 2000, pp. 43-8.

Kuhn, R. 1957. Über die Behandlung depressives Zustande mit einem iminodibenzyl-derivat (G22355), Schweiz. Med. Wochenschr. 87, 1135-40.

Lange C. Om periodiske Depressionstilstande og deres Patagonese. Copenhagen; Jacob Lunds Forlag; 1886.

Lehmann HE, Hanrahan GE. Chlorpromazine. New inhibiting agent for psychomotor excitement and manic states. Arch Neurol Psychiatry 1954; 71:227-37.

Leonhard K. Episodische Dämmerzustände (Kleist) mit gleichartiger Vererbung. Monatschr f Psychiat 1931; 81:226.

Leonhard K. Atypische endogene Psychosen im Lichte der Familienforschung. Z f Neurol 1934; 149:520.

Leonhard K. Die Defektschizophrenen Krankheitsbilder. Leipzig: Thieme; 1936.

Leonhard K. Erbbiologie der Katatonien. Allg Z f Psychiat 1943; 122:39.

Leonhard K. Grundlagen der psychiatrie. Stuttgart: Enke; 1948.

Leonhard K. Aufteilung der endogenen Psychosen. Berlin: Akademie Verlag; 1957.

Leonhard K. Aufteilung der Endogenen Psychosen. 3 Aufl. Berlin: Akademie Verlag: 1965.

Leonhard K. Aufteilung der Endogenen Psychosen. 4 Aufl. Berlin: Akademie Verlag: 1968.

Leonhard K. Classification of Endogenous Psychoses (translated from the 5th edition of the German original by Berman R). New York: Irwington Press; 1979.

Leonhard K. Aufteilung der endogenen Psychosen. Berlin: Akademie Verlag; 1986.

Leonhard K. Differenzierte Diagnostik der endogenen Psychosen unter Anlehnung an einem Symptomenkatalog. Psychiatr Neurol Med

Psychol 1990; 42:136-45.

Leonhard K, Trostorff S. Prognostische Diagnose der endogenen Psychosen. Jena: Fischer; 1964.

Maggs R. Treatment of manic illness with lithium carbonate. Br J Psychiatry 1963; 109:56-65.

Mayer-Gross W, Slater E, Roth M. Clinical Psychiatry. Second edition. London: Cassell & Company; 1960.

Mendels J. Lithium in the treatment of depressive states. In: Johnson FN, editor. Lithium Research and Therapy. New York: Academic Press; 1975, pp.43-62.

Menninger K. Mayman M, Pruyser P. The Vital Balance. The Life Process in Mental Health and Illness. New York: The Viking Press; 1968.

Merikangas KR, Cui L, Kattan G, Carlson G, Youngstrom EA, Angst J. Mania with and without depression in a community sample of US adolescents. Arch Gen Psychiatry 2012; 69:943-51.

Merikangas KR, Cui L, Heaton L, Nakamura E, Roca C, Ding J, Quin H, Guo Y, Yao-Shugart Y, Zarate C, Angst J. Independence of familial transmission of mania and depression results of the NIMH family study of affective spectrum disorders. Mol Psychiatry 2014; 19:214-9.

Meynert T. Psychiatrie. Lehbruch der Erkrankungen der Vorhirnes, begründet auf dessen Bau, Leistungen und Ernährung. Vienna: Braumuller; 1884.

Montagu KA. Catechol compounds in rat tissues and in brains of different animals. Nature 1957; 180:240-1.

Neele E. Die phasischen Psychosen nach ihrem Erscheinungs und Erbbild. Leipzig: Barth 1949.

Indications

Noack CH, Trautner EM. The lithium treatment of maniacal psychosis. Med J Aust 1951; 2:219-22.

Noyes R Jr, Dempsey GM, Blum A, Cavanaugh GL. Lithium treatment of depression. Compr Psychiatry 1974 15:187-93.

Nyiro Gy. Psychiatria. Budapest: Medicina; 1962.

Pacheco Palha A, Arrojo A. Clinical aspects of unipolar mania. In: Figureira ML, Akiskal H, editors. Clinical Aspects of Mania. Alphen an den Rijn: Wolters Kuwer Health; 2009, pp. 47-52.

Perris C. A study of bipolar (manic-depressive) and unipolar recurrent depressive psychoses. Acta Psychiatr Scand 1966; 42:1-189.

Pethö B. Development and structure of the DCR Budapest-Nashville. Psychopathology 1990; 23: 316-30.

Pethö B, Ban TA in collaboration with Kelemen A, Ungvari G, Katczag I, Bitter I, Tolna J (Budapest), Jarema M, Ferrero F, Aguglia E, Zurria GL, Fjetland O (Nashville). DCR Budapest-Nashville in the Diagnosis and Classification of Functional Psychoses. Psychopathology 1988; 21: 153-240.

Pethö B, Ban TA, Kelemen A, Ungvari G, Karczag I, Bitter I, Tolna J. KDK Budapest. Kutatasi Diagnosztikus Kriteriumok functionalis psychosisok korismezesehez.. Ideggyogyaszati Szemle 1884; 37: 102-31.

Pichot P. A Century of Psychiatry. Paris: Roger Dacosta; 1983.

Schou M, Juel-Nielsen N, Strömgren E, Voldby H. The treatment of manic psychoses by administration of lithium salts. J Neurol Neurosurg Psychiatry 1954; 17:250-60.

Shorter E. Historical Dictionary of Psychiatry. Oxford: Oxford University Press; 2005.

Stokes PE, Shamoian CA, Stoll PM, Patton MJ. Efficacy of lithium in acute treatment of manic-depressive illness. Lancet 1971; 1:1319-25.

Teichmann G. The influence of Karl Kleist on the nosology of Karl Leonhard. Psychopathology 1990; 23:267-76.

Twarog BM, Page IH. Serotonin content of some mammalian tissues and urine and a method for its determination. Am J Physiol 1953; 175:157- 61.

Vogt M. Concentration of sympathin in different parts of central nervous system under normal conditions and after administration of drugs. J Physiol 1954; 123:451-81.

Vojtechovsky M. Zkusenosti s lecbou solemi lithia. Problemy Psychiatrie v Praxi a ve Vyzkumu. Prague: Czechoslovak Medical Press; 1957, pp. 216-24.

Weber MM, Engstrom EJ. Kraepelin's diagnostic cards; the confluence of clinical research and preconceived categories. History of Psychiatry 1997; 8:375-85.

Wernicke C. Der aphasische Symptomen complex. Eine psychologische Studie auf anatomischer Basis. Breslau: M.Crohn und Wegert; 1874.

Wernicke C. Diskussionsbeitrag auf dem 59. Treffen des Vereins ostdeutscher Irrenarzte. Leubus, 19. Juni 1892. Allgemeine Zeitschrift fur Psychiatrie und psychisch-gerichtliche Medizin 1893: 486-9.

Wernicke C. Grundrisse der Psyhiatrie. In Klinischen Vorlesungen. Leipzig: Barth; 1896.

Wernicke c. Ueber die Klassifikation der Psychosen. Breslau; Sclettersche Buchhandlung; 1899.

Wernicke C. Grundrisse der Psyhiatrie. In Klinischen Vorlesungen. Leipzig: Barth; 1900.

Winokur G, Clayton P, Reich T. Manic Depressive Illness. Saint Louis; Mosby: 1969.

Woodruff RA, Goodwin DW, Guze SB. Psychiatric Diagnosis. New York: Oxford University Press; 1974.

World Health Organization. International Classification of Diseases. Ninth Revision. Geneva: Word Health Organization; 1977.

Wundt W. Grundzüge der physiologischen Psychologie. Leipzig: Engelsman; 1874.

Wundt W. Grundriss der Psychologia. Leipzig: Engelsman; 1896.

Yazici O, Cakir S. Unipolar mania: A distinct entity or characteristic of manic preponderance. Turk Psikyatyri Derg 2012; 23:201-5.

Young AH, Marek S, Patterson RM. Unipolar mania. In: Figueira ML, Akiskal H, editors. Clinical Aspects of Mania. Alphen an den Rijn: Wolters Kuwer Health; 2009, pp. 39-4.

Ziehen T. Psychiatrie für Ärzte und Studierende. Berlin: F. Wreden; 1894.

April 21, 2016

EDWARD SHORTER'S INTRODUCTORY COMMENT

INTRODUCTION TO LITHIUM IN PSYCHIATRY

Thomas A. Ban

IN HISTORICAL PERSPECTIVE

The story of lithium is really the story of everything that's wrong with psychopharmacology. It was difficult to get lithium accepted. It has been difficult to keep lithium on the radar. Yet it is the most powerful form of pharmacoptherapy that psychiatry has on offer. Possibly the most effective drug treatment for mood disorders ever introduced, lithium was systematically shoved aside in graduate training and marginalized in clinical use, so that more profitable – but less effective – "mood stabilizers" carried the day and lithium found itself in the rear of the van. The whole story documents the inadequacy of psychiatry's efforts to become a clinical neuroscience.

Preamble: Lithium had a long "folkloric" existence

At some point, Senator Tom Connally of Texas asked Morris Fishbein, longsttanding editor of the Journal of the American Medical Association and a leader in the campaign against quackery of the 1920s and '30s, if Fishbein couldn't possibly interest the FDA in the "Crazy Crystals" of Texas, evidently containing lithium. Fishbein dismissed the notion[1]. But there is some evidence that the lithium springs had an impact on mental illness and in 2014, on the basis of these lithium-water stories, the New York Times headlined, "Should We All Take a Bit of Lithium?" (Sept 13). The effectiveness of lithium in spring water holds up in a statistical analysis: The 27 Texas counties where lithium in the water ranges from 70-170 micrograms/L have significantly lower levels of suicide, homicide and rape than do the low-or no-lithium-counties.[2]

Lithium inserted itself rather insidiously in American culture in the

---

[1] Interview with Morris Fishbein, "History of the U.S. Food and Drug Administration," transcript in National Library of Medicine, History of Medicine Division, FDA Oral History Collection, 99. Mar 12, 1968.

[2] Schrauzer GN, Shrestha KP. Lithium in Drinking Water and the Incidence of Crimes, Suicides, and Arrests Related to Drug Addictions. Biol Trace Elem Res. 1990; 25:105-13.

1930s and '40s. The soft drink "7-Up" was advertised as "lithiated lemon soda" from its launch in 1929 until 1950[3]; ads featured happy babies consuming bottles of it[4]. So the notion that lithium was somehow beneficial infiltrated popular culture before medical culture. Various medical efforts in the 19th century to use lithium therapeutically in psychiatry may be noted[5]. All remained curiosities of the literature and had no impact. John Cade, in any event, had probably never heard of any of it and deserved, as Carroll puts it, "a pass, in recognition of the distractions of WWII and the concentration camp. Then after the war, he was a man in a hurry to make up for lost time."[6]

Rise

As is well known, in the mid-1940s Cade discovered the efficacy of lithium in mania and published in 1949 one of the most famous articles about it in the history of psychiatry[7]. In today's lingo Cade's patients, in Carroll's view, were probably "rapid cycling bipolar" rather than

---

[3] Aita JF. 7-Up Anti-Acid Lithiated Lemon Soda or Early Medicinal Use of Lithium. Nebraska Medical Journal. 1990; 75:277-80.

[4] http://time-warp-wife.blogspot.com/2010/09/vintage-humor-what.html?m=1.

[5] For a careful review, see Demling JH. Lithium – Irrtümer, eine Wiederentdeckung und ein Goldstandard. Schriftenreihe der Deutschen Gesellschaft für Geschichte der Nervenheilkunde. 2014; 20:227-43.

[6] Carroll B. personal communication, July 16, 2017.

[7] Cade JF. 1949. Lithium Salts in the Treatment of Psychotic Excitement. Med J Austr, 36: 349-352. On these events, see Johan Schioldann, History of the Introduction of Lithium into Medicine and Psychiatry (Adelaide: Adelaide University Press, 2009); Walter Brown, Lithium: A Doctor, A Drug, and a Breakthrough (Toronto: Penguin/Random House Canada, 2019); also De Moore, Gregory, et al. 2016. Finding Sanity: John Cade, Lithium and the Taming of Bipolar Disorder. Sydney: Allen and Unwin. See on this rapildy growing literature Barry Blackwell, "Comments," http://inhn.org/cn/publications/books/walter-a-brown-lithium-a-doctor-a-drug-and-a-breakthrough-reviewed-by-walter-a-brown/barry-blackwells-comment.html.

"chronic mania" and very lithium-responsive[8]. There have been several recent histories of this epochal discovery, including Walter Brown's Lithium: A Doctor, A Drug, and a Breakthriough (2019). Yet Cade's initial patient died of a lithium overdose; Cade turned his back on the treatment and, as Sam Gershon points out, it was the 1951 paper of Charles Noak and Edward Trautner at the University of Melbourne[9] that, as Gershon put it, "did much to stem the flight from interest in exploring lithium in psychiatry."[10]

This Noak-Trautner study was the first in the world to monitor lithium levels with the newly developed flame photometer. And it was in fact this photometer that made possible the expansion of lithium therapy because the ion was otherwise too tricky to use.[11] It was impossible to obtain blood levels and overdoses could easily be fatal.

At the instigation of his chief Erik Strömgren at the University of Aarhus, in 1954 Mogens Schou published the first of a series of papers on lithium based on randomly controlled trials. These were among the first RCTs in psychiatry.[12] The story was so good it could not possibly be true! A group at the Maudsley Hospital led by psychopharmacologist Michael Shepherd sought to diminish Schou's contribution and to downplay the importance of lithium. Healy writes, "This controversy dragged lithium out of obscurity and made it one of

---

[8] Carroll B. Interview. In: Ban TA. editor. An Oral History of Neuropsychopharmacology, The Frst Fifty Years: Peer Interviews. Brentwood TN: ACNP: V, 100. 2011.

[9] Noack C, Trautner EM. The Lithium Treatment of Maniacal Psychosis. Med J Austr. 1951; 38:219-22.

[10] Gershon S. Lithium Discovered, Forgotten and Rediscovered. inhn.org.archives. August 15, 2013.

[11] Caldwell AE. In: Clark WG, Del Giudice J, Aden GC, editors. Principles of Psychopharmacology, 2nd ed. New York: Academic Press: 1978, pp. 9-40, 30.

[12] Schou M Juel-Nielsen N, Strömgren E, Voldby H. The Treatment of Manic Psychoses by the Administration of Lithium Salts. J Neurol Neurosurg Psychiatry. 1954; 17:250-60.

the stars in the psychotropic firmament."[13]

Yet it has been a controversial star. Among authorities on "bipolar disorder," the lack of enthusiasm for lithium has been palpable. In 2007, Guy Goodwin at Oxford and others, in an ECNP "consensus meeting on bipolar disorder," essentially give lithium the back of their hand and concluded that "positive findings seem to many authorities to... support the addition of lamotrigine during or after the resolution of a depressive or manic episode to prevent further depressive relapse."[14] A patent-protected remedy of indifferent clinical application – What a recommendation!

What could explain such foot-dragging in the presence of unquestionable data on the efficacy of lithium in treating and forestalling mood disorders and in suicide prevention? First, there was the Zeitgeist argument. Psychiatry was just emerging from its entombment in psychoanalysis.

Then, Sam Gershon ventured the "complexity" explanation: "The clinical monitoring for lithium usage is too complicated for psychiatrists and [they are] better off using antipsychotics or anticonvulsants. The other attraction is that for the latter drugs you do not need to carefully make a diagnosis, which may take a couple of visits. So educational instiutions are actively contributing to these decisions because it's quicker and cheaper for the instiution, but does lifelong harm to the patient."[15]

Other explanations spring readily to mind: clinicians drowning in the torrent of Pharma literature praising patent-protected "mood stabilizers" and so forth. But the phenomen of lithium-aversion remains puzzling; the ion gave clinicians the means of actually saving

---

[13] Healy D. Mania: A Short History of Bipolar Disorder\. Baltimore: Johns Hopkins University Press, 2008, p. 122.

[14] Goodwin GM, Anderson I, Arango C, Bowden CL, Henry C, Mitchell PB, Nolen WA, Vieta E, Wittchen HU. ECNP Consensus Meeting. Bipolar Depression. Nice, March 2007. Eur Neuropsychopharmacol. 2008;18(7):535-49.

[15] Gershon S. personal communication, May 5, 2017

lives – 70% of suicides are caused by serious depressive illness, which responds readily to lithium. Why would doctors not rush to take advantage of it?

Schou coined the term "mood stabilizer" in 1963,[16] by which time he had become the most enthusiastic academic authority on lithium and, to be sure, on lithium in all mood disorders, not just acute mania. So, at the beginning, the concept of "mood stabilization" was a portmanteau term for any agent affecting mood.

Prophylaxis

The notion that lithium could be prophylatic rather than merely therapeutic had been in the air yet without garnering much support. Jules Angst later said, "I remember one CINP meeting in Munich in 1962, at which Mogens Schou stood up in a discussion dominated by talk of neuroleptics and antidepressant drugs and spoke about the prophylactic properties of lithium and was greeted with loud laughter. People simply didn't believe that lithium was active."[17]

Then in 1963, with anecdotal data, Geoffrey Hartigan at Queen Square observed that lithium "has repeatedly shown its worth in the prophylaxis of manic-depressive and manic states," and the few cases that he presented suggested that once again.[18]

In 1967 Schou and fellow psychiartrist Poul Baastrup reported lithium prophylaxis in an open trial of 88 female patients at the Glostrup Psychiatric Hospital. The authors concluded, "Lithium is the first drug for which a clear-cut prophylactic action against one of the major psychoses has been demonstrated... Lithium seems to be of

---

[16] Schou M. Normothymics, "Mood Stabilizers": Are Lithium and the Imipramine Drugs Specific for Affective Disorders? British Journal of Psychiatry, 1963; 109:803-9.

[17] Angst J. Interview. In: Healy D, editor. The Psychopharmacologists. London: Chapman and Hall, I: 1996, p. 290.

[18] Hartigan GP. The Use of Lithium Salts in Affective Disorders. Br J Psychiatry. 1963; 109:810-4.

unusual potential value for reserarch on manic-depressive psychosis." (The authors meant manic-depressive illness in the Kraepelinian sense of all mood disiorders, not in the DSM sense of "bipolar disorder.")[19]

The demonstration of lithium prophylaxis of mania and depression was eye-opening. Heinz Lehmann, chief of the Douglas Hospital in Montreal, said in 1978, "Perhaps the most important new development during the last decade has been contributed by Baastrup and Schou with the lithium maintenance treatment of affective disorders. A number of studies in several countries have demonstrated reliably that continuous lithium treatment, carried on over the years, can prevent many recurrences in patients who previously were periodically disabled and endangered by frequent arttacks of depression or mania."[20]

Lehmann was prescient: Lithium became significant only when Baastrup and Schou found it useful in "preventing recurrences of affective disorders," as Linford Rees, who virtually initiated controlled trials in psychiatry, put it.[21] In a discussion at an FDA approvals committee in 1995, Dennis Charney, then at Yale University, seconded this point, "The miracle of lithium was not its trteatment of acute mania. Neuroleptics, even high-dose benzodiazepines, are quite effective for the treatment of acute mania. And neuroleptics may even be superior to lithium in the treatment of acute mania. The issue is prevention of relapse."[22]

In 1971 Alec Coppen at West Park Hospital in Epsom and

---

[19] Baastrup P, Schou M. Lithium as a Prophylactic Agent. Its Effect Against Recurrent Derpressions and Manic-Depressive Psychosis. Arch Gen Psychiatry. 1967; 16:162-72.

[20] Lehmann H. Discussion, In: Lipton MA et al. eds. Psychopharmacology: A Generation of Progress. New York: Raven Press. 1978, p.15.

[21] Rees L. Interview. In: Healy D. The Psychopharmacologists. London: Chapman and Hall, II. 1998, p.176-7. (My italics.)

[22] Charney D. Discussion, FDA Psychopharmacologic Drugs Advisory Committee, transcript of proceedings, Feb 6, 1995, 135; obtained through Freedom of Information Act.

colleagues published in The Lancet an RCT of 65 patients with recurrent depression. The results were striking: "Patients receiving lithium had very significantly less affective illness than patients receiving placebo tablets... No patient on lithium was given electroconvulsive therapy (E.C.T.), whereas 43 percent of the placebo group received one or more courses of E.C.T." Coppen said that his research affirmed Schou's conclusion "that lithium has a definite prophylactic action in recurrent affective disorders."[23] (Coppen remembered, at a meeting of the "Denghausen Group" on some Caribbean island, "Ted [Edward] Hare coming along with his colleague Ramon Gardner and he said that this can't be right. He and Gardner went through the results but they couldn't find any fault with them."[24]). Coppen strengthened doubts about bipolar and unipolar depression as constituting two separate diseases when, at a symposium in St. Moritz in 1972, he said that his group could detect no difference in the lithium prophylaxis of depressions of either polarity.[25] (With time, belief in the separateness of unipolar depression ["major depression"] and "bipolar disorder" became an article of faith.)

International Spread

The global progress of lithium following its introduction in Australia was swift.

In France there had been a long history of using lithinated spa waters, including such venerable remedies as "Les Lithinés du Docteur Gustin," in the treatment of gout.[26] In 1951, two French investigators

---

[23] Coppen A, Noguera R, Bailey J, Burns BH, Swani MS, Hare EH, Gardner R, Maggs R. Prophylactic lithium in affective disorders. Controlled trial. Lancet. 1971; 2(7719):275-9.

[24] Coppen A. Interview. In: Healy D, editor. The Psychopharmacologists. London: Chapman and Hall: 1996, pp. 272-3.

[25] Coppen A. Discussion. In: Kielhoz P. États Dépressifs: Dépistage, Évaluation, Traitement. Berne: Huber: 1972, p. 36.

[26] See Raynal C. Un Exemple d'Eau Minérale Artificielle à Reconstituer Chez Soi:

reported on 12 psychiatric cases treated with lithium citrate, of whom three had "chronic mania." All three did well and the authors concluded, "The use of lithium in the manic phases of manic-depressive psychosis seems particularly effective."[27] French clinicians used lithium citrate, which enjoyed a momentary vogue until the introduction of chlorpromazine 1953.[28] By 1958 the firm Laboratoire T.E. in the Rue Ste Anne was indicating lithium benzoate for "the biological treatment of anxiety and anxious insomnias."[29] Not quite mania yet, but getting close.

In Britain, in 1966 the Drug and Therapeutics Bulletin praised the use of lithium in the treatment of mania and said it could be prophylactic against recurrent depression and mania: "Because there is a delay of two or three days in onset, a major transquilliser should be given parenterally at the start."[30] Yet it was unhelpful that Aubrey Lewis, professor of psychiatry at the Institute of Psychiatry at the Maudsley Hospital – the primary training center in England – thought lithium "dangerous nonsense."[31]

In 1968 Curt Rossman at the Women's Clinic of the Uppsala

Les Fameux "Lithinés du Dr Gustin." Revue d'Histoire de la Pharmacie. 2007; 356:505-18.

[27] Despinoy M. Romeuf J de. Emploi des Sels de Lithium en Thérapeutique Psychiatrique. Rapports et Comptes Rendus, Congrès des Neurologistes et Aliénistes de Langue Française. 1951; 49:509-15. See also Reyss-Brion R. Grambert J. Essai de Traitement des États d'Excitation Psychotique par le Citrate de Lithium. Journal de Médecine de Lyon, 1951; 32:985.

[28] Reyss-Brion R. Discussion. In: Sutter J-M, editor. VIes Journées d'Information Psychiatrique de Marseille.. L'Encéphale. 1973; 62 supp:64-5. (The conference was in 1972.)

[29] Vidal L. Dictionnaire de Spécialités Pharmaceutiques. Paris: Office de Vulgarisation Pharmaceutique, 1927.

[30] Lithium in mania and depression. Drug and Therapeutics Bulletin, 1966; 4:103-4.

[31] Post F. Reminiscence. In: Wilkinson G, editor. Talking About Psychiatry. London: Gaskell: 1993, pp. 157-77.

Academic Hospital in Sweden reported good results with lithium in the treatment of premenstrual syndrome. The eight women were said to have "severe premenstrual conditions with aggressiveness, irritability, emotional lability and listlessness as well as marked water retention." At serum levels between 0.4 and 0.7 mg/Eql "in all cases the result has been good or very good and the patients have all been satisfied. All mental symptoms have been alleviated."[32]

The US story

It was a trainee of John Cade, Sam Gershon, who brought lithium to the United States in 1959 when he accepted a post in the "Schizophrenia and Psychopharmacology Joint Research Project" of the University of Michigan. One of the program's clinical arms was at Ypsilanti State Hospital – financed by a program grant from John Cole's Psychopharmacology Service Center at NIMH – and there Gershon would, according to Cole, buy lithium "by the kilo from a chemical supply store and then get a drug store pharmacist to put it into capsules."[33]

Barry Blackwell writes of Gershon's migration, "He would have more to do with lithium there [in the US], and became an evangelist, preaching its virtues to the non-believers until the Americans eventually re-entered the fray – like their entry into both world wars – late."[34]

Gershon and Arthur Yuwiler reported in 1960 – in anecdotal form

---

[32] Rossman C. Discussion. In: Diding N, Ottosson JO, Schou M, editors. Lithium in Psychiatry: Proceedings of a Symposium in Lidingö, Sweden, March 22, 1968. Acta Psychiat. Scand. 1969; suppl. 207, p. 89.

[33] Cole J. Interview. In: Healy D, editor. The Psychopharmacologists. I. London: Chapman and Hall: 1996, p. 254.

[34] Blackwell B. Review. Gregory de Moore and Ann Westmore: Finding Sanity: John Cade, Lithium and the Taming of Bipolar Disorder. Sydney/Melbourne/Auckland/London: Allen & Unwin; 2016. inhn.org.biographies. February 2, 2017.

Indications

– the results of their lithium trials at Ypsilanti State.[35] At the same time, Edward Kingstone – or "Eddie" as he styled himself in the title – reported an open trial that he had conducted, under the supervision of D. Ewen Cameron, the directior of the Allan Memorial Institute in Montreal.[36] (Kingstone said he was first to write. Yet publication was delayed when the American Journal of Psychiatry, under the editorship of Clarence Farrar, turned it down.). Both trials included patients with a variety of diagnoses and highlighted lithium for investigation in North America.

In 1962 George Winokur initiated the use of lithium at Washington University in St. Louis. Paula Clayton, then a resident, recalled their early use: "We had a manic minister, kind of like Elmer Gantry [figure in a novel by Sinclair Lewis]. He'd written bad checks. George [Winokur] read about lithium in The Lancet and after the patient was given multiple ECTs and trifluoperazine, but was still not well, George had the pharmacy make up lithium pills because nobody produced them. We gave lithium to the manic minister and he got better. So we began using lithium for mania in 1962 even though it wasn't marketed and approved by the FDA."[37]

By 1971 four RCTs of lithium had been conducted for acute mania. The average response rate was 71%.[38] These results could not be overlooked. In 1970 the FDA approved simultaneously all three New Drug Applications for lithium carbonate: Pfizer for Lithane, Rowell for Lithionate and Smith Kline and French for Eskalith – all were for

---

[35] Gershon S, Yuwiler A. Lithium Ion: A Specific Psychopharmacological Approach to the Treatment of Mania. Journal of Neuropsychiatry. 1960; 1:229-41.

[36] Kingstone E. The Lithium Treatment of Hypomanic and Manic States. Comprehensive Psychiatry. 1960; 1:317-20.

[37] Clayton P. Interview. In: Ban TA, Gershon S, editors. An Oral History of Neuropsychopharmacology, The First Fifty Years: Peer Interviews. Brentwood TN, ACNP: VII: 2011, p. 95.

[38] Goodwin FK, Jamison KR. Manic-Depressive Illness. New York, Oxford University Press: 1990, pp. 613-14.

"acute manic states."[39] Thus, the US became the 50th country to adopt lithium, a testimonial to the foot-dragging of the FDA in this area.

Yet already in the 1960s a network of US practitioners who prescribed lithium was forming, some of whom had permits to study Investigational New Drugs (INDs) from FDA. (And some didn't, just ordering their lithium from abroad or getting the corner pharmacist to buy some from a chemical supply house and put it in capsules).[40] In 1968 an Ohio physician wrote to an FDA administator saying that he had "a few patients who could definitely benefit from this treatment." But the Ohio doctor knew only of Dr. Arthur Sugerman at the Carrier Clinic in Belle Mead, New Jersey, who administered lithium; yet Ohio patients would need to have their levels checked monthly and New Jersey was a long drive. Were there no Ohio physicians, this doctor asked, who had been approved by FDA?[41]

A member of this network was Paul Blachly at the University of Oregon. And it was partly owing to a campaign organized by Blachly that FDA was finally induced to approve lithium for "acute manic states in manic-depressive psychosis" in 1970[42] (and for "the maintenance" of manic-depressive psychosis in 1974). "The FDA has had no good reason for holding this drug up," Blachly told the press.[43] In 1971 Blachly and his resident Barry Maletzky wrote the first

---

[39] For actual approval, news story, F-D-C Reports ("The Pink Sheet"), Apr 13, 1970, T&G -3.

[40] See Diamond E. Lithium vs. Mental Illness; Lithium vs. mental illness. New York Times, Jan 12, 1969, MagazineSM p. 30.

[41] Basil D Roman to Merle Gibson (FDA), Oct 10, 1968; National Archives, RG88, box 4137.

[42] Schmeck HM Jr. Long-Studied Drug Is Licensed for Treatment of Mental Illness. New York Times, Apr 7, 1970, p. 1.

[43] Unsourced news clipping in the National Archives, FDA RG-88, box 4256, 520. Attached to Gibson to Vacchiano, Oct 6, 1969.

textbook, The Use of Lithium in Psychiatry.[44]

Lithium clinics began opening. Ronald Fieve at the New York State Psychiatric Institute, alerted to the European literature by director Larry Kolb, established in 1966 the first lithium clinic in the US.[45] David Dunner, who was a junior associate of Fieve's in the clinic, said later, "Ron Fieve's major effort was to get wider acceptance of lithium. When patients from our clinic went on vacation, it was difficult to find psysicians they couuld consult who knew about the drug."[46] Fieve said at a conference in 1973 that there was no doubt as to lithium's effectiveness in the prophylaxis of bipolar illness. As well, "Studies to date strongly suggest that lithium alone or lithium plus tricyclics may likewise be the future choice for maintaining unipolar depressives in a lithium clinic."[47]

Further lithium clinics saw the light of day: in 1968 William ("Dutch") Dyson founded one at the Coaldale Mental Hospital in the Delaware Valley; in 1973 Bernard Carroll at the University of Michigan established another. Donald Klein imported lithium to Hillside Hospital, Nathan Kline to Rockland State Hospital. These were the pioneers. By the early 1980s, lithium had been generally accepted as the therapy of choice in mania (except for highly active episodes) and for forestalling the recurrence of depression.

Lithium in depression

---

[44] Maletzky B, Blachly P. The Use of Lithium in Psychiatry. Cleveland CRC Press. 1971, pp. 55-9.

[45] On Kolb's role, see Ivan Goldberg to Edward Shorter, personal communication, Jan 28, 2007.

[46] Dunner DL Interview. In: Ban TA, Gershon S, editors. An Oral History of Neuropsychopharmacology, The First Fifty Years: Peer Interviews. Brentwood TN, ACNP: VII, 2011, p. 166.

[47] Fieve R. Discussion. In: Angst J, editor. Classification and Prediction of Outcome of Depression. Stuttgart: Schattauer Verlag, 1974, p. 113. (The conference took place in 1973.)

Schou had suggested in 1954 that lithium might have antidepressant action but this was not widely taken up. Then, as noted, in 1967 Baastrup and Schou reported that lithium was effective in the prophylaxis of depression as well as in manic-depressive illness.

Lithium changed the diagnostic picture considerably in the 1970s in the US. Under the influence of psychoanalysis, "schizophrenia" had been the favorite diagnosis of analytically-influenced clinicians for patients not suitable for psychotherapy. But once mania and manic-depressive illness became treatable with lithium, much of the previous "schizophrenia" turned into mood disorder. At Mt. Sinai Hospital in New York, in the years 1947 to 1957, 15% of the patients were diagnosed as schizophrenic, only 4% as manic-depressive. This then reversed once lihium was included in the hospital pharmacopeia. At the Payne Whitney Psychiatric Clinic, as staffer Stuart Asch said in 1987, "Every year, as previous schizophrenic patients were readmitted... we have had to repeatedly correct the old diagnosis of schizophrenia to manic-depressive illness."[48]

A substantial literature arose on the use of lithium in the treatment of depression.[49] (See the level-headed assessment in the respected Drug and Therapeutics Bulletin in 1981.[50]) In 1969 Fred Goodwin and colleagues at NIMH became first to document in an RCT that lithium had antidepressant effects outside of the framework of bipolar disorder. There were only five patients in the "noncyclic group" and the study was scarcely definitive.[51] The antidepressive effect of lithium

---

[48] Asch SS. History of the General Hospital Psychiatric Inpatient Unit, 1947 to 1986. Psychiatric Clinics of North America. 1987; 10:155-64. (Also the source for the Mt. Sinai statistics.)

[49] For an overview that includes the older literature, see Mendels J. Lithium and Depression. In: Gershon S, Shopsin B, editors. Lithium: Its Role in Psychiatric Research and Treatment. New York: Plenum Press: 1973, pp. 253-68.

[50] "Lithium Updates," Drug and Therapeutics Bulletin. 1981; 19:21-4.

[51] Goodwin FK, Murphy DL, Bunney WE Jr.. Lithium-Carbonate Treatment in Depression and Mania. A Longitudinal Double-Blind Study. Arch Gen Psych.

was confirmed in 1972 by Joseph Mendels and William ("Dutch") Dyson at the University of Pennsylvania; the authors said their finding "raises the question of whether lithium carbonate might be effective in the treatment of selected depressed patients."[52] (The University of Pennsylvania became a fortress of the study in lithium in bipolar illness, led by Dyson's successor Jay Amsterdam at the Depression Research Unit.[53])

Paul Janssen, who founded Janssen Pharmaceutica and counts as one of the epoch's great drughunters, advocated lithium in depression rather than one of his own drugs. He described disagreements within his lab: "In our laboratory I have always fought the idea of some of the old pharmacologists who claimed to be interested in making antidepressants – my question has always been: What is an antidepressant? Because the best treatments that I know of for endogenous depression are electroconvulsive therapy and lithium. For me these two modes of treatment are clinically far more obviously effective than imipramine-like tricyclics."[54] The use of lithium in depression has been a turning point at which the conventional wisdom failed to turn, for even today lithium is considered a bit experimental in the treatment of unipolar depression.

Resistance

Things got off to a bad start. In 1955 the second edition of Goodman and Gilman, the stanard guide to pharmacology, said, "The

---

1969; 21:486-96.

[52] Mendels J. Secunda SK. Dyson WL. A Controlled Study of the Antidepressant Effects of Lithium. Arch Gen Psych, 1972; 26:154-7.

[53] See for example, Amsterdam JD, Rybakowski JK. Pharmacotherapy of Bipolar Disorder. In: DeRubeis RJ, Strunk DR, editors. The Oxford Handbook of Mood Disorders. 2016.

[54] Janssen Paul. Interview. In: Healy D, editor. The Psychopharmacologists. London. Chapman and Hall. II: 2011, p. 63.

lithium ion has no therapeutic application."[55] The third edition in 1965 was scarcely more enthusiastic but did note without comment Schou's work.[56]

In the 1960s there was a whole scientific climate of opinion that pushed back against lithium. After the discovery of amine neurotransmitter reuptake at the National Institutes of Health in the late 1950s, the field focused laserlike upon drugs with differing reuptake profiles. It was clear that serotonin and norepinephrine were the key to some kind of antidepressant effect. But a drug that was simultaneously antimanic and antidepressant? That did not fit well within the theoretical framework and so, as a a result, it didn't exist. Goodwin, then at NIH, later recalled, "One of my patients was on lithium and I felt both the patient's depression and mania was getting better, which was counter to the prevailing wisdom of the time; the amine hypotheses were dominant and it was incomprehensible to have a substance that combined antimanic and antidepressant effects."[57]

Lithium treatment is not innocuous. From the beginning it was known that lithium, excreted in the kidneys, could cause renal damage. This was nailed in 1977 by a team of pathologists and clinicians at the University of Aarhus who, in renal biopsies of fourteen patients on long-term lithium treatment who had been admitted for acute lithium intoxication, found twice the amount of damage in interstitial renal connective tissue as in controls. As well, "The number of sclerotic glomeruli was five times as great as in controls."[58]

---

55 Goodman LS, Gilman A. The Pharmacological Basis of Therapeutics. 2nd ed. New York: Macmillan: 1955, p. 817.

56 Goodman LS. Gilman A. The Pharmacological Basis of Therapeutics. 3rd ed. New York: Macmillan: 1965, p. 805.

57 Goodwin FK. Interview. In: Ban TA, editor. An Oral History of Neuropsychopharmacology, The First fifty Yeaars: Peer Interviews. Brentwood TN, ACNP: V, 2011, p. 157.

58 Hestbech J, Hansen HE, Amdisen A, Olsen S. Chronic Renal Lesions Following Long-term Treatment with Lithium. Kidney Int. 1977; 12(3):205-13.

Indications

Bernard Carroll later commented, "Australians are very pragmatic and all through the 1950s, lithium was widely used in Australia and was picked up in England through Mogens Schou in Scandinavia and later in Europe in the 1950s and the 1960s. The resistance to lithium as a clinical agent was centered mostly in the United States."[59] Why so much resistance in the US?

It was a mixture of commercial rivalry and psyhchoanalysis. The spirit of the times in psychiatry in the 1950s and -60s was psychoanalysis. Alec Coppen, the very image of a bioloical psychiatrist, said "A lot of people who are in psychiatry are not really interested in the medical model. They went into psychiatry to get away from it."[60] Clearly, those who sought the origin of illness in "the unconscious" would be skeptical of lithium.

As for commerce, there is a fine line between documenting side effects and counter-detailing on the part of commercial competitors. As one psychiatrist in a small town in Wisconsin told his listmates in 2008, "Under Abbot Labs coaching, I switched many lithium patients to valproate starting in the 1980s, and well, yes, it was better for several years. And now it is not in way too many patients . . . [Valproate] has at least as many cognitive difficulties as lithium, and is unacceptable in women aged 16 to 50."[61]

A whole subculture arose around the supposedly severe side effects of lithium treatment. Goodwin and Kay Redfield Jamison described in 1990, "The antagonism towards lithium... on the part of some mental health workers, who may subtly or overtly sabotage drug compliance."[62]

---

[59] Carroll B. Interview. In: Ban TA, editor. An Oral History of Neuropsychopharmacology, The First Fifty Years: Peer Interviews. Brentwood TN: ACNP: V, 2011, p. 99.

[60] Coppen A. Interview. In: Healy D, editor. The Psychopharmacologists. London: Chapman and Hall, I: 1996, p. 274.

[61] [Name redacted]. Aug 3, 2008 to psycho-pharm@psycom,.net.

[62] Goodwin FK, Jamison KR. Manic-Depressive Illness. New York, Oxford

At the request of Abbott, Charles Bowden, at the San Antonio campus of the University of Texas, led in 1994 the first RCT of valproate versus lithium and placebo in the treatment of mania (48% of the divalproex [Depakote] patients improved, 49% of the lithium patients; 25% of the placebo patients)[63]. Bowden's lack of enthusiasm for lithium was palpable. He told an interviewer in 2003, "Lithium is a very poorly tolerated medication. I think the evidence increasingly is that it worsens depression more often than it helps depression (sic)." He added a bit later in the interview, "Valproate has its own side effects but was generally much more tolerable [than carbamazepine or lithium]. It also seemed to have a broader spectrum of efficacy."[64] Bowden continued to work closely with Abbott. (Valproate was not universally admired. George Simpson, a longtime clinician with Nate Kline at the Rockland State asylum in New York State, said, "When valproate came, they sold it to everybody saying it was the most efficacious treatment for bipolar patients, which is clearly untrue. Its never ben proven; the more serious studies suggest lithium is still the drug to beat and I would agree with that. I also think that the side effects of lithium are somewhat exaggerated.")[65]

It was Abbott's promotion of valproate that led to the concept of "mood stabilizer," given that few knew of Schou's earlier usage.[66]

University Press: 1990, p. 749

[63] Bowden CL, Brugger AM, Swann AC, Calabrese JR, Janicak PG, Petty F, Dilsaver SC, Davis JM, Rush AJ, Small JG, et al. Efficacy of Divalproex vs Lithium and Placebo in the Treatment of Mania: The Depakote Mania Study Groiup. JAMA. 1994; 271(12):918-24.

[64] Bowden CL. Interview. In: Ban TA, Gershon S, editors. An Oral History of Neuropsychopharmacology, The First Fifty Years: Peer Interviews. Brentwood TN, ACNP: IV, 2011, p. 62.

[65] Simpson G. Interview. In: Ban TA, Gershon S, editors. An Oral History of Neuropsychopharmacology, The First Fifty Years: Peer Interviews. Brentwood TN, ACNP: IX, 2011, p. 305.

[66] See on this Harris M, Chandran S, Chakraborty N, Healy D. Mood-stabilizers: the archeology of the concept. Bipolar Disord. 2003; 5(6):446-52; Grof P. "Mood-

Indications

Carroll was scathing on the subject of Abbott's promotion of valproate (Depakote). He called Pharma influencing medical practice "a familiar story – look at how Abbott badmouthed lithium to promote Depakote (aided and abetted by venal KOLs [key opinion leaders], of course."[67]

Ads for the mood stabilizers made no secret of the superiority of their products to lithium. Abbott Labs trumpeted in 1995, apropos its drug Depakote (divalproex sodium), "Significantly superior to placebo in patients intolerant or not responsive to lithium."[68]

Lithium was not driven entirely out. DSM-III in 1980 abolished Kraepelin's "manic-depressive illness," a basin that included all mood disorders, and replaced it with unipolar depression ("major depression") and "bipolar disorder," a quite separate illness, said the Manual. Yet such was the purchase that manic-depression had in psychiatric practice, that companies manufacturing lithium continued to promote it for "manic-depressive illness" long after 1980.[69] (Other companies did, however, switch their lithium indications over to "bipolar patients" – SmithKlineBecham 1993). Manic-depression was thus a trailing edge rather than a leading one. But it was a powerful edge.

The contagion spread. American drug companies producing "mood stabilizers" had no interest in promoting lithium and, just as with electroconvulsive therapy, it was hoped this was a treatment that would die in silence. Mogens Schou said in retrospect, "The industry was never really interested in lithium because of the lack of opportunity to make money from it... Students and young physicians [in the United

---

stabilizers: the archeology of the concept"--by M Harris, S Chandran, N Chakraborty and D Healy: a commentary. Bipolar Disord. 2003; 5(6):453-5.

[67] Carroll B. personal communication, May 28, 2013.

[68] Depakote ad, 1995. AJP. 152.

[69] See for example Solvay Pharmaceuticals ad for "Lithobid" (lithium carbonate) in the American Journal of Psychiatry, 151 (1994), ad pages. Solvay acquired the license for Lithobid from Ciba in 1993.

States] hear exclusively about the anticonvulsants and nothing about lithium, and that of course gives a bias."[70]

Much was made of the "triad of toxicity": tremor, desequilibrium and confusion. Of course all drugs have side effects. Important is the balancing of the risk/benefit ratio and increasingly this ratio was made to move to lithium's disfavor. The alternative "mood stabiliozers," such as lamotrigine and valproic acid, were presented as much more appealing. So successful was this campaign that many trainees and younger clinicians removed lithium from their personal pharmacopeias. And even among lithium fans, there was a lively awareness that supposedly subtherapeutic doses of lithium could have toxic effects. In 1994 Jonathan Himmelhoch, at the University of Pittsburgh (who had trained at Yale in the 1960s), cautioned against "the failure to recongize lithium failure."[71]

Experienced old hands pushed back, pooh-poohing the renal toxicity alarm. Ivan Goldberg in New York City had been treating patients with lithium since 1962.[72] He had been on staff at Columbia-Presbyterian Medical Center and by 2008, as a very experienced senior figure, told colleagues on a list-serve, "I'd estimate the percent with renal impairment sufficient to require the discontinuation of lithium being in the 5-10 percent range."[73] This was not a forbidding number. He continued in another note, "Over the years I have treated about 400 patients with lithium. I know of four patients who required dialysis... While I suspect there are people who progress to total renal failure with no risk factors other than long-term lithium treatment, I

---

[70] Schou M. Interview. In: Healy D, editor. The Psychopharmacologists London: Chapman and Hall, 1998: II, 1996, pp. 276-7.

[71] Himmelhoch J. On the Failure to Recognize Lithium Failure. Psychiatric Annals. 1994; 24(5):241-50.

[72] Goldberg I to Shorter E. Personal communication. Jan 26, 2007.

[73] Ivan Goldberg to psycho-pharm@psycom.net, Aug 13, 2008.

have not seen such a patient as yet."[74]

Senior clinicians, generally speaking, were lithium fans. Said one, "For you young ones on the list whose pharma-company-sponsored teachers brainwashed you against Li, I have not seen any other medication than Li fully normalize the mental status of a severely disturbed patient."[75]

But the battle was largely lost. In 2017, Olga Zivanovic at the Univeresity of Novi Sad in Serbia reached the discouraging conclusion, "Despite abundant evidence regarding the efficacy of lithium in the treatment of bipolar disorders, its use is declining at the beginning of the 21st century." It was, she said, necessary to remind the field of this again and agin, so that lithium "should once again become the first-line treatment for bipolar disorders." Jay Amsterdam, who led the Mood Disorders Unit of the University of Pennsylvania, asked rhetorically in 2017, "Who do you know in the US since 2008, who actually applies lithium as a first-line therapy for bipolar disorder (whether manic or depressed), when the de jour treatment-of-choice in the US is 'anything but lithium.'"[76]

The indictment of the nay-sayers by Bernard Carroll in 2017 is interesting. He told Sam Gershon, "I remain deeply wary of the anticonvulsant Mafia. What they did to lithium use and education was terrible. Full disclosure: John Cade was one of my teachers in Melbourne."[77] As indeed Cade had taught Gershon.

Pushback

A page was turning. Paul Grof at the University of Ottawa said in 2014, "Voices have now arisen suggesting that lithium may actually be

---

[74] Ibid., Mar 17, 2008.

[75] David M Tobolowsky (Miami), ibid., Aug 13, 2008.

[76] Amsterdam J. Nov 18, 2017; personal communication.

[77] Bernard Carroll to Sam Gershon, personal communication, Gershon threat dated Feb 15, 2017.

the only true mood stabilizer, as it demonstrably acts against both polarities of manic-depressive disorders."[78] He himself helped lead the comeback.[79]

The pushback against the patented mood stabilizers in favor of lithium commenced around 2000. It was precisely in 2000 that a group of investigators at the Free University in Berlin conducted a "withdrawal" study to assess the effectiveness of lithium in the continuation phase of a trial for depression. The technique: in phase I a group of 75 depression patients were placed in an open trial of lithium + antidepressant. In phase II, the 29 responders from phase I were randomly assigned to antidepressant + placebo or antidepressant + lithium for four months; in the placebo group, the lithium was then tapered early. The results were significant. In the lithium-taper group one of the patients committed suicide, several other experienced severe relapses. Evidently, it was the lithium, not the "antidepressant," that had kept everyone well in phase I. The authors concluded, "Substitution of placebo for lithium medication resulted in a rapid return of severe symptoms in a significant number of patients who were euthymic during the week lithium was withdrdawn. One-third of the patients suffered a depressive relapse after they had entered the placebo phase of the study but none of the patients who were randomly assigned to receive active lithium medication did so."[80]

Then it was discovered that lithium responsiveness may cluster in families – and thus have a genetic basis. This goes back to the work of

---

[78] Grof P, Angst J. Reply to Barry Blackwell. Comment by Paul Grof and Jules Agnst.
The Lithium Controversy: Somewhat Different Hindsights inhn.org.controversies. November 1, 2014.

[79] Grof P, Müller-Oerlinghausen B. A Critical Appraisal of Lithium's Efficacy and Effectiveness: The Last 60 years. Bipolar Disorders. 2009; 11:10-19.

[80] Bauer M, Bschor T, Kunz D, Berghöfer A, Ströhle A, Müller-Oerlinghausen B. Double-Blind, Placebo-Controlled Trial of the Use of Lithium to Augment Antidepressant Medication in Continuation Treatment of Unipolar Major Depression. AJP. 2000; 157:1429-35.

Paul Grof and colleagues in 2002. Finding a genetic basis for anything is rare enough in psychiatry and the discovery that 67% of the relatives of bipolar lithium-responders – as opposed to 35% of contrrols – had an "unequivocal" prophylactic lithium response was an important advance.[81]

As for looking at lithium versus the on-patent mood stabilizers, in 2003 a study led by Frederick Goodwin at George Washington University comparing the prevention of suicide and suicide attempts in bipolar disorder at treatment centers in Washington DC and California, concluded that lithium had a superior efficacy to divalproex. The authors commented rather ironically, "This evidence of lower suicide risk during lithium treatment should be viewed in light of the declining use of lithium by psychiatrists in the Unites States, particularly among recently trained psychiatrists."[82]

In a meta-analysis of eight studies, Francesca Guzzetta at the University of Bologna, and Ross Baldessarini at McLean Hospital and colleagues confirmed this finding in 2007 for unipolar depression: "Antisuicidal effects of lithium in recurrent major depressive disorder [are] similar in magnitude to that found in bipolar disorders."[83]

There was a continuous string of findings. A large trial in 2010 known as BALANCE and led by John Geddes at 41 centers in the UK, France, Italy and the US, found lithium more effective than valproate in preventing relapse in bipolar disorder. Most effective was a lithium-valproate combination.[84]

---

[81] Grof P, Duffy A, Cavazzoni P, Grof E, Garnham J, MacDougall M, O'Donovan C, Alda M Is Response to Prophylatic Lithium a Familial Trait? J Clin Psych. 2002; 63:942-947.

[82] Goodwin FK, Fireman B, Simon GE, Hunkeler EM, Lee J, Revicki D. Suicide Risk in Bipolar Disorder During Treatment with Lithium and Divalproex. JAMA. 2003; 290(11):1467-73.

[83] Guzzetta F, Tondo L, Baldessarini RJ. Lithium Treatment Reduces Suicide Risk in Recurrent Major Depressive Disorder. J Clin Psych. 2007; 68: 380-3.

[84] BALANCE investigators and collaborators, Geddes JR, Goodwin GM, Rendell J, Azorin JM, Cipriani A, Ostacher MJ, Morriss R, Alder N, Juszczak E. Lithium plus

A nationwide registry-based prospective study in Finland in 2015 of suicide in bipolar patients found that, among mood stabilizers, lithium was the only one associated with a significant reduction in suicide mortality. The authors concluded, "Maintenance therapy with lithium, but not with other medications, is linked to decreased suicide and all-cause mortality in high-risk bipolar patients."[85]

These were powerful moments in the lithium comeback, conducted by seasoned investigators at leading institutions. They were seen essentially as a poke in the eye to antipharmacotherapy groups such as the Critical Psychiatry Network in the UK that denied that pharmacotherapy had any disease-specific action.

In sum, lithium responsiveness opens the question of what Donald Klein called a "pharmacological torch" in the area of bipolar disorder. There is a small group of these patients who respond beautifully to lithium. As Martin Alda at Dalhousie University in Halifax puts it, "Compared to other psychiatric conditions, lithium-responsive bipolar disorder appears to be a narrower, more homogeneous and highly heritable phenomenon... The excellent responders are a reminder that there is a group of patients for whom lithium is not only the best but perhaps the only treatment option."[86] That would make lithium-responsive bipolar disorder, or even better, lithium-responsive mood disorder, a separate disease.

In historical perspective, it is difficult to disagree with Gershon: "Lithium was the first unlikely salvo in the revolution of

---

valproate combination therapy versus monotherapy for relapse prevention in bipolar I disorder (BALANCE): a randomised open-label trial. Lancet. 2010; 375:385-95.

[85] Toffol E, Hätönen T, Tanskanen A, Lönnqvist J, Wahlbeck K, Joffe G, Tiihonen J, Haukka J, Partonen T. Lithium Is Associated with Decrease in All-Cause and Suicide Mortality in High-Risk Bipolar Patients: A Nationwide Registry-Based Prospective Cohort Study. J Affect Disord. 2015; 183:159-65.

[86] Alda M. Who Are Excellent Lithium Responders and Why Do They Matter? World Psychiatry. 2017; 16:319-20.

psychopharmacology in psychiatry."[87]

August 27, 2020

COMMENTS

ROBERT HAIM BELMAKER'S COMMENT
A SAGA OF LITHIUM RESEARCH 1975-2020

CLINICAL LITHIUM RESEARCH:

The Jerusalem Mental Health Center, where I was Director of Research (1974-1984), was a hospital of about 300 beds with a catchment area of Northern Jerusalem. The first clinical trial I planned was with a young resident in psychiatry named Joseph Biederman. I gave him the task of seeing whether there was a cut-off at a particular place along the dimension between bipolar disorder and schizoaffective disorder where lithium ceased to work. The design was a double-blind "add-on" of lithium or placebo to haloperidol-treated, acutely psychotic patients. Some of the patients were bipolar manics; others were schizophrenic patients with "excited psychosis." Most patients were excited schizoaffectives. The findings of that first study were published in the Archives of General Psychiatry in 1979 (Biederman, Lerner and Belmaker 1979). There were about 35 patients included in it. We found highly significant benefits for lithium without any difference between the bipolar manics and other patients. It was infrequently quoted, perhaps because DSM-III diagnoses were

---

[87] Gershon S. Lithium Discovered, Forgotten and Rediscovered. inhn.org.archives. August 15, 2013.

introduced soon after and became an inclusion criterion for review articles. Another possible reason for this study's obscurity is that it was an "add-on" study and at the time "add-on" studies were considered uninformative about basic psychopharmacological questions. Lithium added benefit whenever there was an affective component; it really didn't matter whether the patients met DSM-III criteria for bipolar disorder or schizoaffective disorder or schizophrenia. That conclusion might have been hard to accept for all those of us who hoped that lithium would allow a biochemical dissection of bipolar disorder.

We did another "add-on" study to test indirectly the specificity of the lithium effect which was also published in 1984 in the Archives of General Psychiatry (Klein, Bental, Lerer and Belmaker 1984). It was "add on" of carbamazepine or placebo in haloperidol-treated patients with "excited psychosis" done by Ehud Klein who was a young psychiatry resident then. Again, we found benefit of carbamazepine without any relationship to strict bipolar diagnosis.

LABORATORY LITHIUM RESEARCH:

The laboratory at the Jerusalem Mental Health Center was headed by Richard Ebstein, PhD. He set up an assay for measuring cyclic AMP in human plasma, based on a paper by Sutherland (Ball, Kaminsky, Hardman et al. 1972). Sutherland demonstrated that if one gives a dose of epinephrine, in a dose equivalent to that given in those days in an asthma attack subcutaneously, and takes blood samples every 10 minutes from an indwelling venous catheter, one sees a rise in cyclic AMP, exactly the same as occurs inside cells in response to stimulation of the adrenergic receptor. We were able to show that in euthymic patients on lithium at therapeutic doses the cyclic AMP response to epinephrine was completely blocked, compared to controls (Ebstein, Belmaker, Grunhaus and Rimon 1976). This was an early translational research study where a finding in basic science that lithium affects second messengers was replicated in humans. A finding that might have been put aside as occurring at non-therapeutic concentrations was shown to work in patients.

Indications

Vetulani and Sulser (1975) published findings that turned the old catecholamine hypothesis on its head, saying antidepressants induce postsynaptic sub-sensitivity rather than an increase in synaptic monoamines. Salbutamol had just been released for clinical use in the treatment of asthma. We hypothesized that salbutamol should increase plasma cyclic AMP just like other adrenergic agonists. Bernard Lerer, a young resident at the time, tested depressed patients at baseline for cyclic AMP response to salbutamol, then again after a month of treatment and then treated for depression. We were then able to demonstrate in vivo in humans the sub-sensitivity of the ß-receptor second messenger response (Lerer, Ebstein and Belmaker 1981). This seemed to connect the effect of lithium on the second messenger cyclic AMP system to that of unipolar acting antidepressants (Belmaker 1981). With a new post-doctoral fellow, Michael Newman, we tried to examine the mechanism of lithium's effects on the cyclic AMP generating system using tools such as forskolin that bypass the adrenergic receptor. We found definite effects of lithium distal to the receptor, consistent with developing concepts in basic science revealing that the receptor is G-protein coupled (Newman and Belmaker 1987)

In 1985 I moved to the Beersheva Mental Health Center of Ben Gurion University and began working with Gabriel Schreiber MD, a psychiatry resident, and Sophia Avissar PhD, a post-doctoral student. They developed a receptor binding assay for G-protein activation and we found that lithium could block the receptor activated increase in G-protein binding in tissue from rat brain (Avissar, Schreiber, Danon and Belmaker 1988). The effect has since been found to be dependent on magnesium concentration in the experimental medium and not clearly relevant to human therapeutic conditions. As a result, I became interested in looking at lithium effects on a newly emerging second messenger system, phosphatidyl inositol (PI), and inspired by the work of Michael Berridge (Berridge, Downes and Hanley 1989) who received the Wolf Prize in 1994 for his work in the Israeli Knesset. Our first efforts were behavioral, working with a young post-doctoral fellow at the time in our lab, Ora Kofman PhD, and a young resident in psychiatry at the time, Yuly Bersudsky. The work was based on the 1980 serendipitous finding by Hallcher and Sherman that lithium at therapeutic concentrations inhibits inositol monophosphatase, the final step in the dephosphorylation of a key product in the PI cycle. Sherman and colleagues Honchar and Olney (1983) found that lithium in rats hugely potentiated the effects of cholinergic agonists to cause a peculiar limbic seizure syndrome and connected this convincingly to inositol depletion. While lithium was not thought to have cholinergic mechanisms, this effect was the most powerful behavioral effect of lithium I had seen before or since. I spent the summer of 1989 in Sherman's lab at Washington University in St. Louis to acquaint myself with this phenomenon. Sherman was a great scientist and teacher, an organic chemist, as he said it, "for an organic psychiatry department." Ora set up the lithium-pilocarpine model in our lab in Beersheva and we soon proved that the lithium effect was stereospecifically reversed by the natural isomer of inositol (Kofman and Belmaker, 1993) but Yuly found that inositol, unfortunately, was not an antidote to lithium toxicity in general (Bersudsky, Vinnitsky, Ghelber et al. 1993). When Haim Einat that joined us as a doctoral student we found that, as with the cyclic AMP effects of lithium described above, the effects of lithium on PI could be joined to the effects of inositol and the PI cycle in depression models and treatment more generally (Einat and Belmaker 2001). This theme of lack of specificity of lithium effects in humans to the specific narrow diagnosis of bipolar disorder and the lack of specificity of lithium mechanisms to any unique system in biochemistry has run throughout my years of research, much against my hopes and inclinations in the direction of Occam's razor. Galila Agam joined the team as a biochemist in the 1990s and some of our exciting new approaches to lithium and the PI cycle involved knockout mice (Agam, Bersudsky, Berry et al. 2009). The inositol monophosphatase-1 knockout mice have pilocarpine sensitivity and behave on the Porsolt forced swimming test as if the animal is taking lithium.

Indications

Most recently, Nisha Singh, a doctoral student from Grant Churchill's lab at Oxford in the UK, came to our lab in Beersheva to study ebselen compared to lithium in the pilocarpine potentiation model. Ebselen is a compound developed for treatment of inflammation found to be an inositol monophosphatase inhibitor and to lower brain inositol, both biochemical effects of lithium. It's possible clinical effectiveness will be the ultimate test of the inositol depletion hypothesis, first proposed by Berridge, Downes and Hanley (1989) as discussed above. Unfortunately for the lithium-pilocarpine model, Nisha and coworkers in our lab found that ebselen did not potentiate pilocarpine seizures (Singh, Serres, Toker et al. 2020). This may not be decisive evidence against the inositol depletion hypothesis of lithium action but it is evidence against the generalizability of lithium pilocarpine seizures as a useful behavioral model of lithium-like biochemical effects.

In a 2004 article in the New England Journal of Medicine I developed the concept that lithium research has found effects of lithium in every dominant paradigm in each generation of psychopharmacology. When monoamine metabolites were being investigated, lithium had effects on monoamine metabolites; when receptors were the frontier, lithium had effects on receptor hypersensitivity; when second messengers were at the forefront, lithium was found to have effects on second messengers; and when gene expression was of interest to all, lithium was found to have effects on gene expression. This generational shifting has continued but my strong impression of my own 45 years of work is that we still do not know the mechanism of lithium action and are not even close in lithium research to a concept parallel to the central theme of dopamine blockade in neuroleptic action and monoamine reuptake or MAO inhibition in antidepressants.

EPILOGUE:

I still use lithium in the clinic and find it very beneficial in many patients with bipolar disorder, some with recurrent unipolar disorder and many with schizoaffective disorders; atypical antipsychotics are often but not always equally useful and are very convenient (Osher, Bersudsky and Belmaker 2010). Given the long period of lithium usage in many of my patients, kidney effects including progression to renal dialysis and transplant have become a very real issue (Azab, Schnaider, Osher et al. 2015). Basic research on the mechanism of lithium action has not led to application of Occam's razor; but clinical usage surely justifies the adage that there is no free lunch.

References:

Agam G, Bersudsky Y, Berry GT, Moechars D, Lavi-Avnon Y, Belmaker RH. Knockout mice in understanding the mechanism of action of lithium. Biochem Soc Trans. 2009; 37(Pt 5):1121-5.

Avissar S, Schreiber G, Danon A, Belmaker RH. Lithium inhibits adrenergic and cholinergic increases in GTP binding in rat cortex. Nature. 1988; 331(6155):440-2.

Azab A, Schnaider A, Osher Y, Wang D, Bersudsky Y, Belmaker R. Lithium Nephrotoxicity. Int J Bipolar Disord. 2015; 3:13.

Ball JH, Kaminsky NI, Hardman JG, Broadus AE, Sutherland EW, Liddle GW. Effects of catecholamines and adrenergic-blocking agents on plasma and urinary cyclic nucleotides in man. J Clin Inves.1972; 51(8):2124-9.

Belmaker R. Bipolar Disorder. N Engl J Med. 2004; 351(5):476-86.

Belmaker R. Receptors, adenylate cyclase, depression and lithium. Biol Psychiatry. 1981; 16(4):333-50.

Berridge MJ, Downes CP, Hanley MR. Neural and developmental actions of lithium: a unifying hypothesis. Cell. 1989; 59(3):411-9.

Bersudsky Y, Vinnitsky I, Ghelber D, Kofman O, Kaplan Z, Belmaker R. Mechanism of lithium lethality in rats. Journal of Psychiatric Research. 1993; 27(4):415-22.

Indications

Biederman J, Lerner Y, Belmaker R. Combination of lithium carbonate and haloperidol in schizo-affective disorder: a controlled study. Arch Gen Psychiatry. 1979; 36(3):327-33.

Ebstein R, Belmaker R, Grunhaus L, Rimon R. Lithium inhibition of adrenaline sensitive adenylate cyclase in humans. Nature. 1976; 259:411-13.

Einat H, Belmaker R. The effects of inositol treatment in animal models of psychiatric disorders. J Affect Disord. 2001; 62(1-2):113-21.

Hallcher L, Sherman W. The effect of lithium ion and other agents on the activity of myo-inositol-1-phosphatase from bovine brain. J Biol Chem 1980; 255(22):10896-901.

Honchar MP, Olney JW, Sherman WR. Systemic cholinergic agents induce seizures and brain damage in lithium-treated rats. Science. 1983; 220(4594):323-5.

Klein E, Bental E, Lerer B, Belmaker RH. Carbamazepine and haloperidol v placebo and haloperidol in excited psychoses: A controlled study. Arch Gen Psychiatry. 1984; 41(2):165-70.

Kofman O, Belmaker RH. Biochemical, behavioral and clinical studies of the role of inositol in lithium treatment and depression. Biol Psychiatry. 1993; 34(12):839-52.

Lerer B, Ebstein RP, Belmaker RH. Subsensitivity of human-beta adrenergic adenylate cyclase after salbutamol treatment of depression. Psychopharmacology (Berl). 1981; 75(2):169-72.

Newman ME, Belmaker RH. Effect of lithium in vitro and ex vivo on components of the adenylate cyclase system in rat cerebral cortex membrane. Neuropharmacology. 1987; 26:211-7.

Osher Y, Bersudsky Y, Belmaker RH. The new lithium clinic. Neuropsychobiology 2010; 62:17-26

Singh N, Serres F, Toker L, Sade Y, Blackburn V, Batra SA, Saiardi A, Agam G., Belmaker RH, Sharp T, Vasudevan SR, Churchill G. Effects of the putative lithium mimetic ebselen on pilocarpine-induced neural activity. European J of Pharmacology. 2020; 883:173377.

Vetulani J, Sulser F. Action of various antidepressant treatments reduces re-activity of noradrenergic cyclic AMP generating system in limbic forebrain. Nature. 1975; 257: 495-6.

September 24, 2020

WILLIAM E. BUNNEY JR'S COMMENTS
CONTRIBUTIONS TO PSYCHIATRY RESEARCH
WITH LITHIUM

In 1871 William Hammond, Professor of Diseases of the Mind and Nervous System at the Bellevue Hospital Medical College in New York, became the first physician to prescribe lithium for mania. In 1894 Danish psychiatrist Frederick Lange used lithium in the treatment of depression.

However, lithium was not referred to until 1949 when John Cade from Melbourne successfully treated manic patients. In 1951 C. H. Noack, also in Melbourne, conducted an open trial of over 100 patients in the treatment of mania. In 1952 Danish psychiatrist Mogens Schou conducted a randomly controlled trial of lithium in mania and published the results in 1954. He showed that many patients could be kept in a normal state by administration of a maintenance dose. In the United States the use of lithium was studied in the 1960s; Samuel

Indications

Gershon published the first paper on the use of lithium and the treatment of mania. In 1962 George Winokur utilized lithium in the treatment of mania at Barnes Hospital, St. Louis.

I became actively involved with Fred Goodwin, John Davis and Jan Fawcett at the Intramural Program of the NIMH in clinical trials of lithium in mania and depression and published more than 20 papers investigating the mode of action of lithium over the next two decades (two of these papers were published in Science and two were published in Nature.

In the mid-1960s, while I was still at the Intramural Program of the NIMH, along with Ron Fieve at New York Columbia Presbyterian Medical Center, we initiated studies using lithium in manic-depressive illness. In 1968 Fred Goodwin and I conducted a longitudinal double-blind study of two manic patients treated in a random fashion with lithium carbonate and placebo. Daily ratings of mania were recorded independently by a trained psychiatric nursing team and by a psychiatrist. The major finding was a definite increase in mania, reflected in the daily ratings, during placebo periods within 24 hours of the withdrawal of lithium. Placebo was substituted for lithium on five occasions, resulting in a rapid increase in mania. Then lithium was administered and there was a complete decrease in manic symptomatology. This publication on the double-blind consistency of the repeated relapses of manic symptoms on placebo and the subsequent therapeutic response on lithium, along with the research of Gershon and Fieve, helped convince many clinicians and researchers in the United States of the efficacy of lithium in the treatment of mania (Bunney WE Jr, Goodwin FK, Davis JM, Fawcett JA. A behavioral-biochemical study of lithium treatment. Am J Psychiatry. 1968; 125:91-104).

Published Papers on the Clinical Use of Lithium in the Treatment of Mania and Depression, and Studies of the Mechanisms of Action of Lithium

1. **Colburn RW, Goodwin FK, Bunney WE Jr, Davis JM. Effect of lithium on the uptake of noradrenaline by synaptosomes. Nature 1967; 215:1395-8.**
   The effect of lithium on NE is several-fold. We demonstrated that acute lithium treatment increases labeled NE update by rat brain synaptosomes.

2. **Greenspan K, Goodwin FK, Bunney WE Jr, Durell J. Lithium in retention and distribution. Patterns during acute mania and normothymia. Arch Gen Psychiatry. 1968; 19:664-73.**
   Unlike the phenothiazines, Lithium is believed to control the mood state at plasma levels which do not cause general sedation, and which have virtually no subjective effects in normal subjects. This high degree of specificity suggests that lithium salts will prove to be important pharmacological tools for the study of the pathophysiology of manic-depressive disorders. We embarked on studies of the mechanism of action of the lithium salts, and confirmed that acutely manic patients retain more lithium ion than normal subjects.

3. **Goodwin FK, Murphy DL, Bunney WE Jr. Lithium-carbonate treatment in depression and mania. A longitudinal double-blind study. Arch Gen Psychiatry. 1969; 21:486-96.**
   This paper presented the clinical results of an intensive longitudinal double-blind study in 30 manic-depressive and depressed patients. The therapeutic use of lithium-carbonate in affective disorders has recently been the focus of considerable interest, particularly in light of clinical evidence that it may have beneficial effects not only in mania but also in some cases of depression. We showed that the unique feature of this drug in these patients demonstrates long-term mood-stabilizing properties when used prophylactically.

4. **Murphy DL, Goodwin FK, Bunney WE Jr. Aldosterone and sodium response to lithium administration in man. Lancet. 1969; 2:458-61.**
   Administration of lithium carbonate to 16 manic-depressive and depressed patients was found to lead to an initial 1-2 days of sodium

and water diuresis. In the subsequent 4-5-day period of treatment, sodium retention associated with a 50% increase in aldosterone excretion occurred. In the next several days there was a return towards pre-lithium levels. These changes occurred in all patients and were apparently not related to the initial clinical state of the patient nor the presence or absence of symptomatic improvement with lithium.

5. **Murphy DL, Colburn RW, Davis JM, Bunney WE Jr. Stimulation by lithium of monoamine uptake in human platelets. Life Sciences. 1969; 8:1187-93.**

Blood platelets share with monoamine-containing nerve endings from brain and peripheral organs the capacity to transport and store serotonin. In vitro, platelets concentrate serotonin up to 1000-fold from the incubation medium. The amine concentrating mechanism in both platelets and nerve endings depends on metabolism, exhibits saturation kinetics, and is inhibited by ouabain and other drugs including the tricyclic antidepressants. In addition, there are morphological similarities between platelets and nerve endings in that they both contain amine storage vesicles and mitochondria enclosed within a limiting membrane. Pretreatment with lithium was found to increase the uptake of noradrenaline into nerve endings (synaptosomes) isolated from rat brain. In the present study platelets obtained from manic-depressive patients receiving lithium showed a similar increase of monoamine uptake.

6. **Murphy DL, Colburn RW, Davis JM, Bunney WE Jr. Imipramine and lithium effects on biogenic amine transport in depressed and manic-depressed patients. Am. J. Psychiatry 1970; 127:339-45.**

It is often risky to extrapolate to man the results of animal studies on the mechanism of action of psychoactive drugs. In this study, platelets obtained from patients before and during treatment with imipramine and lithium were used to determine whether the effects of these drugs suggested by animal studies to be involved in cell membrane transport could be identified in these human cells.

Imipramine was found to inhibit and lithium to stimulate amine transport in platelets. confirming that the cellular effects of these drugs in man are similar to their effects on brain cells from animals.

7. **Murphy DL, Goodwin FK, Bunney WE Jr. Leukocytosis during lithium treatment. Am J Psychiatry. 1971; 127:1559-61.**

An increase in circulating leukocytes accompanied lithium treatment in 28 consecutively studied manic-depressive patients. Acutely manic patients showed the most marked changes and maintained leukocyte counts of 10,000 to 14,000 during the first two to four weeks of lithium administration. Leukocyte counts returned to pre-lithium levels within one week after discontinuation of the drug. In 11 patients receiving lithium for longer periods the elevation in white cell count persisted throughout treatment.

8. **Murphy DL, Bunney WE Jr. Total body potassium changes during lithium treatment. J Nerv Ment Dis. 1971; 152:381-9.**

Total body potassium decreased after 2 weeks of lithium administration in 12 of 13 depressed patients but increased in 6 of 7 manic patients treated with lithium under identical conditions. These opposite changes were statistically significant for each group of patients. In a smaller group of depressed patients followed for longer periods during lithium treatment, the potassium levels returned to pre-lithium values. The dependence of the direction of potassium change on the clinical state of the patient may be related to some previously described differences between manic and depressed patients and also to differences in the therapeutic response to lithium between the two groups.

9. **Goodwin FK, Murphy DL, Dunner DL, Bunney WE Jr. Lithium response in unipolar versus bipolar depression. Am. J. Psychiatry. 1972; 129:44-7.**

The antidepressant effects of lithium carbonate were evaluated in a group of 52 hospitalized depressed patients, using a longitudinal double-blind design that involved alternating drug and placebo periods in the same patient. Thirty-six of the 52 patients showed some improvement on lithium, including 15 who had complete remission of symptoms. Virtually all of the antidepressant responses occurred in patients with a past history of mania or hypomania.

10. **Bunney WE Jr, Murphy DL. Neurobiological considerations on the mode of action of lithium carbonate in the treatment of affective disorders. Pharmakopsychiatr Neuropsychopharmakol. 1976; 9:142-7.**

The effects of lithium on membrane function and cellular processes are considered in relation to lithium's physiochemical properties. Several cellular regulatory functions, including cyclic AMP formation and metabolism and biogenic amine neurotransmitter metabolism, are examined as possible mechanisms whereby lithium might exert its mood stabilizing actions. The necessity for understanding lithium's interactions with "receptors" - the molecular sites affected by lithium - in considering its pre-and post-synaptic effects in stressed.

11. **Jasinsky DR, Nutt JG, Haertzen CA, Griffith JD, Bunney WE Jr. Lithium: Effects on subjective functioning and morphine-induced euphoria. Science. 1977; 195:582-4.**

The therapeutic usefulness of lithium in decreasing the euphoria and other symptoms associated with manic behavior and the hypothesis of a common final mechanism for elevations in mood have led to speculation that lithium may block the euphoria induced by drugs of abuse. In this study, lithium alone was anti-euphoric in drug-free opiate addicts and, further, did not block morphine-induced euphoria.

12. **Gallager DW, Pert A, Bunney WE Jr. Haloperidol-induced presynaptic dopamine supersensitivity is blocked by chronic lithium. Nature. 1978; 273:309-12.**

Several groups have theorized that alterations in catecholamine receptor sensitivity may be a factor in the etiology of affective disorders, especially manic-depressive illness. As lithium therapy has been shown to be effective in preventing recurrent episodes of mania and depression in manic-depressive illness, it is of interest to determine whether, at the level of individual DA neurones in the CNS, chronic lithium treatment could also affect the development of presynaptic supersensitivity. We provide here electrophysiological evidence for the blockade of presynaptic supersensitivity development following chronic lithium treatment.

13. **Pert A, Rosenblatt JE, Sivit C, Pert CB, Bunney WE Jr. Long-term treatment with lithium prevents the development of dopamine receptor supersensitivity. Science. 1978; 201:171-3.**

Long-term treatment of rats with haloperidol produced an increased sensitivity to the locomotor and stereotypic effect of apomorphine. This behavioral dopaminergic supersensitivity was accompanied by increased binding of [3H] spiroperidol in the striatum. Rats treated concurrently with lithium and haloperidol failed to develop both behavioral sensitivity to apomorphine and increased striatal dopamine receptor binding. The ability of lithium to prevent recurrent manic-depressive episodes may be related, in part, to its ability to stabilize dopaminergic receptor sensitivity.

14. **Rosenblatt JE, Pert CB, Tallman JF, Pert A, Bunney WE Jr. The effect of imipramine and lithium on alpha- and beta-receptor binding in rat brain. Brain Res. 1979; 160:186-91.**

Lithium is an efficacious prophylactic agent for preventing unipolar and bipolar mania and depression. Its mechanism of action is unknown, but it is assumed to interact at cellular sites normally designated for sodium. A recent proposal is that lithium's action is due to its ability to stabilize and, hence halt the development of receptor super- and subsensitivity which is postulated to accompany the various psychotic states. We have recently tested this hypothesis in an animal model in which chronic haloperidol treatment was used to induce dopamine receptor supersensitivity. In that study, we found that lithium administered concurrently with haloperidol blocked the development of haloperidol-induced dopamine receptor supersensitivity as measured both behaviorally and biochemically.

Chronic treatment with lithium rather than acute exposure of rat brain membranes to lithium ion appears to be responsible for the effects we have observed. Acute exposure of rat brain membranes to lithium concentrations ranging between 0.03 and 3.0 mM, the concentrations of lithium expected to be carried over into the test tube from the brain levels which we have routinely noted, failed to alter the binding to either a-, fl- or dopamine receptors. However, we found that lithium is able to block the supersensitivity of a-and fl-receptors which develops after 6-hydroxydopamine lesions.

This was the first report of lithium's ability to alter the sensitivity of adrenergic receptors in brain. Could this be due to a non-specific 'toxic' effect of lithium? Rats maintained on lithium for 3-5 weeks in our laboratory show a 15 ~ weight loss but no overt differences in behavior from controls. The effects of lithium on adrenergic receptors are highly reproducible, but it is impossible to rule out a 'stress' effect. These alterations in receptor sensitivity may relate to lithium's therapeutic effect. It will be important to demonstrate concomitant behavioral alterations in receptor sensitivity accompanying the biochemical changes observed here.

15. **Alexander PE, van Kammen DP, Bunney WE Jr. Antipsychotic effects of lithium in schizophrenia. Am. J. Psychiatry. 1979; 136:283-7.**

The lithium carbonate therapy of 13 psychotic schizophrenic patients was evaluated in a placebo-controlled three-week study that was double-blind. Seven of the 13 patients were less psychotic while receiving lithium; 4 of these 7 patients relapsed after lithium withdrawal. Patients who improved during the third week on lithium could be differentiated from nonresponders on the basis of their improvement during the first week. Clinical factors such as diagnosis, prognosis, and symptoms failed to predict responders from nonresponders. To the authors' knowledge, this is the first controlled study to yield positive results with schizophrenic patients treated with lithium alone.

16. **Gallager DW, Bunney WE Jr. Effects of chronic lithium administration on the development of supersensitivity in CNS**

amine systems. A microiontophoretic study. In: Usdin E, Kopin, IJ, Barchas JD, editors. Catecholamines. Basic and Clinical Frontiers. New York. Pergamon Press, 1979, pp. 669-71.

A supersensitive response of the activity of DA-containing cells in the zona compacta of the substantia nigra to microiontophoretically applied DA and to intravenously administered apomorphine was produced by chronic haloperidol treatment in rats. Animals treated concurrently with lithium and haloperidol failed to develop this presynaptic DA supersensitivity. However, lithium's ability to block the development of supersensitivity in the DA system may not be generalized to other amine systems since chronic lithium treatment did not prevent the development of supersensitivity to 5HT in hippocampal pyramidal cells following chronic tricyclic antidepressant administration.

17. Pert CB, Pert A, Rosenblatt JE, Tallman JF, Bunney WE Jr. Catecholamine receptor stabilization. A possible mode of lithium's anti-manic action. In: Usdin E, Kopin IJ, Barchas JD, editors. Catecholamines. Basic and Clinical Frontiers. New York. Pergamon Press, 1979, pp. 583-5.

Chronic administration of lithium to rats treated with repeated doses of haloperidol prevents the dopamine receptor supersensitivity that normally develops when haloperidol is administered alone. Lithium's prevention of dopamine receptor supersensitivity has been documented by behavioral, neurophysiological, and biochemical receptor binding techniques. Chronic lithium treatment alone in rats has small but reproducible effects: an increase in α-receptor binding, a decrease in β-receptor binding and no alteration in dopamine receptor binding. In preliminary experiments, lithium is able to block the development of the α- and β receptor sensitivity that normally accompanies brain norepinephrine depletion by 6-hydroxydopamine.

18. Bunney WE Jr, Pert A, Rosenblatt J, Pert CB, Gallager D. Mode of action of lithium. Some biological considerations.

Arch Gen Psychiatry. 1979; 36:898-901.

This communication will review some of the properties of lithium and four possible cellular sites of interaction between lithium and other cations. It will emphasize the observation that lithium interacts with cyclic adenosine monophosphate (AMP)-mediated processes and, finally, will review a hypothesis that the onset of mania may be associated with the development of supersensitivity of catecholamine receptors. New evidence will be reported that lithium can block the development of supersensitivity in CNS neuronal receptors in rats.

19. **Rosenblatt JE, Pert A, Layton B, Bunney WE Jr. Chronic lithium reduced [3H] spiroperidol binding in rat striatum. Eur J Pharmacol. 1980; 67:321-2.**

The efficacy of lithium in the acute treatment and prophylaxis of mania is well established. Although the mechanism of lithium's anti-manic effects is not entirely understood, it is thought to involve central nervous system catecholamine neurotransmission. Recently we reported that lithium prevented development of both the behavioral supersensitivity to apomorphine and the increase in [3H] spiroperidol binding following chronic haloperidol treatment in rats. We confirmed these findings with electro- physiological techniques. In the present study we report that chronic treatment with lithium alone decreases dopamine receptor density in the corpus striatum in a rapidly reversible manner.

20. **van Kammen DP, Alexander P, Bunney WE Jr. Lithium treatment in post-psychotic depression. Brit J Psychiatry. 1980; 136:479-85.**

Six of eleven drug-free schizophrenic patients who were depressed following remission of their illness showed a significant decrease in their depressive symptomatology during a double-blind, placebo substitution lithium trial. Traditional indicators of prognosis did not predict lithium response in this small sample; the schizophrenic patients tolerated the lithium well. Lithium should be studied further in a larger patient sample as an adjunct in the treatment of post-psychotic depression, which frequently is treatment resistant.

21. **Bunney WE Jr, Garland BL. Possible receptor effects of chronic lithium administration. Neuropharmacology. 1983; 22(3B):367-72.**

Evidence suggests that lithium pretreatment might be effective in blocking the development of pharmacologically-induced behavioral dopamine supersensitivity although alterations in receptor binding may not be directly correlated to behavioral changes. Experimental results indicate that the effect of lithium may not be consistent throughout the brain, may be related to specific methods of sensitivity-induced alterations and may simultaneously alter several receptor systems.

22. **Bunney WE Jr, Garland BL. Lithium and its possible modes of action. In: Post RM, Ballenger JC, Uhde TW, Bunney WE Jr, editors. Neurobiology of the Mood Disorders. Baltimore. Williams and Wilkins, 1984, pp. 731-43.**

This review covers biological effects of lithium electrolytes, the neurotransmitters dopamine, norepinephrine and serotonin, acetylcholine, c-AMP, effect of lithium on receptor sensitivity, cholinergic muscarinic receptor binding, and GABA.

23. **Cohen IM, Bunney WE Jr, Cole JO, Fieve RR, Gershon S, Prien RF. The current status of lithium therapy. Report of the APA Task Force. Am J Psychiatry. 1975; 132:997-1001.**

In 1969 the American Psychiatric Association appointed a Task Force on Lithium and assigned to it the charge of providing "an appraisal of current knowledge about efficacy and safety of lithium therapy in psychiatry." In its report to the Council on Research and Development in the 1970s, the task force recommended that APA continue to critically evaluate lithium therapy; this resulted in the appointment of the present task force in 1973. The following report responds to the charge given to this task force to reappraise lithium therapy after it had been generally available for several years. In it the task force proposes to assess the value of lithium in the indications that have been suggested

Indications

for its use, to describe and explain the procedures used in administering it therapeutically and prophylactically, to review the undesirable effects and complications of the treatment and their significance and management, and to bring to the attention of the membership those issues about lithium therapy that remain unresolved.

Note: Lithium was approved by the FDA for the treatment of mania in 1970.

October 22, 2020

**THOMAS A. BAN, EDITOR.
LITHIUM IN PSYCHIATRY IN
HISTORICAL PERSPECTIVE
BERNARD CARROLL INTERVIEW
BY LEO HOLLISTER AND THOMAS BAN***

LH: *In knowing the history of Australian neuropsychopharmacology from early on did you ever have occasion to meet the most famous Australian psychopharmacologist, John Cade?*

BC: John Cade was one of my teachers in psychiatry.

LH: *Did he teach at the medical school?*

BC: He did. I knew him well. His son, David, was in my medical school class and his other son, John, was two years ahead of us in medical school. I knew the Cades and I knew John; in clinical psychiatry we were taught at the Royal Park Psychiatric Hospital, the inner-city State hospital where John Cade was director of. We would go, as medical students, to the auditorium on Saturday mornings where John Cade would teach us psychopathology and his style was very Kraepelinian. He was up on stage with two chairs, one for the patient and one for him. An assistant would be hovering around and the patients would be lined up off stage. He would signal to stage right for a patient to be brought in and would say, in a very Edwardian authoritarian manner, "Ladies and gentlemen, I'm now going to demonstrate a patient with schizophrenia." The patient would be brought and John Cade would put the schizophrenic patient through his hoops, send the patient off stage left, signal again to stage right and say, "Ladies and gentlemen, I'm now going to demonstrate a patient with mania so you should pay close attention to the differences between them." His style was very autocratic and old fashioned, but in many ways, effective.

LH: *Better than learning from a textbook.*

BC: Much better. Then, in my psychiatry training, I had more encounters with Dr. Cade. I learned he had what can be called a divergent manner of thinking, a cognitive style with lateral and not always linear thinking. He published a paper in the Australian Medical Journal, on his theory of the etiology of schizophrenia. This, is in the late 1950s, was that schizophrenia was a disease that resulted from a deficiency of stone fruit such peaches and plums. An epidemiological study in the State of Victoria found that most acute schizophrenics were admitted to the receiving hospital from the densely populated parts of the city. They had the lowest density of fruit trees. That's very similar in style to the thinking that led to his discovery of lithium. He had this weird idea that some toxin in the urine of manic patients was responsible. He thought it was a urate salt. Needing a soluble urate salt, he got onto lithium urate. And his one good scientific question was to ask was it the urate or was it the lithium? And the rest is history.

Indications

LH: *When he was teaching you had he already made that discovery?*

BC: He had.

LH: *Why did it take so long to catch on? Was it because he had a reputation of being a wild thinker and nobody believed him?*

BC: No. Australians are very pragmatic and all through the 1950s, lithium was widely used in Australia and was picked up in England through Mogens Schou in Scandinavia and later in Europe in the 1950s and the 1960s. The resistance to lithium as a clinical agent was centered mostly in the United States.

LH: *That was due to its earlier use as a salt substitute for congestive heart failure and deaths due to toxicity before blood levels were available.*

BC: Exactly, and that's all being written up in Frank Ayd's book, Discoveries in Biological Psychiatry. I now have in my possession glossy photograph copies of John Cade's original case notes of the first patients he treated with lithium and I will donate them to the ACNP Archives. They are very, very interesting.

LH: *How was he lucky enough to pick the right dose?*

BC: The dose was known, because lithium had been used for epilepsy and gout, so people knew t lithium was safe. John's description of his IND process, shall I say, was that after he'd completed his guinea pig experiments he did a Phase 1 clinical trial on himself and the determining factor, when he treated himself with lithium for two weeks, was whether his wife, the long suffering Mrs. Cade, noted any difference. She did not notice, so he proceeded to treat a group of patients who were essentially chronic residents of the hospital. Today, we would call those patients, looking at the case notes, rapid cycling bipolar. They were in and out of manic and depressive phases of bipolar illness and to everybody's astonishment, they were all discharged within about four months of starting on lithium, so they truly were stabilized. John had complete freedom to do whatever he wanted in those days. There was no drug regulatory agency.

LH: *He was the superintendent of the hospital.*

BC: He lived on the hospital grounds. I remember going to his house to visit with his sons, who were in medical school with me, going in by the back gate from the hospital grounds to the superintendent's house. There was a basket on the gate that was replenished every day with vegetables from the patients' garden for the consumption of the superintendent and his family.

LH: *This is really old style, isn't it?*

BC: He was a beloved figure in the hospital and a very conscientious clinician.

LH: *That's a new element to your Australian training.*

TB: *So, you were in medical school about ten years after his publication on lithium, in the late 1950s?*

BC: I entered medical school in 1958.

TB: *Just ten years after.*

BC: That's correct.

TB: *Some clinicians had already picked up lithium?*

BC: Sam Gershon was using lithium in Australia and in the pharmacology department in Melbourne a number of basic studies of lithium kinetics and distribution were under way and were published during the 1950s. Sam Gershon was already publishing his work on lithium.

LH: *I think Gershon came to this country around the early 1960s.*

BC: Correct. I was with him in 1961 and he came to America in 1957-1958, came back in 1959-1961 to Melbourne and in 1962, returned to the United States.

LH: *Sam would talk lithium to the sceptics over here. I remember saying, "Lithium, that's a good thing to kill you," because I had fresh in my mind toxicity in cardiac patients.*

BC: The last time I saw John Cade was at a very important event. It was the 1979 International Conference on Use of Lithium in New York and John was the featured person at that meeting, along with Schou. I remember being at the hotel, walking across the lobby the day the meeting was getting underway, and I saw John wandering around in a dazed and confused way. I knew immediately what the problem was. He was in his late seventies and terribly jet lagged. I went up to him and I said, "John, how are you?" And, he said, "I'm alright, Barney, leave me alone." That was his usual style but I went on, "John, you look as though you're not very well." He replied, "All I need is a little sleep." I asked, "Where have you been?" and he said, "I just got off the plane from Australia." So, I said, "John, do you mean to tell me you didn't break the journey anywhere between Melbourne and New York?" He said, "No, I just flew straight here." I admonished him but he was in a travelers' delirium with severe jet lag and disorientation. So, we got him to his room and he slept that off was back to his happy self for the rest of the meeting. I take credit for helping to get John settled down in time for his public appearance.

LH: *Well, that's an interesting side light on an aspect of major importance in the history of psychopharmacology. Thank you, then.*

BC: Thank you.

LH: *I'm glad we caught that.*

> *Extracted from the interview of Bernard J. Carroll by Leo E. Hollister and Thomas A. Ban conducted for the Oral History series in Las Croabas, Puerto Rico, at the Annual Meeting of the American College of

Neuropsychopharmacology on December 17, 1998. The edited interview was first published in Samuel Gershon, editor. Neuropsychopharmacology, in Thomas A. Ban, series editor: An Oral History of Neuropsychopharmacology The First Fifty Years Peer Interviews. Volume 5. Brentwoood: American College of Neurosychopharmacology; 2011, pp. 85 -101.

April 2, 2020

AITOR CASTILLO'S COMMENT
WALKING WITH LITHIUM IN PERU

This story began on a distant gray morning during a cloudy winter at Lima city at the end of the '70s. There was a large auditorium in the very ancient psychiatric hospital "Victor Larco Herrera" (100 years old), surrounded by antique buildings and romantic gardens, occupied by a group of medical students who were attending their course of psychiatry organized by a local university. Every week we gathered there to listen to some talks and perform some clinical practices with patients.

I enjoyed going to that particular psychiatric hospital because, at the very beginning, it was pretty close to my beloved Pacific Ocean and also because I could walk along wide roads under tall trees full of peace while being away from the noisy and busy city. However, I have to say that those psychiatric lessons were not very interesting, even though I was considering entering a residency training program in psychiatry when I finished my studies. The lectures used to be boring and the faculty spoke in such very low voices that the only thing one could hear were the sound of the waves coming from the sea. Maybe more important, the concepts were pretty abstract and difficult to understand.

On that cold morning, the students were silently listening to the teacher who was standing up there on the stage dreaming, maybe, of being a rock star. I was among them accomplishing the same routine duty. Suddenly, the teacher, whose name and face I do not remember now, mentioned something about a medicine that apparently could help some special patients. He mentioned a kind of stone, a molecule, an ion, something that could change the way the brain works. Its name was lithium. Then, after the class was over, I left the room with that name echoing in my head. I thought that maybe this mineral could show me the way to understand all those patients who were talking to themselves, smiling without reason and behaving in such strange ways. Then I told myself, this issue is related to all these people around us who are waiting for something to help them leave this big impersonal hospital.

Finally, a couple of years after finishing my medical studies, I entered the psychiatric residency training program of the Universidad Nacional Mayor de San Marcos in Lima city, Perú. While there, the old mineral name came back to my memory. In this way, lithium started to become some kind of a special hope for helping people during my professional life. I studied it, I prescribed it to my first appropriate patients and I realized that apparently we could do more personalized psychopharmacology. It was clear that lithium required a dose titration until reaching a therapeutic concentration level that helped me feel more confident about my medical skills. In some way, lithium could let me anticipate the therapeutic results. At the same time, it helped me keep updated regarding my knowledge about pharmacology and pharmacokinetics, neurological, renal and thyroid functions among others, and integrate them with pharmacodynamics and clinical psychiatry.

In parallel, step by step, I started to notice that, in general, lithium increased concerns among doctors and patients. They imagined lithium to be a sort of toxic monster reserved only for lost causes. Some of them believed (and still do) that lithium only works in people "who lack it inside their bodies." For that reason, the first step in the treatment strategy is to educate people that there is no evidence that bipolar patients (or any person) have a lithium deficit in their organisms.

A few years ago, as a very interesting anecdote, during an electoral campaign conducted in Perú a very charismatic presidential candidate known by the nickname of "crazy horse" was asked on a television program interview if it was true that he was treated with lithium. Obviously, the answer was negative but most of the public was convinced that he really took lithium. Curiously enough, he won the election with an ample margin. Although there never was any evidence about his medical treatment with lithium, he was really a very clever, ingenious and emphatic person. Regretfully, he committed suicide in 2019 while on the verge of serious judicial affairs. In the field of private practice, many patients did not want to be identified with him when I suggested lithium for them and refused the prescription.

Now, I must go back to my wonderful training period with Tom Ban at the Tennessee Neuropsychiatric Institute in Nashville during 1978-1979. I remember my conversations with Stuart Berney, who was at that time the head of the laboratory there, about the methods to measure the blood levels of psychotropic drugs in order to get a more personalized treatment for the patients. During the following couple of years I continued my training at the Institute of Experimental Medicine in Caracas-Venezuela with Luis Ordoñez and at the Psychiatric Research Institute of Tokyo-Japan with Takashi Moroji where I had the opportunity to get deep insight about psychopharmacology and biological psychiatry.

By 1982 I had returned to Perú and joined a very small group of senior people in order to develop the country's National Institute of Mental Health. I want to be honest and say that it was a kind of political-academic agreement between the governments of Perú and Japan, taking into account that the Japanese International Cooperation

Agency donated a lot of money for the implementation of the project. I was then named head of the Biological Psychiatric Laboratory, where one of the first pieces of equipment that arrived at my lab from Tokyo was an Atomic Absorption Spectrophotometer.

The institute was administered by the Peruvian Ministry of Health and served a vast economically deprived population from northern Lima city, but, at the same time, was a reference center for the rest of the country. Beside some administrative, academic and research duties, this institution faced a huge amount of clinical work with psychiatric out- and in-patients.

Regarding the measurement of lithium plasma levels, we were the only public facility in the whole country able to do that in the context of very low prices. So, I decided to study how long a sample of lithium serum arriving from a distant health center would be available for doing such work. The study results were published in Anales de Salud Mental (Castillo and Miyahira 1986), in a paper whose title translated to "Stability of serum lithium under ambient conditions." The abstract reads:

> "Serum samples from 52 out-patients treated with lithium salts were studied in order to assess the stability of the ion under ordinary laboratory conditions. Aliquots were taken on day 0 and kept in the laboratory at room temperature. The analyses were performed on days 0, 7, 14, 21 and 30 using a standard atomic absorption spectrophotometric technique. The lithium concentrations remained constant throughout the study period. No significant differences were found among the evaluations. The results show that it is possible to handle and send serum samples for lithium analyses from distant places to the appropriate laboratories without any special care."

Sure, this was a very simple study, but let me encourage doctors to prescribe lithium with the support of the laboratory assuring them of a correct approach to dose titration.

As the years went by, I always kept in contact with the world of lithium. I used to give lectures from time to time about lithium and put special emphasis on it during my seminars in psychopharmacology for first-year residents at Universidad Nacional Mayor de San Marcos psychiatric training program. Very often, I try to create a real-life atmosphere for the audience by remembering the tragic suicide of Kurt Cobain, lead singer of the rock band Nirvana, who wrote a song called "Lithium" but, apparently, never tried it as a part for his treatment of bipolar disorder.

I have also observed that most doctors still do not use lithium with confidence. Anticonvulsants used to be their first choice, maybe following the American psychiatrists' practice. I understand that in Europe lithium is given greater consideration. As a matter of fact, I have to recognize that sometimes I lost some patients in my private practice when I suggested they take lithium for their bipolar disorders. They simply ran away. To the best of my knowledge, lithium is not a panacea but still it is the gold standard for the treatment of bipolar disorder, especially as expressed in the classic manic-depressive clinical presentation.

Lithium continues guiding my interest in trying to understand the complexity of brain function and I share the naive experience of Aretaeus of Cappadocia in those ancient times when he observed the cyclical mood fluctuations of people living together in the mountain caves in order to survive (Tekiner 2015). In those times, obviously they did not have lithium and their suffering remained unrelieved.

References:

Castillo A, Miyahira A. Estabilidad del Litio Serico en Condiciones Ambientales. Anales de Salud Mental, 1986; 2:67-71.

Tekiner H. Aretaeus of Cappadocia and his treatises on diseases. Turk Neurosurg. 2015; 25(3):508-12.

July 2, 2020

REID FINLAYSON'S COMMENTS
A LIFE ON LITHIUM AND LESSONS LEARNED

Tom Ban invited me to contribute a "comment" to a prospective INHN publication on "Lithium in Historical Perspective" in which I will present my observations/findings and/or life-time personal experience with the substance. I accepted the invitation and in the following I will give an account and reflect on my life prior to and after I was prescribed lithium. I will present my life experience in chronology but bring to attention in advance that after 20 years of treatment with lithium I made an impulsive choice to test my diagnosis of manic depression during a mid-life crisis by reducing my lithium dose. The experiment led to personal acceptance and deeper appreciation of the reciprocal interactions between bipolar illness and substance use disorders. Ultimately, in my work as an addiction psychiatrist, I am grateful to have the opportunity to apply my "inside-out" knowledge and experience in working with patients and colleagues who struggle with similar issues.

Part I – What it was like before lithium

I was perplexed and still vaguely angry that Easter Sunday morning. Awaking slowly and hazily I remembered having been wrestled to the floor by a sea of faces dressed in white who held me on the floor and injected my buttocks with sedating drugs, against my will. The reality of my plight began to slowly infuse my mind. That morning I came to in a hospital room on the seventh floor of the Clarke Institute of Psychiatry on College Street in downtown Toronto. It was the 14th of April 1974. It was about five months before my 30th birthday and I was a psychiatric resident, both literally and figuratively. It was nine months into my first year of psychiatric residency training, and I had been hospitalized, involuntarily.

The decision I had made to leave a thriving family medicine practice and begin a four-year training program to become a psychiatrist was complicated. Early in medical school, it was surgery that first appealed to me. I had spent a lot of time in the lab and operating room with Dr. Robert McFarlane, a prominent hand and plastic surgeon at The University of Western Ontario (now Shulick) School of Medicine. He was kind enough to recognize my contribution to a study he published (1968). The technical surgical skills I was taught allowed me to perform appendectomy and cholecystectomy under close and direct supervision, but I had a tendency to occasionally lose focus briefly during long, difficult procedures. I might need to break scrub for a few minutes rest or have a coffee. I also felt light-headed when I donated blood, so I ruled out training to be a surgeon. Dr. Ramsey Gunton, our much-admired professor, and chair of medicine invited me to specialize in Internal Medicine, but I decided to complete a rotating internship at Toronto Western Hospital in 1970, which at that time was enough to qualify me to be a practitioner of medicine, surgery and midwifery in the province of Ontario. As a third-year medical student, I was 23 when I married Mary. She was the daughter of a doctor with a prosperous general practice who also practiced anesthesia. Our son was born before I graduated and our daughter the following year, just after we had arrived in Owen Sound to begin family medicine practice.

I established a successful family medicine practice in Owen Sound, Ontario, in a happy and successful partnership with my late friend and colleague, Dr. Ralph Bunston. We met during my internship in Toronto and agreed to practice family medicine together for just three years because we both considered returning to complete more postgraduate education. During those three years, the practice of family medicine seemed routine and didn't challenge me enough. I pursued training as a private plane pilot and was drawn to become Jail Surgeon, providing medical care to the prisoners in the Grey County

Jail, and the patients at the local provincial psychiatric hospital. The pathology lectures of Dr. Marvin Smout at Western had been fascinating, as was the sensational career of the Chief Coroner, Dr. Morty Shulman in Toronto, plus I was a fan of the television show Quincy (Jack Klugman in the title role played a medical examiner). So, I volunteered to become the youngest coroner in the province.

Being a coroner was more challenging than I expected. Tragic child deaths, accidental deaths, murders and suicides which I was called upon to investigate were often very disturbing. My stress was compounded by the responsibility to speak with the bereaved families. In this area my medical training had been woefully deficient, leaving me ill-prepared to cope with the fallout from unexpected deaths and with insufficient training to counsel shocked families. Psychiatry seemed to offer me an opportunity to increase my knowledge, understanding and to enhance my ability to communicate.

There were personal considerations too. Another reason I chose psychiatry was to follow in the footsteps of my father. I have always admired my father. He served in the British Royal Navy Volunteer Reserve during World War II and was at sea when I was born in Glasgow in 1944. Father had a difficult time finding work as a doctor in post-war Britain while the National Health Service was being organized. He was persuaded that more opportunities would be available in Canada for our family, so we immigrated to Canada in 1952. My father passed the Medical Council of Canada requirements for licensure while working at the Ontario Hospital School, Orillia, and went on to train in psychiatry at the University of Toronto in the mid-1950s. We moved many times as a family, I had attended eight different schools before my graduation from the University of Western Ontario (Schulich) School of Medicine in 1969. My father the psychiatrist, would sometimes invite troubled colleagues to visit with him in our family home because for them, it avoided the embarrassment of seeing him at the hospital or in his office. As a family doctor, I had been a volunteer participant, available to answer calls for the Ontario Medical Association's physician helpline, for doctors in distress, which was an early precursor to Ontario's Physician Health Program.

My wife was reluctant for me to leave family medicine to return to postgraduate training after three years. My father-in-law, a prosperous general practice anesthetist, had invited me to join his practice. The University of Toronto immediately offered me a training position, but I was more attracted to the new Department of Psychiatry at McMaster University in Hamilton, where the emphasis at the time was on family therapy. Inviting Mary to come to an interview with the training director was, in retrospect, a sign of my immaturity because Dr. Nahum Spinner sensed her indecision and suggested that I seek some therapy before deciding to start the program. The stress of changing careers was less obvious to me but a Scottish psychoanalyst in Toronto listened patiently and perceived no problems with my proposed career plan and we determined that I was sufficiently interested to accept the position in Hamilton.

My first training rotation in psychiatry was on an inpatient service at the Hamilton Psychiatric Hospital with Dr. Paul Cakuls, a friendly and supportive teacher. I enjoyed learning with colleagues and also from our patients. Dr. Paul Grof, a brilliant young Czech psychiatrist, worked on an adjacent ward. He was very interested in the new and exciting lithium treatment for manic-depressive illness. At that time, he was researching the various side effects of lithium dose levels, and unaware of my future, I volunteered to be a research subject. I took lithium under carefully monitored experimental conditions for a few weeks, completed questionnaires on its effects and provided samples of blood and urine for the study. Little did I imagine that lithium might become a lifetime medication for me.

My first summer in psychiatry residency was a great experience. I worked hard, read and tried new approaches to working with patients. We purchased a home in Hamilton's Westdale area, and the children attended nursery school. It was fun to meet new neighbors and friends. By winter of that year I began to feel depressed. My wife was unhappy with the move, which strained our relationship and my spirits sank further. I returned to the psychoanalyst I had spoken to about my career change and we began psychotherapy. With each visit, my mood seemed to decline further. I remember in one session recalling my family's departure from Scotland when I was seven-years-old. I cried as I described my aunts, uncles, grandparents and cousins waving us away tearfully on the dock at Millport, singing, "Will ye' no come back again." Through my tears, I had the perception that my analyst's eyes welled with a tear. He prescribed an antidepressant for me, protriptyline, and suggested that I begin to take it.

Although I felt despondent, it was not easy to accept that I might be clinically depressed. I thought of my symptoms, which were poor sleep, decreased appetite with mild weight loss, plus some hopelessness, as the result of events outside myself. Even years later it has been difficult to accept that the changes in mood might originate from within myself.

Within three days of starting daily protriptyline, I felt excited, confused and restless. The irritability was out of character for me. I had returned to my Scottish analyst and offered him my perception that my tearful reminiscence of leaving Scotland might have affected him, but that, he responded, had not been the case. And I remember thinking (rather grandiosely for my first year of residency training) and making a note to myself that I was already as capable as any psychoanalyst. It was a passively aggressive expression of my disappointment with him. Later I came to understand that the antidepressant, protriptyline, had precipitated a sudden, severe change in my mood, within several days of starting treatment for depression. Dr. William E Bunney first described this behavioral switch process in 1970 (Bunney, Murphy, Goodwin and Borge), recognizing that a few patients, most often those with manic depression or bipolar illness, can experience sudden changes into excited, confused manic or mixed states with manic levels of energy while taking antidepressant drugs. This is part of the reason for the black box warning for suicide risk on antidepressant medications now.

By dawn on Good Friday in 1974 I was already awake, and anxious, unsettled and perplexed. I got up early for a walk while deciding to seek help from my program director at McMaster. I arrived at Dr. Nahum Spinner's office unannounced and knocked at his door. He was in the middle of an interview and when we did speak, I don't recall what was said, but he was kind, recognized my distress and arranged for me to accept an injection of haloperidol, a major tranquilizer, and be transported by ambulance to the Clarke Institute of Psychiatry in Toronto. He must have reasoned that it would be wiser to not admit me to one of the Hamilton-area hospitals where I might work again someday. It was quite a different experience, having a psychiatric illness than going to a hospital for surgery. It was also my formal induction into the shame, guilt and stigma of mental illness.

Easter weekend in the emergency admitting area and later on the ward at the Clarke Institute of Psychiatry was quiet at first. I did not want to be there but was persuaded to stay. Understandably, my wife was very concerned. My father visited the following morning and we spoke briefly together with the clinical director, a colleague of his. I still wanted to leave following our discussion, but a certificate for involuntary committal was completed, which meant I was to be confined in the hospital, against my own will, until a board of review could hear my appeal. I was back on the unit when I learned about it and I wasn't going to have that. I became agitated, impatient, angry and tried to leave. A sea of faces dressed in white wrestled me to the floor to inject tranquilizers into my buttocks. And I would not, could not, and did not understand that I needed to be there.

I fantasized my ordeal as being some sort of initiation into becoming a psychiatrist, similar to being initiated into freemasonry or a college fraternity. The ruminative thinking that beset me would often have a religious undercurrent. I was raised in the Presbyterian Church in Scotland. As children in Millport, we had gone to sing hymns at outside services on the sandy beaches accompanied by a portable pedal organ. In Canada, we attended Sunday School each week and sang in the choir. At times of stress, I found comfort in having faith and imagined briefly a career as a minister. But I felt persecuted, righteous and prayed that I wouldn't lose my mind. I can remember lying in bed in the psychiatric unit, in that chemical haze, trying to make sense about what was happening to me. I wondered what God was trying to teach me. It was Easter and I worried that the hospitalization represented personal humiliation and crucifixion. I recall the pathetic fallacy of disappointment and confinement – as if the stone covering my tomb had not been rolled back on that Easter Sunday. The fantasy brought a small measure of comfort temporarily to my confused state.

My attending doctor at the Clarke was polite, confident, but aloof initially and his resident seemed distant and unengaging. For my part, there was anger when my freedom was restricted and I was furious to be confined and drugged against my will.

Medications were the foundation for the beginning of my treatment, but I would look for ways to avoid taking them during my initial hospital stay. I was fearful of the potential side effects and because I wanted to avoid being labeled with a mental illness diagnosis. When the nursing staff might be trusting and inattentive around medication times, I would put the pills in my hand, under my tongue or in my cheek, then later discard them in the toilet because I was appalled and questioned the doses prescribed. Much later it occurred to me that the doses might have been increased because they were not having the expected effect!

The two-week period of commitment in the hospital passed interminably slowly. It was novel to experience being a patient, learning the rituals associated with mealtimes, medications, meetings and spending long hours interacting with other patients. Until I was more able to contain and manage my anger and disappointment about the situation, I was closely monitored by orderlies who were pleasant and sympathetic but unable to negotiate my release. As I began to appear calm and my behavior was more predictable, the difficult adjustment began. It would take years, including many hours in therapy and years of recovery before I was able to more completely accept and even enjoy the harmless "demons" within myself that I was so terrified to face then. The treatment team recommended that I stay on and get more help, but I was afraid to be vulnerable and demanded my immediate release.

My poor judgment resulted in a second hospitalization that followed quickly on the heels of the first. Just after being released, stressed by the fragments of my life, the implications of what had happened and muddled by drugs, I was uncertain about returning to the psychiatry residency program at McMaster. I confess that I had reduced the prescribed doses of my medications to about 25% of what the doctors recommended for me in the hospital. Under the stress of not knowing what was next, plus my wife's extreme level of concern, I decided shortly after being discharged from the Clarke Institute that things might improve if I were to take the full dose of the medications, just as had been prescribed.

Resuming the recommended doses of antipsychotics, I soon became slow, stiff and markedly despondent. My family doctor referred me to Dr. Art Lesser, a psychiatrist who was a family friend and former colleague of my father. I shared my fears about the hospitalization in Toronto and he was the first professional to also listen to my wife's concerns about the situation. He diagnosed clinical depression and recommended that I reduce the high doses of antipsychotic medication and start on the antidepressant amitriptyline (Elavil).

Amitriptyline had a similar effect upon me as had occurred with protriptyline weeks earlier. Within days I became more fearful, confused, irritable and didn't sleep much. I experienced great, lengthy bursts of high energy. Without an appointment, I walked miles from my home in Hamilton to see Dr. Carl Moore again in Dundas. He notified Dr. Lesser, who arranged to meet us at my home. They recognized that I was psychotic and arranged to have me admitted to the psychiatric unit at the Joseph Brant Hospital in nearby Burlington. My wife must have been really upset.

Committed and admitted involuntarily, for the second time within weeks, I became extremely frightened and endeavored to escape. After the first attempt my clothing was removed but I eloped once more and this time made it to the busy highway nearby. I tried to hitchhike but dressed only in an open hospital gown with no shoes, I failed to hitch a ride. A couple of kindly staff caught up and persuaded me to return. They tried to lock me in a seclusion room when we got back to the hospital. My final resistance was to force the door ajar by using the bed on wheels as a battering ram. A sea of faces restrained me again and held me on the floor to administer injectable medicine. Finally, I slept extremely soundly and for a long time when the sedatives and antipsychotic tranquilizers overtook me. I was so sedated I very nearly died, an observant colleague who was there at the time, later informed me. (In retrospect, this may have been due to malignant hyperthermia, a rare reaction to neuroleptic agents whose mechanism is poorly understood to this day.)

A day later I awoke laying wet and naked on the linoleum floor in an empty room, on my urine-soaked gown and sheets, too unsteady to stand up alone. I was stiff, shaking and breathing with difficulty, nearly all due to side effects from the drugs which were used to sedate me. It was like being born again. Within a day or so and while I was still in the process of awakening Dr. Paul Grof (the principal investigator of the lithium study I had been a subject in) came to visit with me in the hospital. He suggested that my diagnosis could be a variant of manic depression (now called bipolar affective disorder). It was on his advice that I again started taking lithium carbonate but as a patient this time instead of a research volunteer. It was a great relief to see him again and his opinion made sense to me. He also suggested to my hospital psychiatrist a gradual reduction of the other drugs, major tranquilizers and anti-depressants and sedatives necessary to calm and sedate me. Quickly thereafter my condition improved substantially. I began to behave more rationally within days and to think more clearly. I was able to relate to other people again. I socialized with the other patients on the floor and remember playing guitar and singing Delta Dawn with them alongside the popular recordings of Tanya Tucker and Helen Reddy at that time. Several of the Joseph Brant nursing staff told me with amazement that they had witnessed my radical transformation and saw me transform into a completely different person – a kind and thoughtful young physician – reminiscent of Dr. Jekyll and Mr. Hyde (Stevenson 1886). It would prove to be more difficult for my wife, Mary, to assimilate the extreme fluctuations in my mood.

Leaving hospital for the second time in as many months, I needed to make decisions about my future. Should I return to psychiatry residency training or look for another career? I was feeling much better, but my wife remained very concerned. I enjoyed being home with the children while I considered whether or not to return to complete my training in psychiatry. My father listened to my ordeal and we discussed the possible options, but, characteristically, he left the decision making to me. I felt I had made the correct choice to train in psychiatry and that I did not wish to start over in another specialty or return to family medicine. If anything, my experience as a patient only heightened my desire to learn more about psychiatry.

A week or two following my discharge from the Joseph Brant Hospital my wife and our young children visited her parents to discuss my decision. My father-in-law had offered to have me join his family practice as an associate and take it over eventually, but I had decided to complete training in psychiatry, if the program would have me back. The events of that day were to have profound effects on my life and eventually on the course of my career. When we arrived at Mary's family home her father, whom I had never known to use alcohol, had an opened bottle of gin or vodka on the shelf. Not only was he drinking, the Doctor's speech was slurred, and he was uncharacteristically garrulous and overly affectionate, much more than usual, with our children.

I was technically off duty on sick leave, but I wanted to talk with him and try to intervene with him and my mother-in-law. His behavior terrified Mary and she insisted that we leave immediately. I have never forgotten that spring day in 1974. Mary and I drove home with our children and as we entered the house, the phone rang with news that Mary's father had been found dead, in his swimming pool beside an empty vial of Demerol and a syringe. I urged Mary that we return to be with her family, but she adamantly refused. His body was quietly buried the following day, but we did return for a memorial service a few days later.

I returned to my second year in the training program and relations at home improved gradually toward normalization. Life was good once again, feeling stable, balanced, back in better control. I resolved to do my best to master the knowledge and practice of psychiatry and to prepare for the Royal College of Physicians and Surgeons of Canada specialty examinations. After three more years of residency training, I became a qualified psychiatrist. The announcement that I had passed surprised me, not only because I learned of my success a few days earlier than we expected to find out. I became completely overwhelmed by an intense rush of feelings of relief, apprehension and experienced a full-blown attack of panic that day.

I was invited to join the faculty at McMaster as a Lecturer in the Department of Psychiatry. My clinical duties included managing the Emergency Psychiatric Service at St. Joseph's hospital, under the guidance and leadership of Dr. Giampiero Bartolucci. I continued my personal and professional interest in family therapy with mentorship from Dr. Nathan Epstein and worked in the Human Sexuality education program with Joyce Asquith, MSW, and Dr. John Lamont. I was also a part-time consultant with the Family Medicine Program. Several small grants were awarded and I began to publish one or two papers.

My wife was less happy with our situation. I had always hoped that she would develop a career interest of her own. She managed a store when our children began school, but it didn't last. I received a small salary increase and we bought a home in nearby Dundas that had a swimming pool. It was a delightful spot for our children, but the marriage continued to strain. Therapy as a couple produced only temporary improvement but I was determined to persist for the children and felt guilt for disappointing her. Our negotiations about nearly every disagreement resulted in questions about the stability of my mood and whether I was compliant with appointments and medication. Reorganizing my life and practice after my episodes of illness and hospitalization had been difficult. Months were required before I was able to return to function at my best. My wife had been severely shaken by what had happened. My behavior, when I was psychotic, must have been terrifying. She tried to be supportive, but Mary grew increasingly wary of any unpredictability and we disagreed about the intensity of my moods. It seemed to me as if she blamed my illness for problems in our marriage.

After a couple of years, I felt the need to move to a higher paying position and so my wife and I relocated to her hometown in Ontario. For 10 years there, I worked in and eventually led the psychiatric clinic which had been created through the University of Western Ontario by Dr. Gil Heseltine, Chairman of Psychiatry.

Following my first hospital episodes in 1974, my wife and I had attended sessions of marriage therapy. I later undertook psychoanalytic treatment with Dr. Johann "Hans" Aufreiter (Naiman 2001), three times a week for nearly five years. The dissatisfaction in my marriage continued. If I did complain, it seemed that my wife distorted it, as if the issues were related to a symptom of my mood disturbance, which was blamed as the cause of the problems. The analytic process slowly allowed me to appreciate myself more fully. Marriage therapy had been unsuccessful, but Mary agreed to attend analytic sessions with Dr. Friedl Aufreiter, the wife of my analyst. After a few months, she decided she had nothing else to discuss and stopped going.

I was again briefly hospitalized, a third time, for an episode of psychosis, possibly triggered by fiberglass resin fumes. I had been repairing a windsurfer in our garage. Dr. Paul Grof arranged to admit me to Hamilton Psychiatric Hospital for a few days while it resolved.

As my analysis progressed my practice was flourishing. I participated in medical organizations and became involved in committee work with the Ontario Medical Association, the Association of General Hospital Psychiatric Units and was eventually elected President of the Ontario Psychiatric Association. I was awarded Fellowship in the American Psychiatric Association, in part for my contribution to rural psychiatry in Ontario and participation in the North of Superior Community Mental Health Program. I also commuted to London, Ontario regularly, per my faculty appointment, to lecture and teach students and trainees.

More than 20 years had elapsed since I had awkwardly arranged to ask the blessing of Mary's parents to marry her, as I began the third year of medical school. Her parents were pleased and supported the marriage, but I could never be entirely sure that being married to me was what Mary wanted for herself. She was much less surprised and upset than were our two children after I found the courage to tell her in 1989 that I was separating and wanted to divorce. More attempts at professional intervention seemed pointless to both of us. I moved into a spare room while we sought legal assistance to separate. Our children were at college. I planned to relocate, away from her hometown and start over.

I joined the faculty at the University of Ottawa and moved there for three years where I enjoyed working with Drs. Edgardo Perez, John Rassell and Doug Wilkins. It was also an opportunity to re-connect with Dr. Paul Grof, who was terrific support for me again as he worked nearby, at the Royal Ottawa Hospital. I attended several of his therapeutic workshops based on holotropic breathwork, a supervised experience that helped me transcend and integrate some traumatic experiences. I agonized over the decision to commit to a long-distance relationship I hoped might work. Then, in 1993 I accepted a position at Homewood Health Centre in Guelph, Ontario, to be the consultant psychiatrist on the Homewood Alcohol and Drug Service.

I had always wondered and gradually persuaded myself that my marriage had contributed to my episodes of mental illness. Somehow, 20 years after my first hospitalization, it seemed to me less necessary to continue taking lithium, my mood-stabilizing medication. I thought that I had been stable for years and I was making a fresh start. Besides that, my episodes of severe psychosis had been chemically triggered. I discussed the idea of stopping lithium with my psychiatrist as we had successfully tried taking closely monitored and seasonally appropriate lithium dose reductions. But I did eventually decide on my own to slowly reduce and stop taking lithium. It was a gamble that made sense to me at that time to put my questions about whether my episodes had been situational and substance-induced to the test. It was a self-imposed experiment whose painful lessons I did not foresee. I doubt that I could have chosen a more difficult time to try being without lithium.

There was an overwhelming degree of stress in my life then, of which I was not aware. Alongside my recent relocation to a brand-new job, plus the stresses of a fledgling relationship, I would have scored at the top of any scale that measured personal stress. Clearly, in hindsight, it was not the time to interrupt my effective mood-stabilizing treatment. At the heart of it, stopping lithium was much like playing Russian roulette. My mood soon began to change from being confidently energetic and expansive to being less energetic, not sleeping well and having ruminative thoughts and indecision. The relationship failed and my feelings of depression intensified. My new psychiatrist prescribed an antidepressant, one of the newer selective serotonin reuptake inhibitor (SSRI) antidepressant medications which are chemically distinct and might have been safer than the older tricyclic agents (protriptyline and amitriptyline) to which I had reacted so badly 20 years earlier. I started taking the prescribed paroxetine (Paxil) but within days symptoms of psychosis necessitated another hospitalization. I was quickly stabilized on risperidone (Risperdal) and started lithium treatment again. I lived with my middle brother's family for a few weeks until I was able to resume working. The new relationship, that had ended with my hospitalization, rekindled as I stabilized and was returning to work.

I had first spoken publicly about my illness, during my term as president, at the Annual Meeting of the Ontario Psychiatric Association. About the same time, I also had the stress of testifying at a murder trial and signing off on the final agreement of my contentious divorce proceedings.

Although I had restarted lithium my mood slipped low and I became more depressed again. My psychiatrist and I felt that another trial of SSRI antidepressant was warranted, but this time with lithium in place. Within a few days of beginning sertraline (Zoloft) it happened again. Confusion and poor sleep quickly led to my fifth admission to a psychiatric unit to be stabilized. I convalesced at the home of my youngest brother and stayed with my parents for several weeks until I was fit to return to my new job at The Homewood, in Guelph, Ontario.

I was to about to learn a great deal more about the frequent associations and interactions between substance abuse and mental illness working at The Homewood from my supervisor, Dr. Graeme Cunningham and the late Dr. Peter Mezciems (1994), among others. My role was to provide psychiatric consultations and treatment to patients on the unit treating alcohol and substance use disorders. The experience considerably deepened my understanding of the frequent mixture of substance use with mood disorders. Nearly two-thirds of patients with bipolar illness experience substance abuse issues and my own life was about to improve significantly.

I had previously seen no clear reason to deny myself the comfort of a glass of wine or a beer now and then because I had always considered myself to be a social drinker. I was raised in a family that celebrated the culture of Southwest Scotland and alcohol use was a daily ritual into which my two brothers and I were slowly initiated after our 16th birthdays. My first real opportunity for unlimited alcohol consumption was on a high school trip to Ottawa – I lost count of the amount of beer I had consumed. I discovered, when it was time to go to the bathroom, that I was completely unable to stand up or balance myself. Crawling, hands and knees on the floor to get to the toilet would frighten most people, I think. But I felt only pleasant bemusement, recognizing that the Glasgow slang term "legless" was appropriately descriptive of my condition. More accurately, what I experienced is described as ataxia caused by potentially fatal alcohol poisoning. What I did not appreciate for many more years was that I had a high tolerance for alcohol, likely genetically determined. I sailed through college and medical school occasionally drinking too much on weekends. I would revel in the Westcoast Scottish accent that I had learned to repress on arriving in Canada.

Working at The Homewood Addiction Division involved teaching patients – among them were many physicians – to stop using alcohol and drugs. Nobody ever seemed to consider me to have any real problems related to my alcohol use, or to be anything more than a social drinker. But I began to notice that my patients at Homewood were being transformed by abstinence and recovery during their treatment on the Addiction Service. Frequently on admission, often arriving there after a crisis, the majority of patients easily met criteria for major depression. But they usually left treatment much brighter, more optimistic and often with restored family relations – without being started on antidepressant medications.

On July 4th of 1994, I awakened one beautiful morning on Georgian Bay. It was a long summer weekend to celebrate Canada Day – visiting at a friend's cottage. I awoke that morning with a headache and the feeling that I had fallen asleep before I had stopped partying the night before – and as was my custom, having a few drinks on such occasions. I was about to take an Aspirin to temper the consequences of my alcohol use, but my conscience replayed the advice I routinely suggested to my patients at my new job. I also recognized that my fuzzy memory might even be a mild blackout. I made a commitment to myself that day to stop drinking alcohol forever and it is remains so to this day – it was the last time I consumed alcohol.

In my late teens I had been a sometime cigarette smoker and continuing to consult at the Addictions Unit I began to obsess about the failure to adequately address tobacco in the program. Dr. Graeme Cunningham, the program director and a fellow Scot, was quite open about his addiction recovery in Alcoholics Anonymous and found the courage one day to question my obsession about patients using tobacco. He wondered whether my behavior resembled that of a "dry drunk," that is being sober, but without benefit of the peaceful serenity that accompanies recovery from alcohol use. It is the same principle, elaborated further by Johann Hari (2015), that the opposite of addiction is not simply abstinence but is the ability to engage in meaningful healthy connections in with other people.

I promptly began following the same directions that I was proposing daily to my patients at The Homewood and began to attend "90 meetings of Alcoholics Anonymous in 90 days." As is typical, it seemed important for me to travel to meetings in a nearby town – to avoid the embarrassment of being recognized, at first! I asked the woman who was chairing the first meeting I attended who might sponsor me and was introduced to her husband Eddie, who agreed to be my sponsor in the program. Eddie taught me how to be peaceful and to enjoy living in the present moment, while we worked together on the 12 Steps of the program. We remained close friends until his death.

Over the seven years at The Homewood I consulted on the assessment team that evaluated physicians, airline pilots and other professionals for substance use and mental health problems. I was also asked to develop and lead a program for patients at risk for compulsive sexual behavior. Men and women in crisis during treatment would occasionally engage in intense relationships with one another that derailed ongoing group therapy and often resulted in discharge and relapses. Although the sexual addiction program demonstrated success (Wan, Finlayson and Rowles 2000), funding for the program could not be continued. Most addiction treatment programs now provide separate therapy groups for each sex to address their intimate, personal issues. Naturally I was disappointed, but it wasn't long before an opportunity arose to work in the United States.

I have been fortunate to have had excellent psychiatric care over the years. Dr. Paul Grof originally made my diagnosis and started prescribing lithium treatment for me in 1974. Dr. Emmanuel Persad treated me when I lived in Guelph, Ontario. After moving to Nashville in 2001, Dr. Ron Solomon and Dr. Bill Petrie were very helpful and have continued to prescribe lithium for me in subsequent years.

Part II – What things are like now - in recovery, on lithium

Dr. Peter Martin became a mentor and friend through our common interests in behavioral addictions (Finlayson, Sealy and Martin 2001) and substance use disorders (Martin and Finlayson 2012). We met at addiction research meetings and he invited me to relocate to Vanderbilt University in Nashville. My children were independent adults by that time and the relocation happened much more smoothly in 2001 than in 1993. I was welcomed to the city and immediately felt supported by my fellowship in Alcoholics Anonymous. In fact, when I crossed the border into the United States immigration officers wanted to know all about me and surprisingly asked me informally and politely about my personal status. They explained that I had been issued a type of US visa that is normally reserved "for individuals with an extraordinary ability in the sciences, education, business, or athletics (not including the arts, motion pictures or television industry)."

Fellowship in Alcoholics Anonymous provided rooms filled with new friends that helped facilitate my relocation to Nashville. My new and current sponsor, Pete, was a terrific resource and guide who also advised me on business matters. With encouragement and support the Vanderbilt Comprehensive Assessment Program was established, grew slowly and has gradually generated a reputation for evaluating troubled physicians from all over the United States and still sometimes from Canada (Finlayson, Dietrich, Neufeld et al. 2013).

It has been both a humbling privilege and a fulfilling experience over the years to participate in the assessment and treatment of many hundreds of physicians with substance use issues, psychiatric disorders and behavioral problems that potentially interfered with their ability to practice medicine with reasonable care and safety. I have had the privilege of working with the late Dr. David T. Dodd, the late Dr. Roland Gray and Dr. Michael Baron in their roles as medical directors of the Tennessee Medical Foundation. I have also had the opportunity over the years to work in a variety of clinical treatment settings, including The Homewood, The Center for Professional Excellence and Journey Pure – rehabilitation centers with a special focus on recovery for physicians. I teach at Vanderbilt Medical School and supervise post-graduate trainees. In 2014 I completed a degree in

Indications

Healthcare Management at Vanderbilt Owen School of Management. In recent years I have been appointed medical director for Vanderbilt Work-Life Connections Employee Assistance Program, for Vanderbilt faculty and physicians. I am grateful to have the opportunity to help others and to repay the care and support that was given to me.

My ex-wife, Mary, died of cancer before I married again in 2006. It seemed to me and without having planned to do so, that I had found peace in my life and career path following my inability to intervene with her father and perhaps prevent his death on that tragic day in May of 1974, those many years before. After being single for 15 years I met a younger Nashville social worker at an agency where we both were practicing. After checking with her supervisor that it was appropriate, I invited Diana for dinner and learned that she was planning to adopt a Chinese orphan as a single mother. The opportunity to be part of a family appealed to both of us. I surprised Diana with a diamond ring. We traveled with her mother to China in July of 2006 to adopt Olivia and married afterward, to avoid having to alter her adoption application. Olivia has been warmly welcomed into both our families as an American citizen. It has now been 15 delightful years together.

Life continues, gratefully I remain healthy and still enjoy working at 75 years of age. I follow the recommendations of my doctors and continue taking lithium and other medications as they are prescribed for me. I look forward to July 4th each year, because I still enjoy pretending that the Independence Day fireworks also celebrate my first day of sobriety!

Psychiatry had begun to change in the early 1970s. The strong influence of psychoanalysis in North America was waning while biological psychiatry, as we now know it, was just beginning. It was a time of psychological and sociological curiosity; interest in the application of family dynamics and family therapy to mental illness was strong. Family therapy might provide new answers for major psychiatric illnesses like depression, schizophrenia and addiction. While working with families can be beneficial, some of the therapeutic zeal of those early days caused family members to feel responsible for symptoms we now believe to have more complex biological, psychological, social and spiritual (how we interact emotionally with others) causation. Also, it is clearer to me now that my interest in family therapy presaged relationship problems that would culminate in separation and divorce. The times and customs of the 1970s and 1980s were different than they are now. Divorce was more frowned upon and unheard of in my family. There was no Oprah show, by which I mean the movement for self-disclosure, self-discovery, self-healing was in the earliest stages. I downplayed the emphasis on my mental illness and believed it was quiescent if I attended appointments, took my lithium faithfully and forged on with life – like the "good little soldier" I had been encouraged to be as child in post-war Scotland.

Denial, pride, shame and fear of stigmatization were all part of my reluctance to look within myself at the outset. There is something more intensely personal about disordered thoughts and the anxious feelings which affect one's internal sense of being, in comparison to the more easily explained reactions to external circumstance or due to an illness that has an understandable cause.

It seems safe to conclude that one's professional status as a physician offers little protection and can sometimes increase the risk from mental disorders. Experience, knowledge and training don't prevent physicians from denying their problems, just as I did, both around alcohol use and the total acceptance of my diagnosis and treatment with lithium. Substance Use Disorders and Bipolar illness are lifelong illnesses that can relapse and significantly interrupt and disrupt life, work and relationships. Fortunately, many helpful forms of treatment and support are now available. Chronic reliance on substances of abuse rarely ends well, especially if used to mask symptoms of trauma or major mental illness.

My personal experiences as a patient have made me much more tolerant, more empathic and wiser than I might ever have become. Even during the worst times, I continued to hope and considered it possible that my experiences as a patient might prove to be an advantage. I recall being attracted to the early thoughts of R.D. Laing, who saw severe mental illness as a transformational experience.

As a result of my illness, I can more readily identify and appreciate the hopelessness, fear, shame, grandiosity and other emotional states which occur in my patients. I had considered studying theology in my teenage years, so the coincidence of Easter with my first hospital stay inflamed fantasies of betrayal, crucifixion and despair but not without hope for resurrection or rebirth. Invariably, my colleagues in psychiatry have been sympathetic, they understood and supported me and my struggles with the illness and provided encouragement when I was well.

I was fortunate to have been raised in a strong family and to have two younger brothers with whom I remain close, many years following the deaths of our parents. Unbeknownst to me at the time, some bipolar illness had been present in our extended family, long before my first episode. One grandmother had several episodes of abnormally elevated mood beginning when she was more than 60 years of age. Tales handed down in the family suggest that others may have had similar difficulties. One of my aunts developed mood swings beginning at the age of 40, another aunt had been treated for recurrent depressions. My family participated in a genetics research study on bipolar illness (Duffy, Alda, Kutcher et al. 2002) at the Royal Ottawa Hospital. Hopefully, such research into diagnosis and treatment will reduce similar suffering for others.

I had no idea previously that I was using alcohol to feel normal in social settings nor that I would begin to feel so much better by simply not using alcohol, until after I had stopped for a few months. "High-bottom drunks" like me are welcomed in AA, because the only requirement to join is a desire to stop drinking. As I began to focus more upon the similarities between myself and other alcoholics and less upon the differences between us, I began to better understand and appreciate how alcohol use had affected my life, my relationships, and my career. Working the 12 Steps with a sponsor, which means working the AA program – in contrast to just attending meetings – has been a remarkably freeing experience. Based on research in psychotherapy (Patterson 1984) and recent scientific validation of the effectiveness of

Alcoholics Anonymous (Kelly JF, Humphreys K, Ferri 2020) plus personal experience, I often recommend the program of AA to my patients as cost-effective psychotherapy.

Some thoughts about lithium

Along with hydrogen and helium, lithium was one of the three elements produced in large quantities by the Big Bang. Lithium is the least solid chemical element, one of the alkali metals; on the Period Table it has the symbol Li and the atomic number 3. The name lithium comes from the Greek word lithos for stone. It was first used medically in the 2nd century AD by the ancient physician Soranus in Ephesus (Purse 2020), who discovered that the waters in his town, which were alkaline due to high levels of lithium, could be used as a treatment for both mania and depression. Johan August Arfvedson, a Swedish chemist, isolated lithium in ore from a Swedish iron mine in 1817 and in 1818 elemental lithium was isolated using electrolysis by William Thomas Brande and Sir Humphry. However, it was John Cade, an Australian doctor, who first discovered the role of lithium in controlling bipolar symptoms. Current information on treatment with lithium may be found in the succinct and easily read, clinical guide (Tondo, Alda, Bauer et al. 2019) for lithium use prepared for the International Group for Studies of Lithium. I recommend it as both an excellent review for prescribers and a valuable information source for patients and their families.

The healing properties of lithium have been extolled for centuries. Bathing in Lithia Springs attracted American pilgrimages to bathe in lithium-rich alkaline waters in Virginia and Georgia – in spas that were recommended by physicians as far away as France – to ameliorate symptoms of excessive uric acid and gout. Various carbonated sparkling water solutions of lithium salts included: Buffalo Lithia Water, Londonderry Lithia Water, White Rock Sparkling Water. Early versions of 7Up were promoted and advertised for improving health. Lithium chloride became a popular sodium chloride/table salt substitute for the dietary treatment of heart failure and high blood pressure until its toxicity was recognized Waldron in 1949.

Lithium occasionally interferes with the functioning of the thyroid gland, which is located at the base of the neck, just above the sternum. My thyroid test results were always fine until an unusual mass on my chest X-ray 10 years ago was biopsied and found to be a goiter growing down into the middle of my chest. It could have been something much more serious. Thyroid cancer cells were found – a common finding in older people – so my thyroid gland was completely removed and I have taken replacement medicine since then.

Doctors have been concerned about the effects of lithium on the kidneys and on the heart. There is no question that excessive intake may result in permanent renal damage or death. There is evidence that renal complications occur more frequently in the presence of other illnesses like high blood pressure and diabetes which are known to interfere with the normal supply of blood to the kidneys. Careful monitoring of my lithium dosing with periodic blood level checks and regular checkups minimized the risk of these side effects for me but inheriting the good health and longevity of my ancestors undoubtedly played a major role.

One of the ironies about lithium is that taking too much of it can be fatal. It is crucial that patients are educated about the importance of maintaining adequate hydration and electrolyte balance to avoid possible toxic effects. Taking more than the prescribed dosage is extremely dangerous. I have felt profoundly depressed and at times briefly hopeless, yet never have I entertained thoughts about suicide or planned to end my existence. Lithium is superior to other medicines in preventing suicide. In areas where increased levels of lithium are found in the groundwater, suicide may occur less frequently. The best outcomes result when treatment with lithium is part of a long-term, well-functioning relationship between the doctor, or lithium clinic, and the patient.

My response to lithium treatment in 1974 was dramatic, but complete acceptance of my diagnosis and the need to continue taking lithium to prevent future episodes, took considerably longer. It was difficult for me to believe that I had a mood disorder and far easier to attribute my symptoms to the antidepressants and untoward external circumstances. I remained in the care of Dr. Paul Grof for many years. He was very supportive, patient and understanding. He negotiated treatment with me, adjusting lithium dose reductions during seasons of low risk, and to boost my mood on long dark Canadian winter nights he suggested light therapy – treatment that is no longer necessary living in the South. He often shared his research ideas, treating me like a colleague. That was a significant boost to my self-confidence, which was always shaken by my psychotic episodes.

I have remained on lithium prophylaxis nearly continuously since 1994 and am convinced that using alcohol even at social levels contributed to poor sleep and mood instability in my case. Occasionally, I have shared parts of my story in my teaching role and sometimes with patients. Lithium has been like a "silver bullet" in my life but successful psychiatric treatment requires multiple biological, psychological, social and, yes, spiritual (the search for meaning) interventions. Bipolar illness is frequently associated with substance use disorders and with a history of adverse childhood experiences. Dr. Vincent Felitti (2003) and others have suggested that addiction be redefined, based upon his large studies relating adverse events during childhood (ACEs) with many illnesses among the Kaiser Permanente patient population.

I have not had many side-effect issues and prefer to think of lithium as a mood-stabilizing salt rather than a psychoactive substance. It occurs naturally in the body where it interacts with other chemicals around and within the membranes of our cells. When calibrated to the range of therapeutic concentration it seems to prevent the drastic mood alterations of manic-depressive bipolar disease. It is the single most effective preventive treatment for suicide. Even the presence of lithium in groundwater may reduce rates of suicide.

Most of us prefer to tolerate and even prefer the expansiveness, mood elevation, energy and the increase in goal-directed activity of hypomania to the dragged down feelings of sadness, low energy and social withdrawal of depressive episodes. For some, the boring sense of near normalcy seems less attractive compared to the grandiose chaos of a manic episode. I have had difficulty persuading several rapidly cycling patients of mine to stop taking the antidepressants which are destabilizing them. The high can be like an addiction. Some patients, on the surface at least, appear to prefer continued chaos over the challenge of accepting life on life's own terms. Facing reality, often necessitates increased levels of care, and considerable support in the early phases as we explore and accept the overwhelming trauma-based fears, guilt and shame, that often rebound when the anesthesia of mood-altering substances, or behaviors ends.

My ordeals have deepened my understanding of the associations and interplay between alcohol, drugs and psychiatric disorders, and to personally address the issue of stigmatization. I have seen both sides of patient coercion, restraint, isolation. I know what it is like to be without judgment, reason and emotional control. But I did not lose my mind, my spirit or my soul. Experience has repeatedly taught me that the most powerful enemy is my own fear. But most importantly, I realize that love and understanding are the most powerful treatments available – for without them, nothing else really works.

References:

Bunney WE Jr, Murphy DL, Goodwin FK, Borge GF. The Switch Process from Depression to mania: Relationships to Drugs Which Alter Brain Amines. Lancet. 1970; 1(7655):1022-7.

Duffy A, Alda M, Kutcher S, Cavazzoni P, Robertson C, Grof E, Grof P. A prospective study of the offspring of bipolar parents responsive and nonresponsive to lithium treatment. J Clin Psychiatry. 2002; 63(12):1171-8.

Felitti VJ. English version of German article: Felitti VJ. Ursprünge des Suchtverhaltens – Evidenzen aus einer Studie zu belastenden. Kindheitserfahrungen. Praxis der Kinderpsychologie und Kinderpsychiatrie, 2003; 52:547-59.

Finlayson AJR, Sealy J, Martin PR. The Differential Diagnosis of Problematic Hypersexuality. Sexual Addiction & Compulsivity, 2001; 8:241-51.

Finlayson AJR, Dietrich MS, Neufeld R, Roback H, Martin PR. Restoring Professionalism: the physician fitness-for-duty evaluation. Gen Hosp Psychiatry. 2013; 35(6):659–63.

Hari J. Chasing the Scream: The first and last days of the war on drugs. Bloomsbury, London, 2015

Kelly JF, Humphreys K, Ferri M. Alcoholics Anonymous and other 12-step programs for alcohol use disorder. Cochrane Database Syst Rev. 2020; 3:CD012880.

Martin P, Finlayson AJR. Pharmacopsychosocial Treatment of Opioid Dependence: Harm Reduction, Palliation, or Simply Good Medical Practice? Dusunen Adam: The Journal of Psychiatry and Neurological Sciences. 2012; 25:1-7.

Mezciems PE, Cunningham GM. Treatment of alcoholism. CMAJ. 1994; 150(9):1383–4.

McFarlane RM, Laird JJ, Lamon R, Finlayson AJ, Johnson R. Evaluation of Dextran and DMSO To Prevent Necrosis in Experimental Pedicle Flaps. Plast Reconstr Surg. 1968; 41(1):64-70.

Naiman J. In Memoriam: Johann Aufreiter 1916-2001. Canadian Journal of Psychoanalysis; Montréal, 2001; 9(1): 117-8.

Patterson CH. Empathy, warmth, and genuineness in psychotherapy: A review of reviews. Psychotherapy, 1984; 21(4):431–8.

Purse M. The Discovery and History of Lithium as a Mood Stabilizer. www.verywellmind.com. 2020

Stevenson RL. Strange Case of Dr. Jekyll and Mr. Hyde. Longman. 1886.

Tondo L, Alda M, Bauer, Bergink V, Grof P, Hajek, Lewitka U, Licht RW, Manchia M, Müller-Oerlinghausen B, Nielsen RE, Selo M, Simhandl C, Baldessarini RJ, International Group for Studies of Lithium (IGSLi). Clinical use of lithium salts: guide for users and prescribers. Int J Bipolar Disord, 2019; 7(1):16.

Waldron AM. Lithium intoxication occurring with the use of a table salt substitute in the low sodium dietary treatment of hypertension and congestive heart failure. Univ Hosp Bull. 1949; 15(2):9.

Wan WM, Finlayson R, Rowles A. Sexual Dependency Treatment Outcome Study. Sexual Addiction & Compulsivity, 2000; 7(3)177-96.

October 8, 2020

LONARDO TONDO'S COMMENT
LITHIUM AND I: CLINICAL EXPERIENCE WITH A REMARKABLE ION

Summary

Lithium as a treatment for mood disorders was introduced in Italy in the late 1960s. Interest in lithium was initiated by Drs. Athanasios Koukopoulos who founded and led the Lucio Bini Mood Disorders Center of Rome from 1974 with Drs. Daniela Reginaldi and Paolo Girardi. I was involved with their clinical and research activities from its founding and later established a second such center in Cagliari, Sardinia, in 1977. These activities include my now 45-year long experience with clinical use of lithium in patients with mood disorders and studies of its effectiveness, limitations, and adverse effects, as well as developing evidence for suicide-preventing effects of long-term lithium treatment. Since the early 1990s, these research activities have been strongly stimulated by an ongoing collaboration with Professor Ross Baldessarini at the Mailman Research Center at McLean Hospital and Harvard Medical School, as part of his International Consortium for Mood & Psychotic Disorders Research. This report summarizes highlights of our work with this important orphan treatment.

- - -

The late Drs. Andrea Dotti (1938–2007) and Athanasios Koukopoulos (1931–2013) introduced lithium in Italy in the late 1960s. Koukopoulos heard of lithium from a patient whom he had treated two years earlier for a severe manic episode. Her husband reported that the patient had been taking lithium for two years, prescribed by Dr. Mogens Schou (1918–2005) in Denmark, and had not had her usual annual illness recurrences since starting this treatment. Koukopoulos called and then met Schou. In Rome, he and Dr. Dotti bought an Eppendorf spectrophotometer to assay lithium concentration in serum and started using lithium following Schou's advice. They successfully treated many patients diagnosed with bipolar disorder, but not without encountering some hostility from colleagues in Rome, who accused them of over diagnosing mood disorders. These skeptics eventually changed their minds after seeing that many patients who had been considered to have "schizophrenia" responded remarkably well to lithium treatment.

In 1973, I started working with Drs. Koukopoulos and Dotti as well as other psychiatrist-colleagues. Among these, Drs. Daniela Reginaldi and Paolo Girardi are still working at the Lucio Bini Mood Disorder Center founded by Dr. Koukopoulos in Rome and named in honor of

Indications

one of the inventors of ECT, Drs. Lucio Bini (1908–1964) and Ugo Cerletti (1877–1963). While I was a medical student, Mogens Schou visited the Roman Mood Disorder Center to discuss research on lithium in the early 1970s. However, those working at the Bini Center did not carry out research with Dr. Schou, possibly because he was more interested in generating interest in the use of lithium rather than in clarifying what lithium did clinically or for whom it was best suited. Nevertheless, Koukopoulos and Reginaldi discussed their research interests with Schou, who proposed an excellent title for one of their early clinical studies: Does lithium prevent depressions by suppressing manias? (Kukopulos and Reginaldi 1973). (Koukopoulos was then using an earlier transliteration of his name from the Greek). In that early report, he and Reginaldi attributed the efficacy of lithium in preventing bipolar depression as a reflection of suppressing manic episodes that often preceded depressions.

Two years later, I participated in a study of effects of lithium on the course of manic-depressive recurrences (Kukopulos, Reginaldi, Girardi and Tondo 1975). We reported that recurring episodes of mania and depression were about 59% shorter (29 weeks before versus 12 weeks with lithium). In particular, reduction of time in manic states was more evident than in the typically longer depressive episodes (62% vs. 50%).

In 1975, we collaborated with Joseph Mendels and Alan Frazer at the University of Pennsylvania to evaluate the significance of intracellular versus circulating concentrations of lithium. We found that, among Lucio Bini Center patients responding poorly to lithium treatment, serum concentrations of lithium were higher than in patients who did well with lithium. Instead, lithium concentrations in corresponding erythrocytes were relatively low in lithium-nonresponders, and the ratio of serum-to-red cell concentrations was higher, even with adjustment for their higher daily doses of lithium carbonate. Of note, however, the ratio of circulating to intracellular lithium was relatively high in the nonresponders, possibly reflecting less efficient entry of lithium into the central nervous system of poor responders (Mendels, Frazer, Baron et al. 1976).

In further studies of serum concentrations of lithium, Koukopoulos noted that the lithium levels tended to decrease in mania and increase in depression—evidently reflecting corresponding changes in levels of arousal, general metabolic activity, and renal clearance (Kukopulos and Reginaldi 1978). Interestingly, they used this finding to improve treatment by predicting imminent changes of mood before they became clinically manifest.

Based on these early studies, Koukopoulos instilled in his colleagues and students consideration of the greater clinical importance of the course of manic-depressive illness than its acute symptomatic presentations. Arising from this interest was an early description of five characteristic course sequences in bipolar disorder: [a] depression–mania–free interval (DMI), [b] mania–depression–free interval (MDI), [c] continuous-circular (CC), [d] rapid-cycling (RC), and [e] erratic or irregular (Kukopulos, Reginaldi, Laddomada et al. 1980; Koukopoulos, Reginaldi, Tondo et al. 2013). These course-patterns had important predictive associations with overall morbidity and treatment responses, notably including less favorable results with DMI than MDI patients.

This work also led to the observation that lithium often failed to prevent mood-disorder recurrences in manic-depressive disorder patients being concomitantly treated with antidepressants, and to the hypothesis that antidepressants may induce mood-switches from depression to hypomania or mania that often were poorly responsive to lithium (Reginaldi, Tondo, Floris et al. 1981).

Long-term treatment with lithium was widely employed by the Lucio Bini group and was found to help many difficult patients, including some who had been hospitalized for years. Lithium treatment also was a prevalent option at a new Lucio Bini Mood Disorder Center, which I co-founded in 1977 in Cagliari, Sardinia. By the 1980s, lithium treatment had become well established internationally, and the research interests of the Rome and Cagliari Centers moved to nosological topics, including the importance of mixed or agitated depression.

Indications

In 1992, I was mentoring Dr. Gianni Faedda at University of Cagliari. After his medical training, he received a fellowship from the Sardinia Region which could be applied for research training only at Harvard Medical School. We contacted Ross Baldessarini who accepted Faedda's candidacy for postdoctoral training in psychopharmacology at the Mailman Research Center at Harvard-affiliated McLean Hospital, initially to pursue laboratory studies of the pharmacology of D1 dopamine receptors.

This development initiated a long and fruitful association with Baldessarini that continues to the present time. I am indebted to him for encouraging discipline in research and rigorous objectivity in the collection, analysis, and interpretation of clinical and research data, and consistent awareness that there were real, suffering persons behind the numbers.

As Faedda's primary interests were clinical, we initiated a study based on patient data from the Bini Center in Cagliari to pursue my idea that the rate of discontinuing lithium treatment might have important clinical consequences. Faedda and Baldessarini noted that patients relapsed much sooner after abrupt or rapid discontinuation of lithium, compared to gradual dose-reduction and discontinuation over at least two weeks. In particular, recurrence rates (new illness episodes per time) were much greater within the initial months following rapid discontinuation of lithium, and risk of recurrences remained parallel (evidently reflecting the natural history of the course of untreated bipolar disorder) but much lower following gradual discontinuation for up to five years of follow-up. This pattern suggested that rapid treatment discontinuation acted as an iatrogenic stressor and that gradual discontinuation not only delayed, but actually reduced risks of later illness recurrences (Faedda, Tondo, Baldessarini et al. 1993). The median time to an illness recurrence was 5.0-times longer following gradual than after rapid discontinuation (20.0 ± 5.8 vs. 4.0 ± 0.7 months; $p<0.0001$), the mean cycling interval also was shorter after rapid discontinuation than before lithium treatment was started (6.3 vs. 14.6 months; $p<0.0001$), adding to the impression that rapid treatment discontinuation was an adjunctive stressor to effects of nontreatment. Over several years of follow-up, patient-subjects remained stable without lithium treatment 20 times more frequently after gradual than rapid discontinuation (37% vs. 1.8% of cases; p<0.0001) (Baldessarini, Tondo, Faedda et al. 1996). This study was replicated with an independent sample of Bipolar Disorder subjects the following year (Baldessarini, Tondo, Floris and Rudas 1997). We also found that Bipolar I disorder patients were 1.5-times less likely than Bipolar II subjects to remain in remission during long-term treatment with lithium, and that the polarity of their first recurrences during treatment was 81% concordant with that of their first-lifetime episode (Faedda, Tondo, Baldessarini et al. 1993).

A related question was whether trials of re-treatment following discontinuation of lithium were less effective, as had been claimed by some colleagues, based mainly on clinical impressions. Instead, we found little difference in average clinical responses between initial treatment and second or even later trials of re-treatment with lithium (Tondo, Baldessarini, Floris and Rudas 1997). Notably, the mean number of episodes/year was similar with first versus second trials of lithium treatment (0.83 vs. 0.94), as was the proportion of time ill with treatment (18.0% vs. 24.2%), with no differences in numbers of manic and depressive episodes, duration of the treatments, interval between treatment trials, or discontinuation rate. However, there was 12.8% more use of adjunctive medication in the second treatment.

We also compared responses to lithium treatment in Bipolar Disorder types I and II patients and found that lithium had superior benefits in type II patients, with significantly greater reduction of episodes per year and a lower percentage of time ill, probably because of a greater effect of lithium on hypomanias (prevalent in Bipolar-II disorder) compared to manias (only in Bipolar-I disorder), whereas reduction of depressive morbidity was somewhat less but similar with both diagnostic types. Moreover, during treatment, Bipolar II patients had 5.9-fold longer inter-episode intervals and were twice as likely as type I patients to have no new episodes (Tondo Baldessarini, Hennen and Floris 1998b).

Following-up on reports that lithium was becoming less effective in recent years, we reviewed published reports on long-term lithium treatment from 1970 to 1996, seeking evidence of a secular decline in response that was not found (Baldessarini and Tondo 2000). We proposed that unfavorable results with any treatment may occur in some settings with heavy representation of patients with complex and less treatment-responsive illnesses, particularly in specialized institutions, but that benefits of long-term maintenance treatment with lithium had changed little in recent decades. We also tested a frequently repeated idea that delay of treatment of Bipolar Disorder results in a decline of effectiveness of treatment and found that latency from illness onset to diagnosis and sustained treatment, though typically delayed for 6–8 years (and longer after juvenile onset), as well as pre-treatment episode counts, were not significantly associated with the quality of clinical responses to treatment with lithium or other mood-stabilizing treatments (Baldessarini, Tondo, Hennen and Floris 1999b; Baethge, Tondo, Bratti et al. 2003; Bratti, Baldessarini, Baethge and Tondo 2003).

We also reviewed studies of the effectiveness of lithium and other treatments in rapid cycling (RC), compared with non-RC Bipolar Disorder patients. We found that 13.7% fewer RC than non-RC patients experienced full protection from all recurrences during maintenance treatment with lithium (Baldessarini, Tondo, Floris and Hennen 2000). Moreover, we compared responses with other treatments among RC (n=905) versus non-RC (n=951) Bipolar Disorder patients in 16 reports involving use of carbamazepine, lamotrigine, lithium, topiramate, or valproate, alone or with other agents, over an average of 47.5 months. Across all treatments, lack of substantial clinical benefit averaged 2.9-times more prevalent with RC than non-RC status. Moreover, contrary to expectation, responses with lithium in RC patients were somewhat greater than with anticonvulsant mood-stabilizers (Tondo, Hennen and Baldessarini 2003). These findings challenged marketing claims that anticonvulsant were more effective than lithium for RC Bipolar Disorder patients.

Noting in the 1990s that patients treated with lithium seemed clinically to have less suicidal ideation and behavior than without lithium or with other treatments, with Drs. Baldessarini and Kay Jamison, we reviewed the then very limited research literature on this topic and found evidence favoring an association of long-term lithium treatment lithium with lower risk of suicidal behavior (Tondo, Jamison and Baldessarini 1997). In 28 research reports based on 17,000 subjects with major affective illnesses, the risk of suicides and attempts averaged 3.2 versus 0.37 per 100 patient-years without versus with lithium—a striking, 8.6-fold difference. The finding encouraged further research on effects of lithium treatment on suicidal risk. These studies included a systematic review on this topic (Tondo and Baldessarini 2000), and a first meta-analysis of research findings (Tondo, Hennen and Baldessarini 2001), as well as reporting of original data from the Centro Lucio Bini Centers (Tondo, Baldessarini, Hennen et al. 1998a).

The original data were based on 5233 patient-years of observation and indicated that of 58 patients who made suicide attempts (8 were fatal), there was a highly significant, 6.4-fold lower adjusted hazard ratio for suicidal acts during treatment with lithium versus before treatment, as well as 7.5-fold greater risk after discontinuing lithium treatment, particularly during the initial 12 months post-discontinuation, with a twice-greater risk after discontinuing abruptly or rapidly (Baldessarini, Tondo and Hennen 1999a). We also reported another review (Tondo, Isacsson and Baldessarini 2003) and another meta-analysis on this topic (Baldessarini, Tondo, Davis et al. 2006) which both supported a substantial reduction of risks of suicide and attempts with long-term lithium treatment. Risk of suicide fatality was lower with lithium than with placebo in several randomized, controlled treatment trials, in which suicidal behaviors were reported passively and incidentally as "adverse outcomes" rather than as a pre-planned and explicitly determined outcome measure (Tondo, Isacsson and Baldessarini 2003; Baldessarini, Tondo, Davis et al. 2006). We also found that risks of suicidal behavior were lower with lithium than during treatment with mood-altering anticonvulsants (Baldessarini and Tondo 2009; Tondo and Baldessarini 2018). In addition, with Dr. Francesca Guzzetta, we extended evidence of an antisuicidal effect of lithium treatment to patients with nonbipolar Major Depressive Disorder (Guzzetta, Tondo, Centorrino and Baldessarini 2007).

In recent years, our research on lithium has included reassessments of adverse effects on renal function. This work included an international collaborative study of 312 patients (mean age, 56 years) who produced 2,669 assays of serum lithium concentration. We found that over 8–48 (mean, 18) years, 29.5% of subjects experienced at least one low value of eGFR (<60 mL/min/1.73 m2), mostly after ≥15 years of treatment and age >55 years; risk of ≥2 low values was 18.1%, and there were no cases of end-stage renal failure (which may well have been avoided by clinically appropriate interventions including discontinuation of lithium before renal dysfunction became severe). Further of note, these encouraging data were obtained in highly specialized clinical settings where the patients were closely followed and monitored and may or may not generalize to other circumstances. Independent risk factors for declining eGFR ranked: longer exposure to lithium, lower lithium dose (probably related to lesser baseline clearance), higher serum lithium concentration, older age, and medical comorbidity. Later low eGFR also was predicted by lower initial eGFR and starting lithium at age ≥40 years (Tondo, Abramowicz, Alda et al. 2017). An important conclusion was that advancing age was a major risk factor confounding the role of lithium in the decline of renal function.

Recently, we collaborated with colleagues from the International Group for The Study of Lithium (IGSLi) to develop a clinical advisory report on use of lithium aimed at guiding patients and prescribing clinicians to its safe and effective use to treat patients with major mood disorders (Tondo, Alda, Bauer et al. 2019).

Having treated approximately 1800 patients with lithium, I understand that it may be not be as easy to use this mood-stabilizer compared to other agents that can be administered without the requirement of monitoring serum drug levels, and assays for renal and thyroid function. However, alternatives have medical risks, too but they do not achieve the same beneficial effects. Mood-stabilizing anticonvulsants can interact with the metabolism of other drugs, and some have extraordinarily high teratogenic risk. Second-generation antipsychotics can increase risk of weight-gain, metabolic syndrome, excessive sedation, and akathisia. Moreover, lithium remains one of the most effective and versatile treatments aimed at long-term mood-stabilization and its evident antisuicidal effect is virtually unique among treatments widely used to treat major mood disorders.

Acknowledgments

The author thanks Ross Baldessarini for helpful comments arising from his careful editing of this manuscript.

References:

Baethge C, Tondo L, Bratti IM, Bschor T, Bauer M, Viguera AC, Baldessarini RJ. Prophylaxis latency and outcome in bipolar disorders. Can J Psychiatry 2003; 48:449-57.

Baldessarini RJ, Tondo L. Does lithium still work? Evidence of stable responses over three decades. Arch Gen Psychiatry. 2000; 57:187-90.

Baldessarini RJ, Tondo L. Suicidal risks during treatment of bipolar disorder patients with lithium versus anticonvulsants. Pharmacopsychiatry. 2009; 42:72-5.

Baldessarini RJ, Tondo L, Davis P, Pompili M, Goodwin FK, Hennen J. Decreased risk of suicides and attempts during long-term lithium treatment: a meta-analytic review. Bipolar Disord. 2006; 8(5 Pt 2):625-39.

Baldessarini RJ, Tondo L, Faedda GL, Suppes TR, Floris G, Rudas N. Effects of the rate of discontinuing lithium maintenance treatment in bipolar disorders. J Clin Psychiatry. 1996; 57: 441-8.

Indications

Baldessarini RJ, Tondo L, Floris G, Hennen J. Effects of rapid cycling on response to lithium maintenance treatment in 360 bipolar I and iI disorder patients. J Affect Disord. 2000; 61:13-22.

Baldessarini RJ, Tondo L, Floris G, Rudas N. Reduced morbidity after gradual discontinuation of lithium treatment for bipolar I and II disorders: a replication study. Am J Psychiatry. 1997; 154:551-3.

Baldessarini RJ, Tondo L, Hennen J. Effects of lithium treatment and its discontinuation on suicidal behavior in bipolar manic-depressive disorders. J Clin Psychiatry. 1999a; 60(Suppl 2):77-84.

Baldessarini RJ, Tondo L, Hennen J, Floris G. Latency and episodes before treatment: response to lithium maintenance in bipolar I and II disorders. Bipolar Disord. 1999b; 1:91-7.

Bratti IM, Baldessarini RJ, Baethge C, Tondo L: Pretreatment episode count and response to lithium treatment in manic-depressive illness. Harv Rev Psychiatry. 2003; 11:245-56.

Faedda GL, Tondo L, Baldessarini RJ, Suppes T, Tohen M. Outcome after rapid vs. gradual discontinuation of lithium treatment in bipolar disorders. Arch Gen Psychiatry. 1993; 50:448-55.

Guzzetta F, Tondo L, Centorrino F, Baldessarini RJ. Lithium treatment reduces suicide risk in recurrent major depressive disorder. J Clin Psychiatry. 2007; 68:380-3.

Koukopoulos A, Reginaldi D, Tondo L, Visioli C, Baldessarini RJ. Course sequences in bipolar disorder: depressions preceding or following manias or hypomanias. J Affect Disord. 2013; 151:105-10.

Kukopulos A, Reginaldi D. Does lithium prevent depressions by suppressing manias? Int Pharmacopsychiatry. 1973; 8:152-8.

Kukopulos A, Reginaldi D. Variations of serum lithium concentrations correlated with the phases of manic-depressive psychosis. Agressologie. 1978; 19:219-22.

Kukopulos A, Reginaldi D, Girardi P, Tondo L. Course of manic-depressive recurrence under lithium. Compr Psychiatry. 1975; 16:517-24.

Kukopulos A, Reginaldi D, Laddomada P, Floris G, Serra G, Tondo L. Course of the manic-depressive cycle and changes caused by treatment. Pharmakopsychiatr Neuropsychopharmakol. 1980; 13:156-67.

Mendels J, Frazer A, Baron J, Kukopulos A, Reginaldi D, Tondo L, Caliari B. Letter: Intra-erythrocyte lithium io concentration and long-term maintenance treatment. Lancet. 1976; 1(7966):966-7.

Reginaldi D, Tondo L, Floris G, Pignatelli A, Kukopulos A. Poor prophylactic lithium response due to antidepressants. Int Pharmacopsychiatry. 1981; 16:124-8.

Tondo L, Abramowicz M, Alda M, Bauer M, Bocchetta A, Bolzani L, Calkin CV, Chillotti C, Hidalgo-Mazzei D, Manchia M, Müller-Oerlinghausen B, Murru A, Perugi G, Pinna M, Quaranta G, Reginaldi D, Reif A, Ritter P Jr, Rybakowski JK, Saiger D, Sani G, Selle V, Stamm T, Vázquez GH, Veeh J, Vieta E, Baldessarini RJ. Long-term lithium treatment in bipolar disorder: effects on glomerular filtration rate and other metabolic parameters. Int J Bipolar Disord. 2017; 5:27–38.

Tondo L, Alda M, Bauer M, Bergink V, Grof P, Hajek T, Lewitka U, Licht RW, Manchia M, Müller-Oerlinghausen B, Nielsen RE, Selo M, Simhandl C, Baldessarini RJ; International Group for Studies of Lithium (IGSLi). Clinical use of lithium salts: guide for users and prescribers. Int J Bipolar Disord. 2019; 7:16-25.

Tondo L, Baldessarini RJ. Reduced suicide risk during lithium maintenance treatment. J Clin Psychiatry. 2000; 61 (Suppl 9):97-104.

Tondo L, Baldessarini RJ. Antisuicidal Effects in Mood Disorders: Are They Unique to Lithium? Pharmacopsychiatry. 2018; 51:177-88.

Tondo L, Baldessarini RJ, Floris G, Rudas N. Effectiveness of restarting lithium treatment after its discontinuation in bipolar I and bipolar II disorders. Am J Psychiatry. 1997; 154:548-50.

Tondo L, Baldessarini RJ, Hennen J, Floris G, Silvetti F, Tohen M. Lithium treatment and risk of suicidal behavior in bipolar disorder patients. J Clin Psychiatry. 1998a; 59:405-14.

Tondo L, Baldessarini RJ, Hennen J, Floris G. Lithium maintenance treatment of depression and mania in bipolar I and bipolar II disorders. Am J Psychiatry. 1998b; 155:638¬-45.

Tondo L, Hennen J, Baldessarini RJ. Lower suicide risk with long-term lithium treatment in major affective illness: a meta-analysis. Acta Psychiatr Scand. 2001; 104:163-72.

Tondo L, Hennen J, Baldessarini RJ. Rapid-cycling bipolar disorder: effects of long-term treatments. Acta Psychiatr Scand. 2003; 108:4-14.

Tondo L, Jamison KR, Baldessarini RJ. Effect of lithium maintenance on suicidal behavior in major mood disorders. Ann N Y Acad Sci. 1997; 836:339-51.

Tondo L, Isacsson G, Baldessarini R. Suicidal behavior in bipolar disorder: risk and prevention. CNS Drugs. 2003; 17:491-511.

July 16, 2020

ANTONIO TORRES-RUIZ'S COMMENT
INTRODUCTION OF LITHIUM IN MEXICO

In the 1960s, and more specifically in 1967, I started my medical residency in psychiatry at the National Institute of Neurology and Neurosurgery (INN), where I met Dr. Dionisio Nieto Gómez, head of the Department of Psychiatry, who had initiated the use of lithium on manic-depressive psychosis in Mexico. He introduced it in 1960, and publicly communicated it for the first time in 1963, in an article entitled "Treatment of Mania with Lithium Carbonate."

It is of interest to note that an important discovery was made by the Australian psychiatrist John Cade in 1949. He observed that lithium had very favorable effects on mania, observations confirmed by Noack and Trautner in 1951. However, systematic employment was promoted by Mogens Schou and his collaborators in Denmark from 1954. Lithium represented a true revolution in psychiatric therapy that also opened new horizons for the investigation of affective disorders. The accurate observation by Schou and other authors that lithium acts as a prophylactic for manic and depressive outbreaks represented an extraordinary step in psychiatric therapy. In 1969, in the journal Neurology-Neurosurgery-Psychiatry, another article by Doctor Nieto was published, entitled "Lithium in Manic-Depressive Psychosis."

The findings of the use of lithium in affective disorders were made public in the 1960s and became widely known in different parts of the Americas. During that time, we were using lithium carbonate in 250 mg capsules, which we ordered as magisterial prescriptions to be prepared in special pharmacies that were able to manufacture them, such as the Valdecasas laboratory in Mexico City. Occasionally, people came to us from other countries, since lithium carbonate did not exist their patent pharmacy until it was approved and used regularly.

We routinely requested serum dosing to maintain lithium levels between 0.5 and 1.2 mEq per liter and retained control over the renal and thyroid functioning. Thus, it was Doctor Dionisio Nieto Gómez and his group of assistants who used lithium carbonate for the first time, as far as we know, in the management of manic-depressive psychosis and in America.

References:

Indications

Cade JFJ. Lithium salts in the treatment of psychotic excitement. Med J.Aust. 1949, 2:349-352.

Nieto D. Tratamiento De la manía con carbonato de litio (Treatment of Mania with Lithium

Carbonate). Neurología, Neurocirugía, Psiquiatría 1963; 4:123-4.

Nieto D. El litio en la psicosis maníaco depresiva (Lithium in Manic-Depressive Psychosis). Neurología, Neurocirugía, Psiquiatría.1969; 10:63-72.

Noack D, Trautner EM. The lithium treatment of maniacal psychosis. Med J Austr 1951; 2: 218-22.

July 2, 2020

ACKNOWLEDGEMENT

The text of this book is based entirely on material posted on INHN's website during the years and I am thankful to Lucrecia Alvarez for rendering it readily accessible in WORD for inclusion in the book. I am grateful to Olaf Fjetland for editing the entire text and for his assistance in converting the material into a format ready for publication.

INDEX

A

B

C

D

E

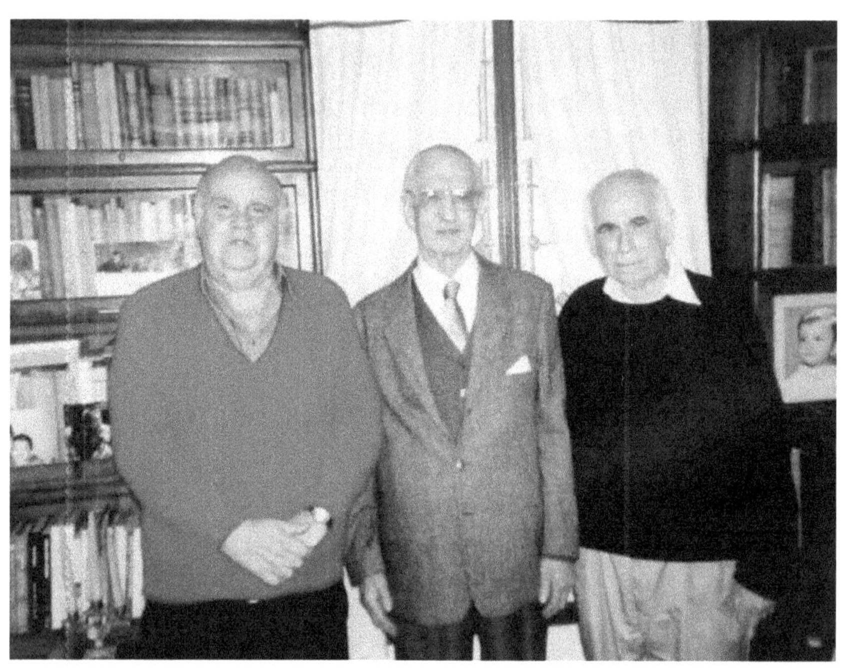

Ronaldo Ucha Udabe, Carlos A. Morra Sr., Thomas A. Ban.
1999
Córdoba, Argentina.